COMPREHENSIVE
CLINICAL SURGERY

COMPREHENSIVE CLINICAL SURGERY

Dr. C. R. Ballal, M.S.

*H.O.D. Dept. of Surgery and
Director of Postgraduate Studies (Retired),
Kasturba Medical College , Mangalore,
Prof. Emeritus Dept. of Surgery (Retired),
K.S. Hegde Medical academy, Mangalore*

Dr. C. Rajesh Ballal, M.S.

*D.N.B. (Gen. Surgery),
Prof. of Surgery,
K.S. Hegde Medical Academy, Mangalore*

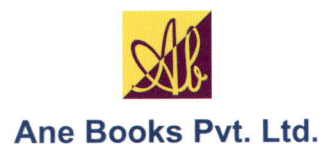

Ane Books Pvt. Ltd.

New Delhi ◆ Chennai ◆ Mumbai

Comprehensive Clinical Surgery

C. R. Ballal and C. Rajesh Ballal

© Authors, **2017**

Published by

Ane Books Pvt. Ltd.

4821, Parwana Bhawan, 1st Floor, 24 Ansari Road, Darya Ganj,
New Delhi - 110 002, Tel.: +91(011) 23276843-44, Fax: +91(011) 23276863
e-mail: kapoor@anebooks.com, Website: www.anebooks.com

Branches

■ Avantika Niwas, 1st Floor, 19 Doraiswamy Road, T. Nagar,
 Chennai - 600 017, Tel.: +91(044) 28141554, 28141209
 e-mail: anebookschennai@gmail.com, rathinam@anebooks.com

■ 138, Chandan Chambers, 1st Floor, Office No. 3, Modi Street, Fort,
 Mumbai - 400 001, Tel.: +91(022) 22622440, 22622441
 e-mail: anebooksmum@mtnl.net.in, anebooksmum@gmail.com

Please be informed that the author and the publisher have put in their best efforts in producing this book. Every care has been taken to ensure the accuracy of the contents. However, we make no warranties for the same and therefore shall not be responsible or liable for any loss or any commercial damages accruing thereof. Please do consult a professional where appropriate.

ISBN : 978-93-8546-280-1

Printed at : Print Creation, Delhi

Foreword

Dr. K. Sridhar

M.S; M.Ch; PGDHHM

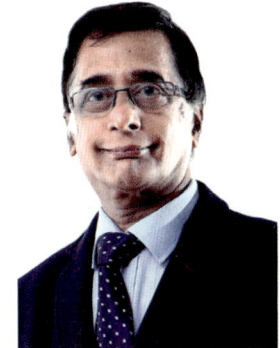

It is very unusual for a student to be invited to write a foreword for a book written by his own teacher (GURU). This is exactly what Prof. C.R. Ballal has done putting me into a predicament which even though is a great honour is also humbling. It also shows the bonding great teachers like him have developed with their students. He has never considered teaching as a profession and has been doing it as a "Dharma" or way of life for many decades. His surgical clinics were one of the most popular ones in the whole country. Students from various parts of the country used to flock to his clinics before their exams. Therefore learning basics from a teacher with a whole life time experience is the best way to learn and live as a good surgeon.

- In Advaya Taraka Upanishad, Sukla-yajuveda, Verses 15,16 says
- The syllable "Gu" in Guru stands for darkness and ignorance (andhakara).
- The syllable "Ru" signifies eradication of darkness or ignorance.

Thus, who-so-ever has the ability to eradicate darkness and thereby bring light into one's life should be called a Guru.

The modern day practice of surgery encompasses various sub specialisations (super specialisation) and the teachings in general surgery get diluted. In this book we can see that more emphasis is given to those topics which normally a modern day general surgeon should manage.

When we go through the book we realise, he has cleared the common doubts that may arise in the minds of students of surgery in the form of question and answers like the dialogues between guru and Sishya with the ancient Vedic wisdom. He has created various clinical situations in an outpatient setting taking the students through a journey from history to treatment protocol.

"It is necessary to watch the patient's expression carefully. The facial expression, the posture adopted may all give important clues". "At times, the answer may appear irrelevant, but the doctor should not show any degree of intolerance" are golden words; clearly underlining the importance of spending sufficient time with the patient, listen to him with patience and gain his confidence.

While reading through the book I felt as if I am attending one of his clinics describing how to examine, why it should be done that way? How we derive inferences from these.

Points to be noted after each section of a chapter helps the student to recapitulate what he has studied until that part. The same way the question answer sessions and MCQ at the end of chapters will help the student to revise the subject and recall the important aspects of examination and investigations.

Salient points in Endoscopy, Radiotherapy, Chemotherapy, FNAC and finer aspects of what to look for an investigation which are normally not covered are explained and it will immensely help the students in their preparation for the examination.

As a former student of his, as a surgeon practicing for the past four decades, as a teacher, and an examiner I could view this master piece from various angles. I have no doubt in stating it is a book which will serve many purposes as a short text book to learn surgery, as a revision manual before examination, a quick reference guide in practice and a step by step manual for common surgical problems. This is a book which must find a place in all medical libraries.

Dr. K. Sridhar

M.S; M.Ch; PGDHHM

Senior Vice president SIMS Hospital,
Former Pro Vice Chancellor (medical) SRM University
Former Member Tamil Nadu State Planning Commission
National President Association of Plastic Surgeons of India -2003

Preface

Comprehensive clinical surgery is a book with a difference. A large number of clinical books are being published across the country. These books focus on a methodical clinical examination with only a brief description of management options. The medical student is faced with the challenge of browsing through voluminous text books to understand the relevance of these investigations and treatment modalities. This book attempts to bridge the vital gap by providing adequate attention to treatment strategies as well

Each chapter starts with a description of a typical patient that a student might find in the wards. This is followed by a logical approach to examination and management of the disease. Certain chapters describe a novel sequence of examination, prioritising those signs that actually help with management. The book encourages students to ask themselves at every step - 'WHY investigate?' 'What happens if I don't treat this patient?'. Such an approach helps build the basic concepts for a complete understanding of the disease.

It is useful for undergraduates as they train to become competent clinicians. Postgraduates will find this book useful in revising their clinical skills and management strategies.

Our thanks are due to Dr. Vidya S. Upadhyaya, Consultant Ultrasonologist, Sengkang Health, Singapore for writing a chapter on Basics of Radiology. We are also thankful to Dr. Krishnaprasad, Prof. Medical Oncology, Kasturba Medical College, Mangalore for writing the chapters on Radiotherapy and Chemotherapy. These subjects have certainly added value to the book.

We thank Prof. K. Sridhar of S.R.M. University, Chennai, Alumnus, Kasturba Medical College Mangalore, who readily agreed to write the foreward when we requested him.

We are very grateful Dr. K. S. Gopinath, Past President, Association of Surgeons of India for providing us with many excellent clinical photographs. We are thankful to Dr. Sandeep Rai and Dr. Raghu Shankar, Dept of Paediatric Surgery K.S Medical Academy, Mangalore for giving us clinical photographs. Many postgraduate students including Dr. Adithya, Dr. Vimal and Dr. Athreya have also helped us in this regard. Our special thanks to all the students.

Ane Books Delhi, our publishers deserve a special word of thanks. Mr. Rathinam at Chennai, Mr. Sunil Saxena and Mr. Kulveer Singh at Delhi have played a special role in getting the book printed and published within a very short period of time.

E-mail: cramakrishnaballal@gmail.com   **Authors**

Contents

Foreword   *v*

Preface   *vii*

 1. **History and Physical Examination**   1–28

 2. **Essentials of Radiology**   29–43

 3. **Basics of Chemotherapy**   45–53

 4. **Diseases of the Thyroid Gland**   55–103

 5. **Diseases of the Salivary Glands**   105–129

 6. **Oral Cancer**   131–152

 7. **Cystic Swellings in the Neck**   153–178

 8. **Abdomen**   179–220

 9. **Obstructive Jaundice**   221–238

10. **Surgical Diseases of the Liver**   239–259

11. **Carcinoma of the Female Breast**   261–293

12. **The Circulatory and Lymphatic Systems**   295–375

13. **Hernias**   377–413

14. **Hydroceles**   415–426

15. **Testicular Tumours**   427–447

16. **Skin and Soft Tissues**   449–487

History and Physical Examination

> *Treat Every Patient as a Fellow Human Being and not as a Case*
> *Have Patience to Listen to your Patients.*

The importance of a good **history** and a **complete physical examination** cannot be **over emphasised**. A **detailed history** will be helpful in arriving at a **diagnosis** in as many as **70% of patients**. Unfortunately, the **advent of sophisticated imaging techniques and laboratory studies** has made the **clinician give less importance** to this **part of the examination**. It must be kept in mind that right through a clinician's career, from a student to a consultant, the proper management of a patient depends on the foundation of taking a good history and a complete physical examination.

HISTORY

It is essential to develop a good rapport with the patient by spending enough time in talking to them. This helps a great deal at the time of physical examination. It makes the patient believe that the doctor is genuinely interested in his/her welfare.

Personal Data

(*a*) **Name:** Asking for the patient's name shows **respect** for the individual and is the **first step** towards building his/her trust in the clinician. It also helps in gathering information and offering advice. In the **West,** it is **customary** to **introduce oneself** before asking **this question**. The name is also **important** for **maintaining a complete medical record**. It is **good practice to remember the name**, as far as possible, and to **recall** the same during the **next visit of the patient.**

(*b*) **Age:**

(*c*) **Address:** A **proper address** must be obtained for the **purpose of maintaining the medical records**. In addition, **certain diseases** are **endemic** to **some areas** and may give a **clue to a diagnosis**. A **classic example** will be that of **Guatemala,** a country nestled in the **Andes Mountains**. When **endemic goiter** was **very prevalent** in **that country**, even the **dolls sold in shops were depicted to have goiters. Another example is the high fluoride content** in the water in many **parts of our country,** which can lead to **numerous health problems**.

(*d*) **Occupation:** A **large number** of **occupational diseases** have been **identified.** In addition, certain **occupations** are **associated indirectly** with a **higher incidence** of a **particular disease**. The **incidence** of **varicose veins** in the **lower limb** is **very common** among **barbers**.

Chief Complaint

This is the **primary reason** for the **patient's** visit to the **doctor**. If there is more than one **complaint**, it **must be recorded** in a **chronological order**. If the **symptoms are vague**, an **attempt must be made** to **clarify the same**.

History of the Present Illness

The **patient** must be given sufficient **time to mention this part of the history** in **his/her own words**. A **study conducted overseas** has shown that the **average time before the doctor intervenes** is **18 seconds**. Therefore, it is **necessary** to be **completely attentive** to the **patients** when they give the

historical **details of their illness.** Although it may be in a **disorderly fashion,** it is best **not to intervene** at this point. Leading questions may be asked by the clinician only when the patien**ts have finished conveying the details of their illness**. The clinician should avoid using **medical terms** as **far as possible. Questions should not be ambiguous**.

Symptomatology

The **symptomatology may** be **grouped** for the **sake of convenience** as **follows:**

(*a*) **Local symptoms:** Symptoms related to the **primary site** of the **disease. Pain, swelling and an ulcer** are the **common presenting symptoms** in a **surgical Patient.**

(*b*) **Regional symptoms: Symptoms occurring** due to **enlargement of the regional lymph nodes** and **distal pressure effects caused by** a **lesion** are to be **noted under this group.**

(*c*) **Systemic symptoms:** It is **impossible** to ask **questions** regarding **all** the **systems in the body** in **every patient**. Hence the **information obtained** in **relation** to the **two groups mentioned above** can help to **decide which systems** need to be **inquired into**. A **lady** with a **lump in the breast** may not **realise** the **significance of back pain**.

Local Symptoms

The **two common symptoms** presenting in the **surgical wards** are **pain and a lump**. Eliciting a comprehensive history in a patient presenting with a lump or swelling is discussed in the next chapter.

The patient's presenting symptoms may be recorded under the following points.

1. **Duration:** It may be noted as **acute, subacute or chronic**, depending on the **time interval**.

2. **Mode of onset:** This could either be **sudden** as in **most acute conditions** or **gradual** as in the **chronic variety**. Some **chronic diseases** may **develop** an **acute complication**.

3. **Rate of progression:** The rate of progression may be **slow or rapid**. In **chronic diseases**, **the rate** may **vary** over a **period of time.**

4. **Pain:** Pain may further be classified as follows:

   (*a*) **Nature of pain:** If the **patient is unable to describe** his **symptoms properly**, it is necessary to ask **leading questions**. The **terms** used are **colicky, pricking, burning, dragging and throbbing types of pain.**

   (*b*) **Intensity** of **pain:** Is the pain **mild, moderate or severe** in nature? An idea about the **intensity** of pain can be obtained by asking the patient whether he is able to **perform** his **daily work**.

   (*c*) **Site of pain:** Many of the **patients will not be able to localise** the **pain** accurately. It is helpful when they are able to point to the site.

   (*d*) **Radiation of pain:** This is usually **referred pain** as per the **segmental nerve distribution**. For example, **pain due** to **gall bladder disease** is **present** in the **right hypochondrium** and is referred **to the right shoulder**.

   (*e*) **Shifting of pain:** This is an **uncommon finding**. In patients with **acute appendicitis**, initially the **pain** is around **the umbilicus**, since the pain is **referred to this region** from structures **developed from the midgut**. But when the **inflammation spreads** to the **parietal peritoneum** the pain **shifts** to the **right iliac fossa**. It is to be **noted that at this stage** the **umbilical area** is **devoid of pain**, thus **differentiating it** from **referred pain.**

(f) **Aggravating and relieving factors: Patients** with **chronic pancreatitis** have pain in the **epigastric region,** relieved by **sitting bent well forwards. Jolting movements** can worsen the **pain** due to **renal calculus.** It is well known that **intermittent claudication** appears on walking a certain distance. It usually **disappears** on **taking rest.** Quite **often, medication** is the **relieving factor.**

(g) Is the **pain severe enough** to **disturb** the **sleep at night**? If the **answer** is **positive it indicates** an **extremely intense type** of pain. **Rest pain** in an **ischaemic limb** is a **classic example.**

5. **Some more points need special mention:** When talking to the patients, the clinician must also **watch their expression carefully.** The patient's **facial expression** as well as **the posture adopted** may **give important clues.** The patient may show a **degree of reluctance** in **answering some questions.** At times, **the answer may appear irrelevant,** but the **doctor should not show** any **degree of intolerance.** Again, **as the physical examination** is being **performed,** it may become **necessary** to ask **more questions.**

Box 1.1:	Points to be noted in history of present illness.

- History of present illness – Eliciting cooperation from the patient.
- Chief complaint – Duration.
- Other complaints in chronological order.
- Pain and swelling – Very common.
- Pain – Site, nature, intensity, radiation, aggravating and relieving factors.
- Local symptoms – Depend on the site.
- Regional symptoms.
- Systemic symptoms.

Past History

History of any **major illness** in the past is **pertinent** at this stage. **Details** may be of **help** in diagnosing the **present condition.** The patient may **not realise the significance** of this **relationship.** Because **diabetes, hypertension** and **tuberculosis** are **very common** in our country, **questions** regarding these **conditions** form an **integral part of past history.** The following **three important questions** must be asked to get a complete **past history.**

1. **History of previous allergy:** If it is **present, i**t must be **written prominently** in the **case paper.**

2. **History of previous surgery:** It **may** or **may not be related** to the **present illness.**

3. In **women of the reproductive age group,** the date of the **last menstrual period** should always be **asked. Many drugs** are **harmful** to the **foetus** during **early pregnancy.**

Box 1.2:	Points to be noted in past history.

- Major illness.
- Diabetes, hypertension and tuberculosis.
- History of allergy.
- History of previous surgery – Related or not related.
- Last menstrual period in women of reproductive age.

Personal History

This should include details regarding **bladder and bowel** habits. **Recent loss** of **appetite and weight** are **significant.** The patient should be asked about **smoking, consumption of alcohol and chewing of tobacco**. All these three **habits are very common** in **most parts of our country. Questions** regarding **exposure to sexually transmitted diseases** and **HIV** quite **often elicit a negative answer** which may **not always be reliable**.

Box 1.3:	Points to be noted in personal history.

- Bowel and bladder habits.
- Loss of appetite and weight.
- Habits – Chewing pan, smoking and consumption of alcohol.
- Drug addiction.
- Exposure to STD – HIV (often not reliable).

Treatment History

Most patients coming to **a tertiary** or a **teaching hospital** would have had **some treatment earlier. Unless inquired into**, the **relevant information may not be forthcoming. Unfortunately,** this **aspect** of the **history** is **underestimated,** with dire **consequences** in **some patients.**

Obstetric and Menstrual History

This should be asked for and recorded in female patients making the process of history taking complete. Thanks to the **time taken for this part,** the **confidence level** of the **patient** reaches a **high grade** and this makes **physical examination much easier**. One of the **primary reasons** for the **rapid increase** in **medical litigation** is the poor quality of history taking and physical examination, owing to **reduction in the time taken for eliciting** the **history** and completing the **physical examination.**

PHYSICAL EXAMINATION

Physical examination can be divided into **general, local, regional and systemic examinations.** This will **ensure** that **a comprehensive physical examination** is conducted in **every patient**.

General Physical Examination

The **first question** to ask oneself is does the patient appear to be in **distress?** If the answer is **positive,** the **rest** of the **examination** is to **be performed** in a **gentle** manner.

The **general part of the examination** consists of a brief **complete survey** of the patient. The focus is on the **build and nutrition**. On the **surgical side** enough **importance** is **not given** to the **nutritional status** of the **patient** in **many instances**. The **skinfold** thickness in **relation** to the **triceps** on the **posterior aspect of the arm** is a **valuable guide. The body mass index (BMI) is to be recorded, giving further information** regarding the **nutritional status**. The measurement of **pulse** and **respiratory rates** along with the **blood pressure** is mandatory for each patient. **Pallor, jaundice, clubbing** of the fingers and pitting **oedema** at the ankle are signs to be looked for. But there should be a **sense of priority** at **this stage. Jaundice** is **significant** if the history is suggestive of **hepatobiliary disease. Jaundice** is to be **examined only** under **natural light,** since **mild jaundice** can easily be **missed in artificial light. Patients** with **carcinoma of the stomach** are often **anaemic**. The **pattern** may vary under **special circumstances. Repeated vomiting** demands a **search for signs** of **dehydration. Evidence of superficial thrombophlebitis** may bring about a **suspicion of cancer of the stomach. Basically, the need is to avoid complacency at this stage**.

Box 1.4:	Points regarding general physical examination are listed.

- Sick patient - Gentle examination.
- Build and nutrition - BMI.
- Pulse rate, rate of respiration and blood pressure.
- Anaemia, jaundice, dehydration.
- Pitting oedema.
- Clubbing of the fingers.

Local Examination

Both the **patient and the doctor** should be in **comfortable positions**. The position of the **patient varies with the region** to be **examined**. There should be **adequate light**. The patient's **privacy** and **dignity** are of **paramount importance**. The **signs differ depending** on the **site of the lesion**. Details are described in individual chapters. The standard pattern consists of the following steps:

(*a*) **Inspection:** The rule is **eyes first and hands next** with reference to the patient. A **lot of information** may be elicited if the **clinician spends enough time** on **inspection**.

(*b*) **Palpation is basically an art:** It can **only improve with experience**. The **quality of a clinician** can be **judged by the degree of success during palpation. Tenderness** demands extreme **gentleness** during palpation. **Most of the physical findings** are obtained at **this stage of examination**.

(*c*) **Special tests** like **fluctuation and transillumination** may be needed in **some patients**.

(*d*) **Percussion: Unlike** the **physicians, surgeons** tend to perform this **part** of examination with a **degree of complacency. Occasionally,** this can **mislead the clinician**.

(*e*) **Auscultation:** It is **not used as**

frequently as in medical wards, but a **bruit** or a **rub** may be **clinically significant**.

(f) **Rectal examination** is to be **performed under particular circumstances**. **Many a clinician avoids this part** of the **examination** and ends up **paying a heavy penalty**.

(g) If necessary, a **pelvic examination** is also performed.

Box 1.5:	Points regarding local examination are mentioned.

- Position of the patient and the examiner.
- Adequate light and privacy.
- Inspection
- Palpation.
- Percussion
- Auscultation.
- Special tests
- Rectal and pelvic examination.

Regional Examination

The following **two examples** demonstrate the **importance of regional examination**. A patient with **melanoma** of the **foot** may have **transit nodules along the limb** with **enlarged inguinal lymph nodes**. A **patient** presenting with **enlarged inguinal lymph nodes** may have a **subungual melanoma** that might have been **missed** during a **cursory clinical examination** A **lesion** in the **supraclavicular fossa** can **produce clinical signs** in the **upper limb** due to **involvement of the nerves and vessels**.

Box 1.6:	Points to be noted on regional examination.

- Regional lymph node enlargement..
- Node enlargement - Catchment area.
- Limb - Distal pressure effects - Artery, vein, lymphatics and nerve.

Systemic Examination

All systems have to be **examined to** make sure that **associated systemic diseases** are **not missed**. **All patients** have to be examined as a **whole**. In addition, **certain systems** are to be **examined in detail** depending on the **nature of the disease**.

CLINICAL DIAGNOSIS

It is **possible** to **arrive** at a **working diagnosis** at the **end of a complete history and physical examination** in most instances. But clinical examination has its own **limitations**. In many instances **investigations** are **performed** to arrive at a **final diagnosis**. The **number and the priority** of the **investigations depend entirely** on the **information obtained** after a **good clinical examination.**

The **tendency** to order a **battery of investigations** in **every patient** is **wrong, both** from the **ethical and economic points of view**. To **conclude,** taking a **detailed history and** performing a **comprehensive physical examination** is a **highly rewarding experience** for a **surgeon**.

EXAMINATION OF A SWELLING

A swelling is defined as an abnormal protrusion identified during a clinical examination. Terms such as 'lump' or 'mass' may cause some confusion, although they carry the same meaning. Conventionally, visible protrusions are called as swellings. The term 'lump' is used for palpable lesions found in the breast, while the terms 'lump' as well as 'mass' are acceptable for palpable lesions in the abdomen.

HISTORY

A set of questions are common for swellings occurring in any part of the body. These are mentioned in detail. But the location of the swelling will decide the specific questions to be enquired into in the history. These are discussed in the later chapters.

1. **Duration of the swelling:** It may be a few days in an inflammatory swelling like a **breast abscess**. The lesion might have been present for weeks or months in many malignant conditions such as **carcinoma breast**. In benign lesions like a **lipoma,** the history may be of several years duration. As per the **time frame**, the swellings can be grouped as acute, subacute or chronic. Most of the **swellings** that are **discussed** in the following chapters belong to the **chronic variety**.

2. **Mode of onset:** It is **sudden** in acute conditions and is more gradual in chronic diseases. Majority of **benign** swellings have an **insidious onset**.

3. **Site of onset:** In swellings which have been present for several years, the patient may **not be able to localize** the site accurately. When **this information is available**, it will help to **suspect** the anatomical origin of the swelling.

4. **Size at onset:** It is surprising that in **our country**, many a **swelling** is **not noticed** by the **patient** until it assumes the **size** of a **lemon** or even of an **orange.** An asymptomatic goiter of a **moderate size** may be **brought** to the **attention** of the **patient** by the relatives. Under **these circumstances**, all the **questions mentioned above** will only get a **negative answer**. When the **size is known**, it helps the **clinician** to proceed with the **next question**.

5. **Rate of growth:** Benign swellings **tend to enlarge** slowly, whereas malignant lesions **increase in size** quite rapidly. When a **benign lesion** undergoes a **malignant transformation,** there is a sudden spurt in the **rate of growth**. A classic example would be a **rapid**

increase in size over a **period of weeks** or months in a **pleomorphic adenoma** of **parotid, which has** been **present for several years**.

6. Presence of similar swellings in other parts of the body. Multiple neurofibromatosis is **the commonest condition** in this regard. Lipomas may also be **multiple.** Sometimes the **patient** may not be aware of **additional swellings** in **other parts** of the body.

7. **Associated pain: Pain precedes** a **swelling** in **inflammatory lesions**. Most benign swellings are painless. **Development** of pain may again herald the **onset of** malignancy in these lesions. A **peripheral nerve sheath** (PNS) tumour is a **good example**. Details regarding pain have been described in the previous chapter.

8. **Associated fever: Acute inflammation** is almost always associated with **fever.** Occasionally, fever may be an **important symptom** in **malignancies** like renal cell carcinoma.

9. **Loss of appetite/weight:** Loss of appetite and significant weight loss over a **short period of time** is often **associated** with **malignant disease**.

EXAMINATION

Inspection

1. **Number:** Most swellings are single. Enlarged lymph nodes are a common example for multiple swellings.

2. **Site and extent:** The **site** is to be described in **detail.** If the site of the lesion is the lobule of **the ear** or the **tip** of the nose, the **description** may be considered as **complete.** But a **swelling** in region of the neck, back or limbs needs to be **defined more accurately**. Both the horizontal and vertical extensions are to be mentioned. **Easily identifiable anatomical** surface landmarks are used for this **purpose**. The **thyroid cartilage**, the **suprasternal notch** and the **two sternomastoid muscles** are **useful surface markings** in the **neck.**

3. **Size:** Both the horizontal and vertical dimensions are to be mentioned in centimetres. It serves as a **preliminary guide** and must be **confirmed** later by **accurate measurements**.

4. **Shape:** It may be spherical or ovoid in shape. **Swellings** that do **not fall** under these **two groups** are said to be irregular.

5. **Margin or border:** In superficial swellings, the **margin** is **clearly made out** and described as distinct. A **sebaceous cyst** has **well-defined margins**. In contrast, deeply **located** swellings may have diffuse margins.

6 **Surface:** It may be smooth as in a **hydrocele.** The term lobular is used if the swelling has a **few elevations** with **slight depressions** in between. **Lipoma** is a good example of a lobular swelling. A nodular surface is **self-explanatory**. **Nodular goiter** and **lymph node swellings** fall under this group. When some of the **nodules are quite large** in size, a term called bosselated can be used, exemplified by a **polycystic kidney**. A granular surface is seen in many of the **macronodular cirrhotic livers**. If the **surface does not fall into any of these categories,** it is called as irregular. Malignant **swellings** often have **an irregular surface**.

7. Skin over the swelling may be normal in many cases. The following changes are to be noted during inspection.

(*a*) The skin may be stretched and shiny. It often indicates a **swelling** that is **rapidly increasing** in **size.** Scaling and **wrinkling** of the **skin** overlying the swelling indicate a **process of resolution**.

This is a **common finding** in **inflammatory swellings following treatment**.

(*b*) It appears red in the presence of an acute inflammation. The skin may also show areas of hyperpigmentation (**varicose veins**) or hypopigmentation seen in relation to scars.

(*c*) The presence of dilated veins suggests **hyperaemia** commonly seen in **superficial** malignant lesions. But there are two exceptions to this statement. In a neonate with a grossly distended abdomen, dilated veins are seen in the subcutaneous plane due to the stretching of the anterior abdominal wall . A similar finding is also seen in the scrotum in a case of a large hydrocele.

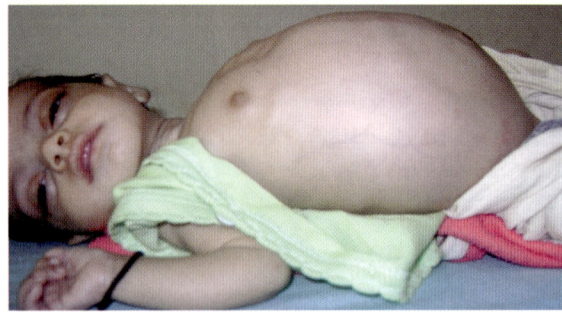

Fig. 1.1: Grossly distended abdomen in an infant showing dilated veins in the abdominal wall.

If the patient has undergone an **operation previously**, a scar is visible over the swelling. A thyroidectomy scar can easily be mistaken for a skin crease. The scar may be clearly made out only when the **patient** is asked to extend the neck. A thin linear scar is the result of healing by primary **intention.** Postoperative infection results in a broad, puckered and **irregular scar** indicating healing by secondary **intention**. When a split-thickness skin graft has been applied over a **wide raw area**, the process is termed as healing by tertiary **intention**. Less commonly, a hypertrophied scar or a keloid may be seen.

(*d*) Presence of sinuses or fistulous openings in relation to a **swelling** are **uncommon** signs. **Tuberculous** lymph nodes in the **neck** may be associated with **sinuses.**

(*e*) Many **patients** reach the hospitals after **certain investigations**. It is **necessary look** to for the puncture mark of a previous FNA or a tiny incision suggesting a **core needle biopsy** (CNB).

(*f*) Absence of hair over the **swelling** may be significant in a **sebaceous cyst** present in the **scalp.**

8. **Surrounding area:** There may be evidence of pigmentation or dilated veins in the **surrounding area.** In the case of **swellings present in the extremities**, changes may be **observed** in the limb distal to the **swelling.** These include **venous or lymph**oedema, **muscular** wasting and signs of ischaemia.

Palpation

1. **Tenderness: Facial expression of pain** also termed wincing, on applying **gentle pressure** over the swelling indicates **tenderness**. Tenderness may be **mild, moderate or even severe,** in which case the term excruciatingly tender is used. Any **effort** to ask the **patient** as to whether he is **feeling the pain** is to be **condemned, as pain is a symptom** and **tenderness** a **sign**. **Tenderness** demands extreme gentleness during **palpation.** This should always be the **first sign to be looked for in palpation**, to **remind the examiner** that the patient is a fellow human being and ought to **be given the care** he/she is **entitled to.** Acute **inflammatory swellings** are **often tender.**

2. **Warmth** over a swelling is **appreciated** by **comparing** the **temperature** on a similar location on the opposite side or in the **nearby sites**. The posterior surface of the fingers are said to **be more sensitive** in this regard. When a swelling is large and superficial, and therefore **easily accessible,**

the palm of the hand can be placed in **contact with the** surface of the **swelling** for the **duration** of about a minute. The transmission of heat from the **swelling to the palm** is **easily sensed.** This sign **has not been described** so far in any of the **clinical books on surgery. Warmth** should be **elicited at this stage,** since there is a **possibility** of the heat from the **examiner's hand** being transmitted to the swelling. In practice, **chances** of this **phenomenon are very low.**

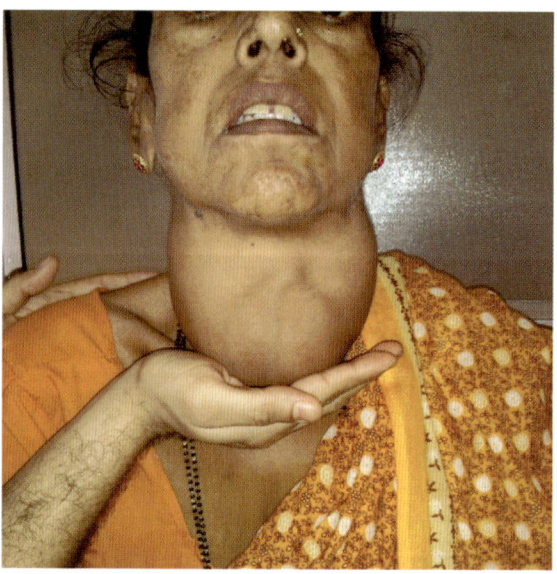

Fig. 1.2: Feeling of warmth in a swelling with the palm.

3. **Size:** Swellings that are deeply situated may be much larger on palpation than when assessed by inspection.

4. **Shape:** The **shape** in **most circumstances** may the **same** as on **inspection.**

5. **Margins or borders:** These are **much better identified** by **palpation**. The difference in the consistency between the swelling and the surrounding region helps **to demarcate the borders accurately.**

6. **Surface:** In deeply **located swellings,** the **surface** is **better** felt on palpation. This is especially **true** of intra-abdominal swellings.

   The **next three signs** are of **paramount importance** in arriving at a **clinical diagnosis.**

7. **Consistency:** It could be soft, firm or hard. The **consistency** of the **lip,** the **cartilage at the tip of the nose** and the **frontal bone** at the forehead are given as **comparisons**. But **during palpation,** a tensely **cystic swelling** may be **felt** as firm or even hard. A hydrocoele is **a perfect example** for this phenomenon. Only **repeated examinations** will reduce the **risk of making this mistake**. Many **additional terms** are used to bring out **subtle changes** in the **consistency**. Lymph nodes in Hodgkin's **lymphoma** are said to be **soft** and rubbery. In a hernia, when the greater omentum forms the content, it is termed doughy and if it is the intestine, **it** is said to be elastic. Hard swellings are further described as stony hard or bony hard.

8. **Fluctuation:** If the consistency is soft, the next step is to decide whether the **contents** are fluid in nature. This is determined by fluctuation. The **test makes use** of **Pascal's law,** which states that when **pressure** is applied to a **fluid medium,** it is **transmitted equally** in **all directions**. Once the swelling is fixed, pressure is applied at one point and the **finger** kept at a point opposite is **raised** by the **transmission** of **pressure across** the **fluid contents**. The test is **repeated** at right angles to the **original direction**. This is to avoid false positive results, which may be **obtained in structures** like the belly of a muscle that may show **movement in one direction** only. It is to be **stressed** that **unless** a **swelling can be fixed**, it is **not possible** to **perform this test.**

(a) *Why fix the swelling before eliciting fluctuation?*

Free mobile swellings produce a false sense of fluctuation by movement of the entire swelling. The best example will be a vaginal hydrocele

Paget's test. When the size of the **swelling is small,** **fluctuation** is elicited by **Paget's test.** Two fingers are used to fix **the swelling**. When **pressure** is applied at the summit with a **finger,** the impulse is felt by the fingers used to fix the **swelling.**

(b) Why is Paget's test used to elicit fluctuation in small swellings?

The **space available** is **so small** that the **conventional method** is **not possible**. **Two fingers** which are used to **fix the swelling** are also used to feel the **impulse** when **pressure** is **applied at the summit**.

(c) What are the circumstances where the consistency of a swelling poses problems?

Tensely cystic swellings may on **routine palpation** feel **firm or even hard**. This is especially true in **hydroceles**. It is therefore safer to **elicit fluctuation** in **most of scrotal swellings**. Again the **consistency** of a **thyroid swelling** is **difficult** to **identify clinically**. **Cystic swellings** may **feel firm** and **solid swellings** may be **interpreted as soft**. It is **not possible** to **fix the swelling** and hence **fluctuation cannot be elicited**. An **US examination** is needed to **demonstrate** a **cystic swelling** in the **thyroid gland.**

9. **Transillumination test:** If **fluctuation is positive,** transillumination is elicited to **determine** whether the fluid is clear or not. **Light always travels in straight lines.** The **test** is either performed in a **dark room** or **extraneous light** is cut off by

the **use** of a **rolled X-ray film** in the form of a **tube.** The light from a **pen torch** is **shone** on the swelling at one end and at a **point exactly** opposite, the transmitted light is **sought for** with this **tube**. If the fluid is clear, a pink glow is seen indicating **positive transillumination**.

10. **Mobility:** Mobility is basically classified as follows.

(*a*) **Intrinsic mobility: Upward movement** of a goiter with deglutition and **downward movement** of the liver with respiration **are two examples** for intrinsic mobility.

(*b*) **Extrinsic mobility:** The clinician tries to move the swelling in relation to the neighbouring structures. This examination is done in both horizontal and vertical directions. Mobility is **closely related** to the **anatomical plane** of the **swelling**. The terms used are free **mobility** (**fibroadenoma of the breast**), restricted **mobility** (**chronic inflammatory** swellings due to **fibrosis**) or fixed to the **deeper structures** (**advanced malignancy**).

(*c*) **Tree top mobility:** It is a **modification** of **restricted mobility.** When a **swelling** is large, the base may not move, but the top may **show** some movement. This is **best demonstrated** with **large and bulky pancreatic tumours.** Pancreas, being a **retroperitoneal organ,** is fixed in the clinical sense. But **being** a **bulky tumour,** a small part may come **in contact** with the **left dome** of the diaphragm. Thus the **swelling shows** some movement with respiration. This is **manifest** when the **patient** is in the supine **position.** But when the **patient is shifted** to the right lateral **position,** this **movement** disappears. This is **comparable** to the top of a tree **moving** with a **strong** breeze.

11. **Anatomical plane: Mobility** and the **anatomical plane** are **inter-related.** For **examination purposes,** the **bone** is **considered** to be a **fixed structure**. A **swelling** may arise from the **skin, subcutaneous tissue, muscle or tendon,** and lastly **bone. Swellings arising** or fixed to the **bone** are totally immobile. Those **arising** or **attached** to the **skin** can **easily be identified. The overlying** skin **cannot** be lifted off the **swelling.**

Most of the **problems** arise in relation to **swellings arising** from either the subcutaneous tissue or the muscle and tendon. The **clinical tests** that are described to **distinguish between the two** are **based** on the **anatomical** principle that a **muscle** has mobility in a **state** of relaxation, but a contracted **muscle** becomes a fixed **structure**. In addition, **maximum force** of **contraction** is present when resistance is **applied** in the opposite direction. To **perform** these tests **properly**, it is **necessary** to **remember** three anatomical facts. These **factors** are the name of the **muscle** in **relation** to the **swelling**, its action and the **method of providing** resistance. **Resistance** can be provided by the **following three methods**.

(*a*) **The examiner provides the resistance:** All the extremity **muscles** can be **examined** in this **manner.** To test the **biceps,** the **patient is asked to flex** his **elbow** and the **examiner** provides resistance at the **forearm.** In addition **muscles of the neck** like **the sternomastoid and trapezius** can also be tested in the **same way**.

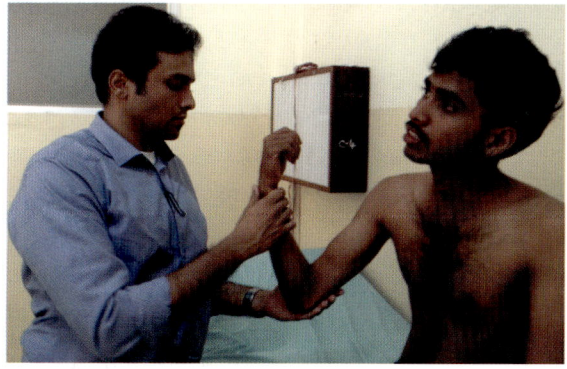

Fig. 1.3: Contraction of the biceps against resistance.

(*b*) **Resistance is provided by gravity:** The test is **useful** to detect the **plane** of an abdominal swelling. The **patient is** made to **lie supine** and **lift his lower limbs** while keeping the **knees extended**. The **contracted abdominal muscles** act **against gravity** to maintain the **limbs in the same position**. The **same result** can be obtained by **asking the patient** to **raise the upper part of the trunk** and the **head without** the **support of the elbows**.

(*c*) **Patient provides the resistance:** Masseter and the pectoralis major are **two muscles** where this **method is employed**. When the **patient clenches** the **teeth,** the **masseter i**s in **a state of contraction**. The **upper jaw** provides the **needed resistance**. Similarly, when the **patient** is asked to **press his hand** against **the hip** with the **elbow in a position of flexion, the pectoralis major** is in a **state of contraction**. **Adduction** of the **shoulder** by the **action** of the **muscle** is prevented by the **resistance** provided by the **flexed elbow.**

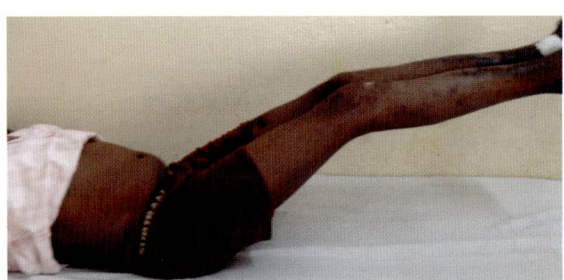

Fig. 1.4: Lower limb raising test to determine the anatomical plane of an abdominal swelling.

The plane of a given **swelling** depends on the **result of these tests**. If the **swelling** is subcutaneous, the mobility remains the same. If the **swellings** are fixed to the muscle, they become less mobile, but **more** prominent. **Swellings** deep to the **muscle** become less mobile and less prominent. Hence a **complete knowledge** of the **relevant anatomy** is a **prerequisite** for an **accurate examination** at this stage.

Examination of the surrounding area may reveal certain abnormalities. These **depend** on the **site** of the **swelling**. A **swelling** may cause compression of the **adjacent structures** and give rise to **certain signs**. If a **swelling is close** to a joint it may result in limitation of **movements** of that joint.

If there is a **swelling** in the limb, one should look for pressure effects in the distal **part** of the **limb**. Lymphatic obstruction leads to **lymphoedema**. **Venous obstruction** leads to **venous oedema**. There may be evidence of **diminished pulsations** or **nerve deficit,** if there is **involvement** of the **artery** or **nerves.**

How is venous oedema distinguished from lymphoedema?

Venous oedema involves the **proximal part** of the **limb** more than the **distal part. Lymphoedema progresses** from the **distal part proximally**. In the lower limb the **thigh segment is not involved** in **most cases**. In the **cases** of **venous obstruction**, the **shape of the limb** is **compared** to that of a **champagne bottle**. The **presence** of **dilated veins** in the **subcutaneous plane points to venous oedema**. These **two types** may **coexist** in a limb. In **such instances**, a **Doppler study** is necessary to **detect the abnormalities**.

Palpation of Regional Lymph Nodes

If the nodes are enlarged, the number, consistency and mobility are to be noted. These **swellings** may be **identified** as **lymph nodes** since they are **present at sites** where **nodes are commonly present** and their **size and shape correspond** to that of **enlarged nodes**. The next proximal group of nodes should also be **palpated**. For example, if the **inguinal nodes** are **enlarged,** the **external iliac group** of nodes must be **palpated**.

If on the other hand, the **swelling comprises** of lymph nodes, the catchment area should be **examined carefully** for a **lesion** that could **be responsible** for the **nodal enlargement**. A classic example would be a patient with a **small subungual melanoma** in one of the **toes,** presenting with **massive inguinal lymphadenopathy.**

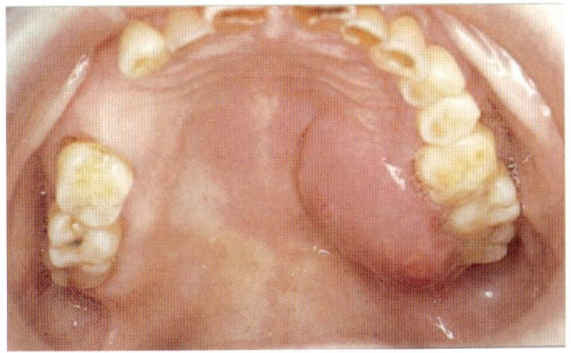

Fig. 1.5: Ectopic salivary gland tumour in the hard palate.

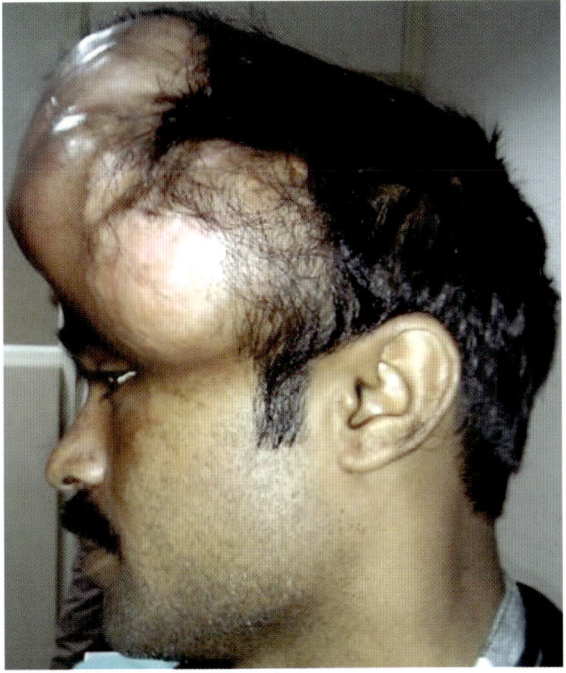

Fig. 1.6: Recurrent malignant soft-tissue tumour in the scalp.

Percussion

Although **presumed** to be **less important** in **surgical patients, and** hence often **conducted** in a **complacent manner,** there are **situations** where percussion **is significant**. In a case of **hernia,** if the percussion **note is resonant**, it indicates **bowel as the content. Dullness** over the **manubrium sterni** suggests a **retrosternal goiter**. In the case of an **epigastric lump**, if the percussion note is **dull** and the **dullness** is **continuous** with that of the **liver,** it suggests an **enlarged left lobe** of the **liver. Lumps** arising from the **stomach** are either **resonant** or show **impaired resonance**, since it is a **hollow organ**.

Auscultation

Auscultation is **needed in some cases. Bruit** in general, is a sign of **increased vascularity**.

EXAMINATION OF OTHER SYSTEMS

The **importance** of this part cannot be **over emphasised**. Despite the presence of a **localised lesion**, the need is to do a **comprehensive examination** of the **whole patient. Loss** of this **concept** has led to **several disasters**.

Rectal and pelvic examinations are **useful** in many **surgical patients**. It should be **explained to the patient in detail** regarding **these two procedures** and **proper consent** must be **obtained**. Both **patients and clinicians** have **suffered** by **not undertaking** this part of the **examination**. It is **important** to **remember** that a **pile**

mass is **not palpable** by a **digital rectal examination**. Since the **mass** comprises of **dilated veins**, **pressure** of the **finger compresses these veins** and the **mass cannot be felt**.

The **common** findings during a rectal examination include the following:

(*a*) **Ulcers–benign or malignant**

(*b*) **Enlarged prostate** in an **elderly male.**

(*c*) **Strictures** (**uncommon**).

(*d*) **Secondary deposit** in the **rectovesical pouch.**

(*e*) **Blood** on the **gloved finger** when it is withdrawn from the rectum, in cases of **malignancy**.

Proctoscopy

Procedure

The **patient** is made to lie in the **left lateral position**. A **well-lubricated scope** is **introduced** into the **anal canal gently** in the **direction of the umbilicus**. Once the **anal canal** has been **passed**, the **direction** of the **instrument** is **changed towards** the **sacrum and pushed inwards**. The **obturator** is **withdrawn** and the **interior** is **inspected** with **good illumination**.

Contraindication

Presence of a **fissure-in-ano** is an **absolute contraindication**. The patient complains of **severe pain during** and **after defecation**. There is an **associated spasm** of the **anal sphincters**. **Attempting** a **proctoscopy** under these circumstances is **extremely painful to the patient**

Piles may be **visualized. Primary pile masses** are seen at **3, 7 and 11 O'clock positions**. An **ulcerated growth** may also be **seen. Biopsy** of suspicious lesions **can be taken**. As the **scope is being withdrawn additional findings** may become visible. They include **secondary piles, internal opening of a fistula,** etc.

EXAMINATION OF AN ULCER

An **ulcer** is defined as a **breach in the continuity** of the **surface epithelium** with **loss of tissue**. A **simple breach** does **not constitute** an **ulcer**. An **incision** carried out by a **laser knife** results in a **breach in the epithelium,** but it **cannot** be **classified** as an **ulcer**. An **ulcer** can only occur in **those** structures having a **lining epithelium**. Thus **skin** and the **epithelial surface** of the **gastrointestinal** tract are **most common sites**. In addition, the **proximal respiratory tract** lined by ciliated **modified stratified squamous epithelium** and the part of the **urinary system** lined by **transitional epithelium** may develop **ulcers.**

The chief complaint is usually the presence of an **ulcer. Chronic ulcers** are seen **more frequently** in the **extremities.** The **distal part of the lower limb** is **one** of the **common sites.**

HISTORY

1. **Duration of the ulcer:** Most ulcers are of **several months** duration.
2. **Mode of onset:** Many patients may give a history of minor **trauma preceding the formation of the ulcer.** Ulcers may arise **spontaneously** following **severe infection,** when the **skin** overlying a **blister gives way.** Ulcers could be part of a **metabolic disease** like **diabetes.** It could be due to a **specific disease** like **tuberculosis.**

3. **Rate of growth:** In the presence of **acute inflammation**, the **ulcer** can **enlarge** in size over a **short period** of time. In **patients** with **chronic ulcers**, the rate of growth is **more gradual**. A **small number of patients** may reach the **hospital** at the **stage** of **healing**.

4. **Pain:** Pain is **severe** in the **acute stage**. Most **chronic** ulcers have **minimal pain**. At times, **the pain** may worsen or **become severe** on **movement**. Pain is **conspicuous** by its **absence** in **neuropathic** ulcers.

5. **Discharge:** In a **healing** ulcer, the **discharge** is **serous** in nature. **Purulent discharge** indicates the **presence** of **infection,** and may often be **foul smelling**. It could be **blood stained** in **malignant ulcers**.

6. **Local symptoms:** They **differ** depending on the **site**. Ulcers located **close to a joint** can cause **limitation of movement** or **deformities.**

7. **Systemic symptoms:** These are present when the ulcers are a part of a systemic disease like **diabetes.**

Box 1.7:	The points to be noted while taking the history.

- Ulcer – Duration.
- Mode of onset and rate of growth.
- Pain.
- Discharge – Purulent – Foul smelling – Blood stained.
- Local symptoms.
- Systemic symptoms.

General physical examination is usually within **normal** limits.

LOCAL EXAMINATION

Inspection

1. **Number:** Most ulcers are **single**. **Tuberculous** ulcers can be **multiple**.

2. **Site and extent:** The **examination is similar** to that of a swelling. The **extent** is mentioned with **reference** to known **surface markings.**

3. **Size:** It is mentioned in both **horizontal and vertical dimensions**.

4. **Shape:** The shape could be **circular**, **oval or irregular**.

5. **Margin:** If the **shape is circular or oval,** the margin is said to be **regular.** Otherwise it is termed as **irregular**.

6. **Floor:** Floor is defined as the **visible area** within the **margins** of the **ulcer**. It is an **important part of inspection**. In most cases, it comprises of **granulation**

tissue. The term is used because it has a **granular appearance**. **Granulation tissue** is **compose**d of a **rich plexus of capillaries** with **actively multiplying fibroblasts** filling the spaces in between. It could either be **healthy** or **unhealthy**. The features of **unhealthy granulation tissue** are as follows:

(*a*) **Paleness:** In **ischaemic ulcers**, the **floor appears pale**.

(*b*) **Presence of slough:** Slough is **dead solid tissue** having a **white or slightly yellow** appearance. **Slough is** formed due to **loss of blood supply**. It is known that **severe inflammation** leads to **vascular thrombosis**. If a **group of small vessels** undergo **thrombosis,** the **part of tissue supplied** by **these vessels dies** and is **invaded** by **bacteria.** Hence **slough denotes severe inflammation with sepsis**. Its **presence prevents complete healing** of **an ulcer**.

(*c*) **Presence of pus:** Pus is the **liquefied material** seen on the **floor.** It contains **dead** and **living bacteria** and white blood corpuscles (**WBCs**) along with **necrotic material liquefied** by the **action** of **macrophages**. Unfortunately, in the **hospital setting, the pus** is **adsorbed** by the **dressings applied** on to the **ulcer**. Hence to **detect** the **presence of pus**, the **dressing** needs to be **examined carefully**. The change in **colour,** and the presence of **smell** if any, will give a clue as to the **nature of the bacterium** present in the **pus.** Thick **creamish yellow** pus suggests infection with *Staphylococcus aureus.* Thick **greenish** pus with a **typical smell** raises a **suspicion of infection by the proteus** group of **bacteria.**

(*d*) **Presence of a biofilm adherent to the floor:** It is **more often** seen in **hospital-acquired infections** and **burns**. A thin **whitish grey film** is seen **covering the floor of the ulcer**. The **film** consists of a **carbohydrate matrix** containing a **colony** of **bacteria linked** to **each other**. These often **represent a group** of **drug-resistant** bacteria.

(*e*) **Uneven appearance:** The **floor** may have **depressions** and **elevations. Pus** may be lurking in the **crevices.** This is of clinical significance because such a **floor** will **not accept a graft**.

(*f*) **Hypertrophic and friable granulation tissue:** The **granulation tissue** appears to be **spreading beyond the margins** and is so **friable** that

bits of **tissue** may be **stuck to the dressing**.

The presence of **any of the factors** mentioned above is an **indication** of a **nonhealing ulcer.**

If **none** are present, the **granulation tissue is healthy** and suggests a **healing ulcer. A skin graft** applied at this stage will **succeed.**

The floor of a **malignant ulcer** poses some **problems.** It has an **appearance** of **granulation tissue.** But the tissue is **malignant.** So the **floor** of a **malignant ulcer** can be described as **reddish-pink nodular or granular** tissue. In addition, **slough** may **be present** on **the floor.** When the **blood supply** is **inadequate** for the **rapidly multiplying malignant cells**, some of the **tumour tissue** undergoes **necrosis. Bacterial invasion** of these tissues results in **slough formation.**

The **level of the floor** in **relation** to the **margin** and the **surrounding area** is **significant.** It could be **elevated.** Such ulcers are **termed** as **proliferative** in **nature.** It could also be **depressed.** These are **excavating** type **of malignant ulcers** and tend to **infiltrate deeper,** thus having a **poorer prognosis**. The **gingivolabial**

sulcus in the **oral cavity** is a **common site** for this type of **malignancy.**

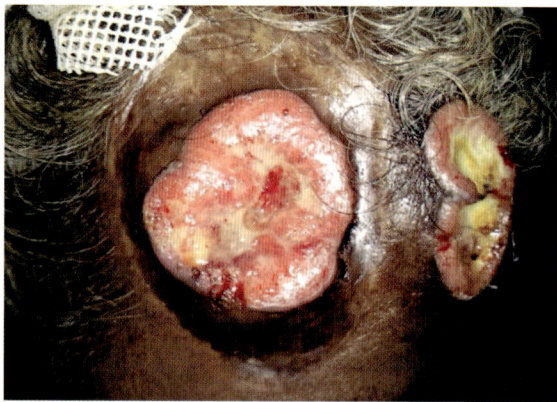

Fig. 1.7: Excavating type of malignant ulcer in the forehead with two satellite lesions, with a depressed floor and raised everted edges.

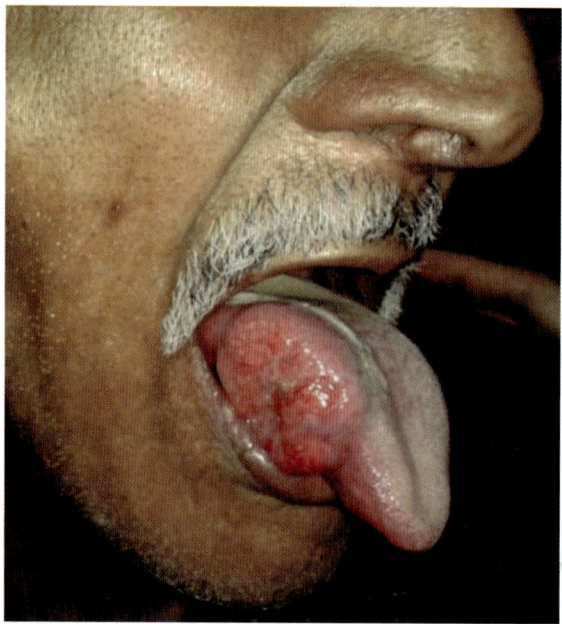

Fig. 1.8: Proliferative type of a malignant ulcer in the lateral margin of the tongue, with a raised floor and everted edges.

7. **Surrounding area:** It may show **pigmentation** (venous ulcer) or **scarring (healing chronic ulcer).**

Box 1.8:	The points to be noted on inspection.

- Inspection
- Number.
- Site and extent.
- Size and shape.
- Margin – Regular or irregular.
- Floor – Granulation tissue – Healthy or unhealthy.
- Floor - Malignancy – Elevated – Proliferative.
  - Depressed – Excavating.
- Surrounding area.

Palpation

1. **Warmth and tenderness:** The surrounding area is checked for change in temperature. **Warmth** is unusual in **chronic ulcers.** An **ischaemic** limb may feel **colder** compared with the **normal.** The presence of **tenderness** demands extreme **gentleness** on the part of the **examiner. Ischaemic** ulcers are **very tender.**

2. **Edge:** Edge is the **three-dimensional structure** that is **felt** between the **border** and the **floor. A gloved finger** is gently **run** from the **margin** till the **floor** is reached. An edge is **better felt than seen.**

   The most frequently seen type is the **sloping edge**. It is a **manifestation** of the **healing process**. The epithelium at the **margin** of an ulcer tends to proliferate. The **cells slide** towards the **floor**, resulting in a **sloping edge**. But the **healing process** will be **completed** only in the presence of **healthy granulation tissue**. Thus an ulcer cannot be **classified** as **healing** in the **presence** of this **isolated clinical finding**.

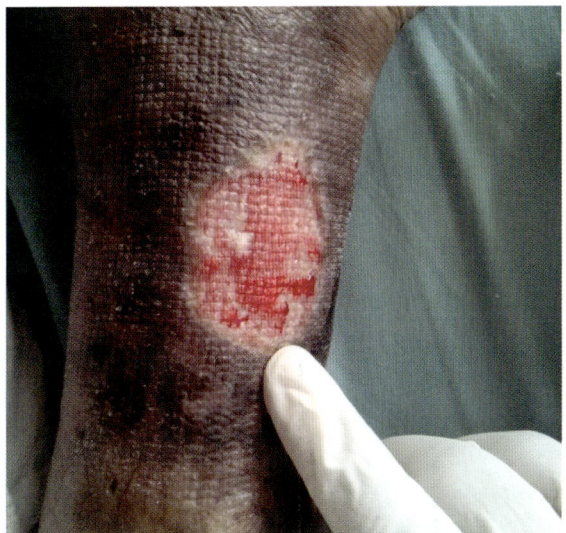

Fig. 1.9: Sloping edge of a healing ulcer with healthy granulation tissue at the floor.

An **undermined edge** is seen in a **tuberculous** ulcer. The skin **overlies** a **part** of the **floor**. A **probe** can be **inserted under the edge** to **demonstrate** this **sign**.

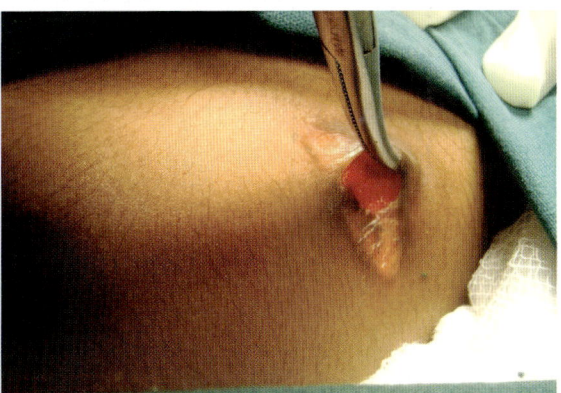

Fig. 1.10: Undermined edge of a tuberculous ulcer.

Raised and everted edges are the hallmark of a **malignant ulcer**. It is also described as **rolled out edges**.

Basal cell carcinoma has **raised** and **beaded** edges.

Punched out edges are seen in **ischaemic** ulcers. They are also **described** in **syphilitic** ulcers, which are extremely rare. A **punched out appearance** may be seen after a **debridement** has been done **surgically.**

3. **Base:** The base is the **tissue** on which the ulcer **rests**. It could be formed by **subcutaneous tissue, muscle, tendon or bone**. The ulcer is **immobile** when the **base** is formed by the **bone.** The **mobility** of an **ulcer** is **restricted** if the **base** is formed by **muscle or tendon,** when **that structure** is put on **contraction against resistance**. The **clinical method** of examination is **similar** to that of a **swelling**.

Induration of the **base** is an **important finding** in a **malignant ulcer**. It is a **feeling** of **hardness** due to a **desmoplastic reaction** on the **part** of the **host** towards the **malignancy**. This is **best exemplified** in **squamous cell carcinoma.**

If the **bone** forming the **base** is **subcutaneous (venous ulcer in relation to the tibia),** it is necessary to **palpate** for **bony thickening**. This can be **identified** by **comparing** the **thickness** of the involved **bone** with that of the **opposite side**. The **thickening** is due to **periosteitis induced** by **chronic inflammation**.

Palpation of Surrounding Area

Chronic ulcers may show **thickening** of the **skin** and **subcutaneous tissue**. In **malignancy**, the **induration** may **extend** over a **variable area beyond** the **edges** of the **ulcer**.

EXAMINATION OF THE REGIONAL LYMPH NODES

Most **chronic ulcers** are **associated** with **enlarged regional lymph nodes**. They may be **soft-to-firm** in **consistency, nontender and mobile**. **Secondary nodes** from **malignant ulcers** are usually **hard,** and they either display **restricted mobility** or are **fixed**.

EXAMINATION OF OTHER SYSTEMS

This part of the **examination depends** on the **anatomical location** of the **ulcer**. Ulcers in **close proximity** to a **joint** may produce **restriction** of **movement** by **extracapsular fibrosis**. These may also result in **deformities**. An **equinus deformity** of **the foot** is a **complication** seen in a **long standing venous ulcer**.

The following systems should be carefully examined while assessing a **chronic ulcer** in **the lower limb.**

Lymphatic System

There may be evidence of **lymphoedema** in the limb. This is **pitting** in **the initial stage,** but later becomes **nonpitting** due to **fibrosis.**

Venous System

Patients develop **venous ulcers** secondary to **idiopathic varicose veins** or due to **deep venous thrombosis (DVT). Varicose veins** should be **looked for** with **the patient** in a **standing position**. The only **evidence of a DVT** may be **swelling** of the **limb.**

Arterial System

Ischaemic ulcers may be **present** with or without **gangrene**. Hence **palpation** of the **peripheral arteries** is an **integral part** of the **examination.**

Nervous System

Peripheral neuropathy is often associated with diabetic **ulcers. Trophic ulcers** occur at pressure points on the **sole of the foot. Joint** and **vibration** sensations are **lost early,** and are **more sensitive** than the **loss of touch** sensation. **Diabetes** as mentioned above is the **common cause** of **neuropathy**. But **Hansen's disease** is still **prevalent** in **certain parts of the country.**

Box 1.9:	Points to be noted during palpation.

- Palpation – Warmth and tenderness.
- Edge – Sloping.
  - Undermined.
- Punched out.
  - Everted or raised.
- Base – Subcutaneous tissue, muscle or tendon and bone.
- Bony thickening – Periosteitis.
- Regional nodes.
- Systems – lymphatic, venous, arterial and nervous systems.

Q. 1. How are chronic ulcers classified clinically?

They are **classified** as **specific and nonspecific. Specific ulcers** have adequate **clinical signs** to identify the **causative organism. Tuberculous, syphilitic** and **actinomycotic ulcers** belong to this **group.** In the case of **nonspecific ulcers**, the **nature of the infective organism** can only be detected by **investigations.**

Nonspecific ulcers include a very **diverse group. Trauma, severe infection and diabetes** are the common causes. **Nonspecific ulcers** are **further classified** into spreading (with inflammatory margins), **healing** and **nonhealing** ulcers. **Nonhealing ulcers** are also known as **callous ulcers. A healing ulcer** is **characterised** by the presence of **sloping edges, serous discharge** and **healthy granulation tissue** at the **floor**.

Q. 2. What are the features of a tuberculous ulcer?

These may be **multiple**. The margin has a **bluish rim** of epithelium**. The floor is comprised of **pale granulation tissue**. The **discharge** is **serous** in nature. The **edges** are **undermined**. The **regional nodes** when **enlarged** show **matting.**

Q. 3. Describe the features of a syphilitic ulcer.

At present they are **uncommon**. They have **punched out** edges. The floor has an appearance of **washed leather slough**. The **regional nodes** are **hard, nontender** and **mobile.**

Q. 4. What are the investigations to be done in a case of chronic nonspecific ulcer?

1. Rule out **systemic diseases** like diabetes and atherosclerosis.

2. **X-ray** of the part if there is evidence of **bony thickening**.

3. **Pus** is sent for **culture** to determine the **causative organism. Sensitivity** tests should be performed to plan the appropriate **antimicrobials**, since the patient would have **received multiple antimicrobials** before admission to the hospital

4. If **malignancy** is suspected, **multiple edge biopsies** are done. **Chronic ulcers** of a **long duration** show some **degree** of **hardness** due to **excessive fibrosis.** This may **simulate induration** and hence **biopsies** are **indicated.**

Q. 5. **What are treatment strategies for a chronic nonspecific ulcer?**

As mentioned earlier, one of the **common sites** for an **ulcer** is the **distal part of** the **lower limb. Rest** to **the affected part** helps **healing. Admission** to the hospital **ensures adequate rest.** If the **floor** contains plenty of **slough,** a **surgical debridement** is performed. The **treatment** then **continues** in the following **order.** The **ulcer** is cleaned with **cetrimide** or normal **saline. Povidone iodine** is applied **locally.** If **culture** shows the growth of ***Pseudomonas aeruginosa,*** silver sulfadiazine is used for **local application.** Systemic antimicrobials are **used** during **surgical interventions only.** In the **presence** of **oedema,** the **limb** is kept **elevated.** Over a **period of time, the slough is completely cleared** and the **floor** is **covered** by **healthy granulation tissue.** A **repeat pus culture** is **done** to **confirm** the **eradication of sepsis.** If the **size** of the **ulcer** is **small, healing** takes place by migration of **epithelium** from the **margins. Larger ulcers** need a **skin cover.** In **most instances,** a **split-thickness skin graft** is **adequate. Complex plastic surgical reconstruction** is used to **cover** the **raw area** in **weight-bearing regions** such as the **sole of the foot**.

Q. 6. **How are malignant ulcers treated?**

The **management** depends on the **site** of the ulcer. **Three-dimensional wide excision** of the ulcer is **commonly performed**. An **excision** performed with a **margin** of about **2 cm** from the **edge** of **induration** will **result** in a **R0 resection**. This would mean that the **margins** of the **resected specimen** do **not show evidence** of **malignancy microscopically.** If the **ulcer** is fixed to the **bone,** an **amputation** becomes **necessary. Metastatic nodes** are **treated** by **radical lymphadenectomy.**

Q. 7. **What is a Marjolin's ulcer? How is it managed?**

Marjolin's ulcer is a **squamous cell carcinoma arising** from a **pre-existing scar.** Here, the **overlying squamous epithelium** is **subjected** to **repeated minor trauma.** This is **likely to occur** when the **scar** is located **around a joint** or on a **weight-bearing** area. As a **result,** the scar **breaks**

down to form an **ulcer,** which **heals** over a **period of time. Repeated episodes** of this **nature result** in a **malignant transformation** of this **fragile epithelium, giving rise** to a **Marjolin's ulcer.** A **burn scar** is described as the **commonest cause** for this **malignancy.** But in **our country**, a very common predisposing cause could be a **chronic ulcer** in **the foot** with **unstable scars** following a **snake bite**.

Clinical Features

Patients give **a history** of a **previous burn injury** or a **snake bite.** The **duration** is of **several years**. Typically, the **scar** has been **breaking down resulting** in an **ulcer** that **heals, only** to **recur** again. But unlike on the earlier **occasions,** the **ulcer** tends to **become bigger** over a **period of time**. But the **fact** that the **patient has had the lesion** for a **long time** is the reason for the **delay** in seeking medical help **at the hospital**.

The **appearance** is that of a **squamous cell carcinoma.** As long as the **growth is confined** within the **limits of the scar, lymphatic spread does not take place**. The **reason** is that the **scar** is **devoid** of **lymphatics.** But **once** the **lesion extends beyond this limit**, it **behaves** like any **other squamous cell carcinoma,** and the **regional nodes** may **harbour metastases**. Hence **lesions within the scar** have a **better** prognosis.

Treatment

A **wide excision** is **usually performed**. In many instances, the **entire scar** has to be **removed. Plastic surgical reconstruction** is **needed** under **those circumstances. Amputation** becomes **necessary** once the malignancy is **fixed** to **the underlying bone. Metastatic nodes** are **removed** by **radical lymphadenectomy** Radiotherapy is contraindicated.

Q. 8. Describe the clinical features and management of a basal cell carcinoma.

Basal cell carcinoma is the **commonest** malignancy arising from the **skin** in the **Caucasian population.** The **cancer arises** from the **cells** of the **basal** layer of the **epidermis. Sunlight** is said to be a **predisposing factor.** A **familial variety** has also **been described.** The **area** of the **face** above the line joining the **angle of** the **mouth** to the **tragus** of **the ear** is the **most common site;** but they are **known** to occur at **other parts** of the **body** as well. These **lesions** present as **ulcers** of a **long duration** with a **slow rate** of growth. They have a pinkish or reddish appearance. In addition, they may appear to be pearly and translucent. Encrustation and raised beaded edges are diagnostic findings.

These tumours are locally invasive, but metastatic spread is extremely rare. The infiltration deep into the tissue resembles the burrowing of a rodent, and hence these are also known as rodent ulcers. When the location is close to vital structures like the eye, it can pose serious problems in management. Microscopically, the palisaded appearance of the cells spreading into the deeper layers is typical. There is minimal myxoid stroma between the clusters of cells. Edge biopsy confirms the diagnosis. Imaging studies are needed for evaluating large and deep lesions that are close to vital structures. Wide surgical excision is the ideal treatment. Attainment of tumour-free margins ensures a good prognosis. In small superficial cancers, it may be about 5 mm from the edges of the tumour, both in the radial and vertical directions. But many of our patients have large tumours infiltrating deep into the adjacent tissues. They need a margin of 2 cm for an adequate clearance. Plastic surgical reconstruction is performed to minimise the cosmetic disfigurement. Recurrent tumours have a poor prognosis.

A well-planned excision along with proper reconstruction is associated with a very good outcome. Radiotherapy is used in advanced and inoperable cases. Many other regimes like cryotherapy, photodynamic therapy and local application of 5-flurouracil have all been described. But surgery remains the best line of treatment.

■■■

Essentials of Radiology

Dr. Vidya S. Upadhyaya

Dr. Vidya S. Upadhyaya, Consultant Ultrasonologist, Sengkang Health, Singapore

2

Radiology plays an essential and integral role in patient care. This introduction to radiology has been kept concise and focusses on the indications and limitations of the various imaging modalities. The basic skills in image interpretation that might be required in patient management will be discussed separately along with the individual cases.

Medical students need **first-hand** experience and should observe radiology departments in action and be **involved** in the **radiological investigations** and **interventions** of their patients. The request for a **radiological investigation** is analogous to a request for a **clinical consultation**. The radiological report is the **end product** of what may have been a **long** and potentially **hazardous** investigation. The **conclusion** expressed in the report is often based on a **detailed interpretation** process and a series of **deductions** based not only on **radiological signs**, but also on **clinical information**.

When planning a series of investigations, it should be remembered that the diagnosis should be reached by the **shortest, safest** and **cheapest** route. Hence a broad knowledge of imaging modalities is very essential.

Basically, the investigations can be divided into two groups: those involving ionising **radiation** and those without their use.

Box 2.1:	Methods using ionising radiation

- Simple X-rays
- Computerized axial tomography (CT)
- Radioisotope scanning — also called nuclear medicine, radionuclide scanning or scintigraphy
- Positron emission tomography (PET)

Box 2.2:	Methods without the use of ionising radiation

- Ultrasound
- Magnetic resonance imaging (MRI)

X-RAYS

These rays are part of the **electromagnetic spectrum**. They are very good at imaging **bones**. They can show some **organs** and **soft tissues**. X-rays are **faster**, **readily available**, and **cost less** than other scans, so they are used to get information quickly. An **X-ray beam** is passed through the patient on to a **photographic plate**. Depending on the **density** of the structures in the body, these get **attenuated** (slowed down). For example, **bones** are very **dense** (more molecules per cu.mm) and hence will **absorb** a lot of X-rays, and they are **visualised** as relatively **white** structures. **Air** will allow a lot of X-rays to pass through, and hence air within bowel or outside it will appear relatively black on the film

Screening and Image Intensifiers

Low-dose X-rays are used **continuously** or intermittently to provide **dynamic** study (over a **period of time**) unlike an **X-ray**, which is a static study (at a **point** of time). The images are observed on the **image intensifier** monitor by the radiologist. This can be recorded on **video** and **recordings** played back as **required**. This is useful in **barium** studies and other **contrast studies**, including conventional **angiographies**.

Contrast Agents in Radiological Investigations

Most body **tissues** have **similar densities**, and therefore **attenuate X-rays** to an **equal extent**. More information can be obtained by **artificially** introducing **high-density contrast** agents into these **organs** either **orally**, by direct infusicn, or through **intravenous** or **intra-arterial** injections. The commonly used agents are listed below.

Barium Sulphate

This salt of the heavy metal barium is used for **gastrointestinal work**. The contrast coats the **intestinal mucosa** well. This along with **air insufflation** distends the bowel to produce the so-called '**double contrast**' examination.

Iodinated Contrast Media

They are **water-soluble salts** and are used for investigating the **urinary** tract (**intravenous pyelography**) and the **cardiovascular** system (**angiography**), in particular. They are also widely used in **CT scans** of the **body** to get more information (contrast-enhanced CT scan [**CECT**]). Adverse **allergic** reactions and even serious fatal **anaphylaxis** is known to occur with their use. At present, the **non-ionic** solutions are used to reduce the frequency of side effects. Since they are **excreted via the urinary system**, they should be used with **caution** in patients with reduced **renal function**, and should be **avoided** in **renal failure** patients.

Air

Air is used as a **negative contrast agent** in **barium studies** as described above. It is also used as the **sole contrast agent** in CT scan for large bowel (**CT colonography**).

Alternative contrast agents are available for use with **MRI** (eg **gadolinium**) and **ultrasonography** (**microbubble** contrast agent).

Box 2.3:	The contrast agents

- Barium sulphate – GI tract + air- double contrast.
- Iodine compounds – ionic and non-ionic – IVP, CT and CECT – urinary tract and the vascular system.
- Gadolinium – MRI.
- Air – CT colonography.

COMPUTERIZED AXIAL TOMOGRAPHY (CT SCAN)

An **X-ray tube** revolves **around** the patient and the **emergent beam** is picked up by detectors. The beam is **attenuated** depending on the **tissue density**, and these are transformed into **images** by the **computer**. In comparison with plain radiographs, the visual grey scale is **enhanced** to improve **organ visualisation** and **definition**. The image can also be **manipulated** to

give **additional detail** about **tissues of widely varying density**, for example, **bone and soft tissues**. Although this data is acquired in the **axial plane**, it can be reformatted in **coronal**, **sagittal** and even **oblique** planes. This data can also be reconstructed to give **three-dimensional** information, for example, by **volume rendering**. Dense **contrast agents** can be used to demonstrate the internal anatomy of structures, and certain organs such as **vascular system**, **urinary** tract and **gastrointestinal** tract.

Box 2.4:	Points regarding advantages

- High-resolution images with good spatial resolution. Bones can be visualized well too (cf. MRI).
- Capability for multiplanar reformatting.
- Very useful in acute setting; good for detection of acute haemorrhage and small perforations.

Box 2.5:	Points regarding disadvantages

- Significant radiation is involved. Hence the examination should be requested with caution.

ULTRASOUND

It uses **sound waves** whose frequency is far **higher** than what a human **ear** can hear. These waves are produced from a **transducer** (containing lead zirconate titanate crystal) and travel through the human tissues. When these reach an **object** or **surface**, the waves are **reflected** back. These **echoes** are again received by the **transducer** and changed into **electric current** and displayed on the **monitor**. The picture on the monitor is studied by the radiologist.

The **choice** of the transducer depends on the **clinical** application with the frequency usually in the range of **2–5 MHz** (convex probe for deep **abdominal** scan) and **5–10 MHz** (linear high-resolution probe for **small parts** and peripheral **vascular** study).

Some of the echo-sounding display forms are as follows:

1. **B mode/Brightness mode:** Here echoes are displayed as **dots** of varying **brightness**.

2. **Grey-scale** imaging is a **refinement** enabling B scan to be scaled in different **shades of grey**.

3. **Real time two-dimensional scanning:** A further advance on grey-scale imaging where images are shown in **real-time**, that is, in actual motion. The commonly used **probes** (transducers) are **linear** probes (for probing **superficial** parts, such as breast, neck and scrotum), phased array **curvilinear** probes (for use in the **abdomen and pelvis**) and **endocavitary** probes (for **endovaginal and endorectal** use).

4. **Doppler:** Using the **Doppler** principle, the **velocity** of the blood flowing **towards** and **away** from the probe can be derived from the **reflected** ultrasound waves. The **Doppler Effect** refers to the change in the **frequency** of a sound **wave** in relation to the **source**. If the wave is moving **towards** the source (**US probe**) there is **enhancement** and an **away** movement **reduces** the frequency. The effect is widely used for **vascular** studies and **foetal** monitoring.

5. **Duplex scanner:** They combine both pulse echo ultrasound and Doppler shift facilities. Both modes are simultaneously recorded.

6. **Continuous wave Doppler:** Uses **two transducer** crystals mounted side by side, one for **transmitting** and the other **receiving** ultrasound waves. It is excellent for **high-velocity flow** and for recording **peak velocities**.

7. **Pulsed Doppler:** Uses a **single** transducer to emit **short bursts** of ultrasound, which are received back by **the same transducer**. This allows **precise** focusing on **small sample volumes**.

8. **Colour-flow mapping:** Is based on **pulsed Doppler** and allows assessment across the **whole field** of a **two-dimensional** image. The results can be coded in colour as **red**, **blue** and varying hues in between.

9. **Availability:** The investigation is available in **most parts** of the **country**. It is also **cost effective**.

It can be **repeated** as and when necessary **without** any **deleterious effects. Pregnancy** is **not a contraindication**.

10. **Limitations:** Ultrasound **beam** cannot **penetrate bone and air**. It is **totally operator dependent**, and hence the **competency** of the ultrasonologist **defines** the **results**.

Box 2.6:	The types of ultrasound

- Grey scale
- Real time two-dimensional scan
- Continuous Doppler scan
- Pulsed Doppler
- Duplex scan
- Colour Doppler scan
- Colour Doppler

MAGNETIC RESONANCE IMAGING (MRI)

It uses **electromagnetic waves** to generate **signals** in a very complex way. The patient lies within a **large circular magnet**, which generates **magnetic field** intensities between **0.2 and 3.0 Tesla** for diagnostic purposes. Under the influence of the **external magnetic forces**, the **hydrogen nuclei** of body fluids **(water and lipids)** behave like **small magnets** that respond to **external** radiofrequencies by producing their own **radiofrequencies**. These in turn are detected by **surface coils** and augmented into **signals**, which are then converted into **images**.

Box 2.7:	Advantages of MRI

- No radiation
- High-resolution images with good contrast resolution.
- Multiplanar capability, i.e images can be acquired in axial, sagittal and coronal planes.

Box 2.8:	Disadvantages of MRI

- Inability to image bone.
- Unsuitable for patients with cardiac pacemakers, old metallic clips and implants, as these can get adversely affected by the magnetic fields. Now newer implants are MRI compatible.
- Relatively long scan time.
- Cost may be a factor with some of our patients.

RADIONUCLIDE SCANNING

Certain **radioactive isotopes** emit gamma rays as they decay. This property is used in **radionuclide imaging**, where isotopes are 'tagged' to compounds that are selectively **concentrated or excreted** by certain **organs. Technetium 99m** is the most commonly used **isotope** and has a **half-life** of only **6 hours**, so that **most of the radioactivity** has **decayed** within an **acceptably short period of time**. This **reduces the radiation burden** to the patient. Gamma radiation is detected over the **surface** of the body by a **gamma camera**, and **images** are produced that represent the **pattern** and the **intensity** of **radioactivity** within an **organ or tissue**. The investigation is also known as **scintiscan**.

POSITRON EMISSION TOMOGRAPHY (PET)

In this **medical imaging** technology the **disorders are imaged** at the **molecular level** before **morphological changes** are visible. It is a **functional imaging** technique that produces a **three-dimensional image** of the **functional processes** in the **body**. A **small** amount of **radioactive** material is necessary to show this **activity**. The **biologically active** molecule chosen for **PET** is **fluorodeoxyglucose (FDG)**. Areas that have **higher** levels of **chemical** activity show increased accumulation of radioactive material. This often corresponds to **areas of disease**, and shows up as **brighter spots** on the **PET** scan. A **PET scan** is useful in evaluating a **variety of conditions** including **neurological** problems, **heart disease** and especially **cancer**. The **response** to **treatment** by the tumour can be assessed by **periodic PET scans**. The presence of **metastases** is identified much **before** symptomatic **secondaries** appear. But the two **limitations** are **availability and cost**.

PICTURE ARCHIVING AND COMMUNICATIONS (PACS)

We often hear the term **PACS** in relation to **radiology**. This system aims at **converting** the conventional **film-based imaging, filing and reporting** in X-ray departments into a **non-film** and **paper free** system based on **digital computing, recording, transporting** and **archiving of images**. It has obvious **advantages**, like **telemedicine**, but the limiting factor is the **high cost**.

BASICS OF RADIOTHERAPY

Dr. Krishnaprasad

Prof. Medical Oncology, Kasturba Medical College, Mangalore

OVERVIEW

Shortly after Roentgen discovered radiographs in 1895, their clinical usefulness as a means of cancer treatment was first appreciated. Since that time, radiation therapy has developed into a recognized medical specialty, and enormous progress has been made to improve the effectiveness of this modality and minimise the side effects.

BIOLOGIC BASIS

The exact mechanism of cell death due to radiation is still an area of active investigation. A large body of evidence suggests that the action is on **double-stranded breaks** of **nuclear DNA** and is the most **important cellular effect** of **radiation**. This breakage leads to **irreversible loss of the reproductive integrity** of the cell and eventual **cell death**. Both **malignant** and **normal cells** in the **treatment field** are subject to the **ionizing effects** of **radiation**. **Normal cells** generally are **better** able to **repair** the **damage** caused by **radiation** at the **cellular level**, using **molecular machinery** that **detects DNA breaks** and **mutations**, and **repairs** them. In contrast, many **malignant cells** lack these **molecular mechanisms**, and therefore are **preferentially damaged by radiation**. However, **normal tissues** have **limits** on the **dose of radiation** that they can **safely withstand**; these limits **determine** the **maximum dose** that can be **safely administered** during a course of treatment.

X-rays and **gamma-ray photons** are part of the **electromagnetic spectrum**.

Radiation dose or **exposure** is measured in **units of absorbed radiation** per unit of tissue. The **Gray (Gy)** unit **represents 1 J/kg of tissue**.

Box 2.9:	Points regarding biological basis of radiotherapy

- Ionising radiation – Damage to the DNA.
- Normal cells – Molecular mechanism for repairs.
- Repair mechanism – Deficient in malignant cells.
- Malignant cells – More susceptible
- Higher dose – Toxicity

EXTERNAL BEAM RADIOTHERAPY (EBRT)

The most common radiation therapy (RT) approach is to **deliver** the radiation from a **source outside** the patient. EBRT machines **produce ionizing radiation** either by **radioactive decay** of a **nuclide** such as **cobalt-60**, or **electronically** by the **acceleration** of **electrons** or other charged particles like **protons**.

In a **linear accelerator**, electrons are **accelerated** to **high energy** and are allowed to either **exit the machine** as an **electron beam** or to **strike a target** that **produces X-rays** (also known as **photons**), which are **directed** at the **tumour**. **Linear accelerators** are relatively **small devices**, and can generate either **photon or electron beams** of various energies; their **output** is managed with **sophisticated computer** controls.

Photons Versus Electrons

Photons are the most **widely used** radiation mode due to their **ability** to **penetrate deeply** and reach **internal organs**. **Electrons** are often used for **superficial targets** such as **skin and breast**, where the **goal** is to **minimise radiation** to **deeper tissues** and **organs**. Clinicians **exploit** the **advantages** of **electrons over photons** when **internal organs** are **not** part of the **treatment target**, and also **better organ sparing** can be achieved with this treatment modality. Often **photons and electrons** can be carefully **mixed** to deliver the **best possible tumour-** and **normal tissue–dose distribution**.

Box 2.10:	Points to be noted regarding EBRT

- Source of radiation is outside of the body.
- Source- cobalt 60 or linear accelerator – High energy electron beam.
- Photons useful for deeply located tumours.
- Electrons for superficial tumours - Skin and breast.
- Both used together for maximum benefit.

Delivery of Therapy

The process of **treatment** calls for integration of the **physical findings** and diagnostic **imaging** information with extensive knowledge of the **pertinent anatomy**, **pathology**, and **natural history** of the particular **tumour type**. The radiation **oncologist** and other members of the **multidisciplinary team** must decide what role **radiation** will play in the **treatment** of the patient. Once the decision is made to **employ radiation**, consideration must be given to whether the **radiation** will be prescribed as **definitive**, **palliative** or **adjuvant therapy**, and whether it will be **integrated with surgery** and **chemotherapy**.

Planning of Radiation Fields

Contemporary treatment-planning **computers** allow the incorporation of **3-dimensional anatomic data** into the planning of **radiation fields**. With **beam's-eye-view technology**, radiation delivery can be planned so as to ensure that the **radiation field** adequately **covers** the **target** and **spares** or **minimises** the **dose** to the **non-target healthy tissues**. **Complex beam** arrangements can be used in the knowledge that a **geometric mis-scan** be **avoided**. An entire **lexicon** of **treatment-planning terminology** has been created as a result. The physician uses the **clinical and radiographic** findings to determine the **gross tumour volume (GTV)**. Next, the **clinical tumour volume (CTV)** is determined, which includes **microscopic extension** of the disease. The **planning treatment volume (PTV)** allows for **day-to-day** variation. To **minimise** any **variation** in **patient positioning**, **meticulous immobilisation** is essential.

Fractionation

Conventional fractionation is considered to be **1.8–2 Gy/day**, administered **5 days** each week for **5–7 weeks**, **depending** on the particular **clinical situation**.

Other fractionation schemes **include hyperfractionation, hypofractionation**, and **accelerated fractionation**. In **hyperfractionated** regimens, the goal is to deliver **higher tumour doses**, while **maintaining** a **level of long-term tissue damage** that is **clinically acceptable**. The **daily dose** is unchanged or **slightly increased** while the **dose per fraction** is **decreased**, and the **overall treatment time** remains **constant**. An **additional rationale** for hyperfractionation is to allow **radiosensitisation** through **redistribution**. With a **greater number** of **fractions**, it is more **likely** that the **tumour** will be in a **sensitive phase** of the **cell cycle** at **some time** during the treatment. This **strategy** invariably **results** in more **intense acute reactions** when compared to conventional treatment.

In the **accelerated fractionation** schemes, the **dose per fraction is unchanged**, while the **daily dose is increased** and the **total time** for the treatment is **reduced**.

Continuous hyperfractionated accelerated radiation therapy (CHART) is an intense schedule of treatment in which **multiple daily fractions** are administered within an **abbreviated period**. An **intense acute reaction** develops in most patients. This reaction usually **limits the total dose**.

Associated Chemotherapy

Chemotherapy can **enhance** the **effects** of **radiation** therapy. Numerous agents have been used either **sequentially** or **concurrently** with radiation. Most studies indicate that the **best results** can be **obtained** with **concurrent radiation** and **platinum**-based **chemotherapy**. Unfortunately, the **concurrent use** of **chemotherapy** also **intensifies** the **acute toxicities** of **treatment**, and **patients** often require **nutritional support** during therapy.

Biologic agents are being studied that may reduce some of **the toxicities** of **combined chemotherapy** and radiation, or may **enhance** the effect of **radiation** therapy.

Conformal Therapy

Conformal therapy is a term that describes a strategy for **matching** ("**conforming**") the **high-dose radiation region** to the **target volume**, while **minimising** the radiation dose to **normal tissues**. This term is typically used when the **target volumes** are defined on a computed tomography (**CT**) or other **high-definition imaging** study used during the treatment planning. Therefore, **3-dimensional conformal RT (3D-CRT)** usually **implies** a **CT- or MRI-based treatment plan**. These plans allow radiation oncologists to **calculate** and **optimise** the **radiation dose** received by the **tumour** as well as adjacent **normal tissues**.

Refinements of 3D-CRT include **intensity-modulated RT (IMRT)** and **image-guided RT (IGRT)**. Conformal therapy has **not been demonstrated** to **improve survival** in the **majority** of **clinical situations**. However, conformal therapy is generally **accepted** as a way to **reduce toxicity**. Furthermore, use of **3D-CRT** has made **retreatment** of **previously irradiated** **area feasible** in **more situations** than were previously possible.

IMRT

This is an **advanced form** of **3D-CRT** that changes the **intensity** of **radiation** in **different parts** of a **single radiation beam** while the **treatment is delivered**.

IMRT relies upon **computer control capabilities** to **maximise** the **delivery** of **radiation** to the **planned treatment volume**, while **minimising radiation** to **normal tissue outside the target**. **Varying the dose** of radiation administered within each beam enables **IMRT** to **simultaneously treat multiple areas** within the **target** with **different dose levels**, thus **providing** a **simultaneous integrated boost**. IMRT results in a **larger volume of normal tissue** receiving **lower doses of radiation** as **compared** with **older techniques**. Another theoretical **disadvantage** of IMRT is the **prolonged time** for **each treatment compared** to **other treatment techniques**, with its **unknown biological impact**. These drawbacks may be particularly important in **children** and other patients with a **prolonged anticipated survival**, where **heterogeneous low-dose** volume may result in **a higher incidence** of **secondary malignancies** or unintended **developmental consequences**.

IGRT

Uncertainty about **patient positioning** requires that **clinicians add extra margins** to the **target volumes**, beyond that based upon the **original imaging of the tumour**. This uncertainty may be due to lack of **precision** in **patient positioning** on a **daily basis** despite **immobilisation** or to **inherent organ motion** (e.g. **respiration**).

Box 2.11:	Points regarding recent advances in EBRT

- Conformal therapy – Maximise dosage to the tumour, with minimal damage to surrounding tissues - 3D-CRT
- IMRT – Refinement in 3D-CRT intensity modulated radiotherapy. Computerised 3-D image of the tumour - High dose to the tumour, sparing the normal tissues
- Disadvantage – Prolonged time - Long-term biological effects not known.
- Children – Risk of second malignancy.
- IGRT- Image guided radiotherapy.- improvement on IMRT.
- Real time imaging – Provides for change in patient positioning and internal movement of organs-eg, during respiration.

Real-time imaging of the **treatment target and normal organs** during each treatment allows for **minimisation of such additional margins** and the **reduction of irradiated volumes**, as it decreases the **chance of missing a target**. This technology is collectively referred to **as image-guided radiation therapy (IGRT)**, and it employs various **methods for real-time imaging** and treatment **adjustment**.

Stereotactic RT Techniques

Stereotactic RT techniques **administer** the **full calculated dose** of **radiation** in **one** or a **very limited number** of **treatment fractions**. Stereotactic techniques typically utilise **photons** that are **generated** by a **linear accelerator** or by a **cobalt-60 source**.

Stereotactic radiosurgery (SRS) refers to the use of this **approach** for **intracranial treatments**, whereas **stereotactic body radiation therapy (SBRT)** refers to the treatment of **extracranial** sites such as **lung**, **spine** or **liver**.

This is in **contrast to conventional EBRT**, which utilises **dose fractionation**, where the **total dose** is **administered** over a **period of many days** to allow **normal cells to recover** between the **daily fractions**. Although these **stereotactic techniques lack** the theoretical **biologic advantages** associated with **fractionation, clinical efficacy** has been **demonstrated** in a variety of settings (e.g. **brain and liver metastases and lung tumours**).

Immobilisation is even **more critical for SRS or SBRT** than for EBRT, in order to achieve **high reproducibility and precision**.

BRACHYTHERAPY

Brachytherapy is a **form** of RT in which a **radiation source** is placed **inside or next** to the **area requiring treatment**. The **radiation emitted** is generally **active over only** a **relatively short distance**. Thus, the **advantage** of **brachytherapy** is the **ability** to deliver **high doses** of radiation to the **tumour**, while **reducing** the **dose** to the surrounding **normal tissues**.

Brachytherapy has **well-defined roles** in a number of **malignancies**. The potential role **of brachytherapy** is illustrated by its use in **prostate cancer**, **gynaecologic malignancies and breast cancer**.

The **advantages** of brachytherapy come at the **expense** of **requiring** an **invasive procedure** to be carried out, and the **benefits** of brachytherapy must be **balanced** against **possible local complications**.

INTRAOPERATIVE RT

Intraoperative RT **(IORT)** is the **delivery of radiation** at the **time of surgery**. Whereas the **dose delivered** by the **EBRT** is **limited by tolerance** of **surrounding normal tissues**, IORT allows **exclusion** of **part** or all **dose-limiting sensitive structures** by **operative mobilisation** and/or **direct shielding** of these structures. A **single fraction** treatment is used, and dose is **limited** by structures (e.g. **nerves**, or **fixed organs**) that **cannot be displaced**.

TARGETED RADIONUCLIDE THERAPY

Highly specific targeting of radiation can also be achieved using **radionuclides** that **decay within the body** in very **specific locations**. These forms of **radiation** can be **based** upon the **specific tissue properties** or by **targeting** the **radionuclide** based upon its **chemical composition** or the ability to **concentrate** the radionuclide.

Examples of these approaches include the following:

1. **Thyroid cells selectively accumulate iodine-131**. The release of **radiation** as the **iodine-131 decays** can be used to **destroy thyroid tissue** and thus treat **thyroid cancer.**

2. **Radioisotopes** that are **accumulated** in **bone** may be particularly **valuable** for the treatment of **bone metastases**. **The isotope** used is **radium 223 which emits alpha particles**, **releasing** its **energy** over a **very short distance**, thus **sparing other organs**. **Radium-223** has been developed as an **important alternative** for patients with **extensive bone metastases** from **prostate cancer**.

Box 2.12:	Points regarding brachytherapy and IORT

- Brachytherapy - The source of radiation is kept inside or next to the tumour.
- High doses to the tumour - Minimal collateral damage.
- Used for cancers of the prostate and breast.
- Disadvantages - Invasive procedure -
- Eg implantation of radioactive iridium pellets.
- IORT - Intraoperative radiotherapy.
- Very high doses to the tumour intraoperatively.
- Exclusion of adjacent structures by mobilisation or shielding.
- Single fraction treatment.
- Disadvantage - Limitation of the dose by the presence of important structures like fixed organs or nerves.

Box 2.13:	Points regarding targeted radionuclide therapy

- Ability of certain cells to accumulate chemicals or isotopes
- High concentration in organs, with minimal absorption in other tissues.
- Thyroid cancer   Radioactive I 131 is selectively taken up by thyroid cells.
- Used in the management of secondary metastases from a differentiated thyroid cancer following a total thyroidectomy.
- Radium 223 - Alpha particles - Energy covers a short distance.
- Selective accumulation in bone.
- Useful for extensive bone metastases from cancer of the prostate.

SIDE EFFECTS OF IRRADIATION

Radiation effects on **normal tissues** are divided into **acute and chronic** (late) effects. **Acute effects** occur during the **course of therapy** and during the **post-therapy period (approximately 2–3 weeks** after the **completion of a course** of irradiation). **Chronic effects** can manifest anytime thereafter, from **weeks to years after the treatment**.

The **acute** effects can be quite **uncomfortable**, but they generally **resolve**. The **chronic** effects can be **devastating, permanent and progressive**.

Acute Effects

Much of the effort that goes into **treatment planning** has to do with **minimising the effects** of treatment on **normal tissue**. The **tissues** that **divide rapidly** (e.g. **mucous membranes**) respond **acutely to radiation** and are responsible for much of the **acute morbidity** of the treatment.

The **mucous membranes** of the **oral cavity** and **oropharynx** respond **early** to **fractionated radiation**. **Erythema** is often evident **after 1 week** of treatment at conventional doses. This condition **progresses over the next few weeks** through various stages of **mucositis**, ranging from **small patches** to **confluent** or even **ulcerated areas**.

Healing begins while the patient is **still undergoing treatment**, but may continue for **several weeks** after radiation **therapy is completed**.

Loss of taste is a common acute effect of treatment. **Taste loss** begins **early** and **progresses rapidly** during the next **2 weeks of treatment**. **Xerostomia** is often present and **exacerbates this loss of taste**. **Recovery** of taste is **slow**, and frequently **incomplete**. Radiation can induce **melanin production**, which is often **first observed** in the **skin follicles** because these **skin invaginations** receive a **slightly higher dose** as the **beam enters tangentially** to the surface. **Sweat glands and sebaceous glands** may **cease functioning**, but the in-field **hair loss is usually temporary**.

Box 2.14:	Points regarding the acute side effects of radiation

- Seen during and up to 3 weeks following treatment.
- Actions temporary - Often full recovery.
- Effects on rapidly dividing cells.
- Mucositis – Ulceration – Mouth and oropharynx.
- Xerostomia.
- Melanin production.
- Atrophy of sweat and sebaceous glands.
- Temporary hair loss.

Chronic Effects

Two major theories are used to explain **late injury**. One theory attributes **chronic injury** to a **damaged microvasculature**, and the other **attributes injury** to **stem-cell depletion**. In either case, **late effects** can be a source of **ongoing morbidity**.

Delayed wound healing can be a consequence of **high-dose preoperative radiation**.

Dry mouth is probably the **most common problem** for patients who receive therapeutic doses of radiation. Some patients use **artificial saliva substitutes**, but most **patients find them inadequate**. Many patients must carry **bottles of water** to provide some relief.

Intensity-modulated radiation therapy (IMRT) is an increasingly available **approach** to the **prevention of xerostomia**. At the **time of treatment planning**, the radiation oncologist uses an **inverse-planning algorithm**, which allows selective **avoidance** of **critical normal tissues without compromising** the **tumor doses**.

Ulceration and bone exposure may develop. If serious injury to the **underlying bone** occurs,

osteoradionecrosis may follow. This complicationwascommonlyseeninthe **past**. **Mandible** was the **bone involved** and **super-added infection** led to the development of **osteomyelitis (septic osteoradionecrosis)**. Fortunately, **this complication** is now **uncommon**. When it **does occur**, **management** of the condition may be **difficult**. Although patience is important, some cases clearly **necessitate intervention**, which includes **antibiotic therapy** and **resection**.

Irradiation of the **spinal cord** may result in a self-limiting **transverse myelitis** known as **Lhermitte syndrome**. The patient notes an **electric shock**–like **sensation** that is **most notable** with **neck flexion**. **Rarely** does this condition progress to a **true transverse myelitis** with associated **Brown-Séquard** syndrome. To **avoid this devastating complication**, the **dose** to the spinal cord must be **limited**.

Chemical **hypothyroidism** is often the **only manifestation of an endocrinopathy**, and is readily treated with supplemental **thyroxine**.

Radiation-induced cancers are, fortunately, **quite uncommon** after **therapeutic doses** of radiation.

Box 2.15:	Points about the chronic side effects of radiation

- More serious and permanent.
- Seen at intervals of weeks to several years after treatment.
- Due to damage to microvasculature or depletion of stem cells.
- Delayed wound healing.
- Dry mouth with Xerostomia.
- Exposure of bone with ulceration – Septic osteoradionecrosis.
- Mandible – Osteomyelitis - Painful with discharging sinuses.
- Transient or permanent transmyelitis.
- Rarely radiation-induced cancers.

Basics of Chemotherapy

3

Dr. Krishna Prasad, M.D.D.M
Prof. Medical Oncology, Kasturba Medical College, Mangalore

The effective use of cancer chemotherapy requires an understanding of the principles of tumor **biology, cellular kinetics, pharmacology**, and drug **resistance.** This chapter focuses on the principles responsible for the development of modern **combination chemotherapy regimens**. This discussion is followed by descriptions of the major classes of chemotherapeutic drugs and their mechanisms of action.

CELLULAR KINETICS

Cytokinetic studies have shown how the kinetics of **cellular growth** define the **characteristics** of **tumor growth,** and in part, explain the **biological behaviour** and **heterogeneity** of tumors.

Normal Cell Cycle

Inherent to **cytokinetic principles** is the concept of the **cell cycle**. Daughter cells formed as a result of **mitosis** consist of **three subpopulations**.

1. Cells that are **nondividing** and terminally differentiated and undergo **apoptosis.**

2. Cells that are continually **proliferating**.

3. Cells that are **resting,** but may be **recruited** into the **cell cycle** (stem cells), and are capable of **proliferating** under special circumstances.

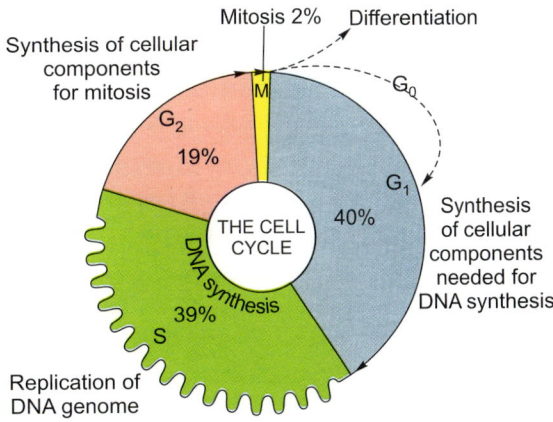

Fig. 3.1: The percentages given represent the approximate percentage of time spent in each phase by a typical malignant cell.

All three populations exist simultaneously in tumours.

Box 3.1:	Points regarding the types of cells seen in a malignant tumour

- Nondividing cells that show terminal differentiation and undergo spontaneous apoptosis.
- Actively dividing cells responsible for proliferation.
- Resting cells that can be recruited into the cell cycle and are capable of proliferation if there is a need.

Cell Cycle

The cell cycle is composed of **four phases** during which the cell prepares for and effects **mitosis.** Cells that are **committed** to **divide again** enter the **G1 phase.** Preliminary **synthetic cellular processes** occur during this phase, and **prepare the cell** to enter the **DNA synthetic (S)** phase. Specific **protein signals** regulate the **cell cycle** and allow **replication of the genome** where the **DNA** content becomes **tetraploid (4N).** After **completion of the S phase,** the cell enters a **second resting phase, G2, prior** to undergoing **mitosis.** The cell **progresses** to the **mitotic (M)** phase, in which the **chromosomes condense** and **separate** and the **cell divides,** producing **two daughter cells.**

Box 3.2:	Points regarding components of a cell division cycle

Cell division by mitosis.
- G1 – Preliminary synthetic processes.
- S – DNA synthetic phase.
- G2 – Resting phase prior to mitosis.
- M – Mitotic phase with cell division.

Chemotherapeutic agents can be **classified** according to the **phase** of the **cell cycle** in which they are **active.** Agents that are **cell-cycle-phase– nonspecific** (e.g., alkylating agents) have a **linear dose–response curve;** that is, the **greater** the **dose** of drug, the **greater is the fraction of cell kill.** However, **cell-cycle-phase–specific** drugs have a **plateau** with respect to **cell killing** ability, and **cell kill will not increase** with **further increases in drug dosage.**

Box 3.3:	Points regarding classification depending on the cell cycle

- Cell cycle phase specific drugs. Increase in dose does not enhance the cell kill activity.
- Cell cycle phase nonspecific drugs - Alkylating agents. Higher dose leads to increased cell kill.

Tumor Kinetics

The rate of growth of a tumor is a reflection of the **proportion** of **actively dividing** cells (the **growth fraction**), the **length of the cell cycle** (**doubling** time), and the rate of **cell loss. Variations** in these **three factors** are responsible for the **variable rates** of **tumor growth** observed among tumors of **differing histologies** as well as among **metastatic** and **primary tumors** of the same histology.

Tumors characteristically exhibit a **sigmoid-shaped Gompertzian** growth curve in which tumor **doubling time** varies with tumor **size.** Tumors grow most **rapidly** at **small** tumor volumes. As tumors become **larger**, growth rates **slow down** based on a **complex process** dependent on **cell loss** and tumor **blood flow** and **oxygen supply.**

Box 3.4:	Points regarding factors influencing cell growth
• Proportion of actively dividing cells – Tumour doubling time. • Quantum of cell loss. • Growth of a tumour - Typical sigmoid curve. • Rate of growth rapid in small tumours - Larger tumours show slower growth rate. • Influencing factors-Blood flow and oxygen supply.	

PRINCIPLES OF COMBINATION CHEMOTHERAPY

Using kinetic principles, a set of guidelines for designing modern **combination chemotherapy** regimens have been derived. Combination chemotherapy accomplishes **three important objectives,** which are **not possible** with **single-agent** therapy:

1. It provides **maximum cell kill** within the range of **toxicity tolerated** by the **host** for **each drug**.

2. It offers a **broader range** of coverage of **resistant cell lines** in a **heterogeneous tumor population**.

3. It **prevents** or **slows** the **development** of new **drug-resistant cell lines.**

Box 3.5:	Points regarding the principles of combination chemotherapy
• Three main advantages: • Maximum cell kill within toxic limits. • Broader coverage in a heterogeneous cell population. • Less chances of drug resistance.	

Selection of Drugs for Combination Regimens

The following principles have been established to guide drug selection in combination regimens:

1. **Drugs known** to be **active** as **single agents** should be **selected** for combinations. Preferentially, **drugs** that **induce complete remissions** should be included.

2. Drugs with **different mechanisms** of action should be **combined** in order to allow for **additive** or **synergistic effects** on the tumour.

3. Drugs with **differing dose-limiting toxicities** should be **combined** to allow each drug to be given at **full** or nearly **full therapeutic** doses.

4. Drugs should be **used** in their **optimal dose** and **schedule.**

5. Drugs should be **given** at **consistent intervals**. The **treatment-free interval** between cycles should be the **shortest possible time for recovery** of the most **sensitive normal tissue**.

6. Drugs with **different patterns of resistance** should be **combined** to minimise **cross-resistance**.

Box 3.6:	Points regarding selection of drugs for combination

- Effective single drug – Aim - Complete remission.
- Combination of drugs with different mechanisms.
- Drugs with differing toxic limits to be combined for limiting toxicity.
- Drugs to be used in optimum dose as per schedule.
- Interval to be adjusted for maximum recovery of sensitive normal tissue.
- Combination to achieve minimal cross-resistance.

Terminology used in Describing Chemotherapy

Chemotherapy is administered with a **variety of treatment schedules** designed according to the **intent and responsiveness** of **therapy.**

Induction: **High-dose**, usually **combination**, chemotherapy given with the intent of inducing **complete remission** when initiating a **curative regimen**. The term is usually applied to **haematologic malignancies,** but is equally **applicable** to **solid tumors.**

Consolidation: **Repetition** of the **induction regimen** in a patient who has achieved a **complete remission** after **induction,** with the **intent of** increasing **cure rate** or **prolonging remission**.

Intensification: Chemotherapy after **complete remission** with **higher doses** of the **same agents** used for induction or with **different agents** at **high doses** with the intent of **increasing cure rate or duration of remission.**

Maintenance: Long-term, **low-dose**, **single or combination chemotherapy** in a **patient** who has achieved a **complete remission**, with the intent of **delaying** the **regrowth** of **residual tumour cells**.

Adjuvant: A **short course** of **high-dose**, usually **combination, chemotherapy**, given with the **intent of destroying** a **low number** of **residual tumour cells to** a **patient** with **no evidence** of **residual cancer** following **surgery** or **radiotherapy** *Neoadjuvant:* Adjuvant chemotherapy given either in the **preoperative** period to **downstage** the tumour or in the **perioperative** period to **destroy residual tumour cells**.

Palliative: **Chemotherapy** given to **control symptoms or prolong life** in a **patient** in whom **cure is unlikely**.

Salvage: A potentially **curative, high-dose**, usually combination, regimen given in a **patient** who has either **failed to respond** or has had a **recurrence** of the malignancy following a **different curative regimen**.

Definitions of Response

Response to chemotherapy is defined precisely as **complete response, partial response, minimal response (stable disease), and progression**.

Complete response is defined as the **disappearance** of **all evidence of disease** and **no appearance of new disease** for a specified interval (**usually 4 weeks**). *Partial response* is defined as a **reduction by at least 50%** in the **sum** of the **products of the two longest diameters** of all **lesions, maintained** for at least **one course of therapy**.

Stable Disease is any response **less than a partial response** and is usually **with no appearance of new disease** reported in clinical trials.

Progressive disease is defined as **growth of existing disease** or **appearance** of **new disease** during **chemotherapy**.

Box 3.8:	Points regarding response to chemotherapy
	• Complete response.
	• Partial response.
	• Stable disease.
	• Progressive disease.

Dose Intensity

Kinetic principles predict that, for **drug-sensitive cancers**, the factor limiting the **capacity to cure** is **proper dosing. Reduction** in dose is associated with a **decrease in cure rate** before a **significant reduction** in the **complete remission** rate **occurs**. A **dose reduction** of approximately **20%** can lead to a **loss of up to 50%** of the **cure rate.** Conversely, a **twofold increase** in dose can be associated with a **10- fold** (1-log) **increase in tumor cell kill** in animal models. The **limiting factor** in most instances is the **associated toxicity**.

Overcoming Chemotherapy Resistance

There are **multiple reasons** for **chemotherapy failure** in cancer patients, involving a **variety of anatomic, pharmacologic, and biochemical mechanisms.** Tumor sanctuary sites (**brain, testes etc.**) and **blood flow** to the tumour represent **anatomic barriers. Pharmacologic and biochemical** explanations include **altered drug activation/ inactivation** in **normal tissues, decreased drug accumulation, increased repair** of **drug-induced damage** to the cell, altered **drug targets**, and most importantly, **altered gene expression.**

Overexpression of the MDR1 (multidrug resistance) gene is the most **notable** mediator of **drug resistance** and encodes a **170-kd transmembrane p-glycoprotein.** p-Glycoprotein is an **energy-dependent pump** that serves to **remove toxins** or **endogenous**

metabolites from the cell. A high level of MDR1 expression is reliably **correlated** with **resistance to cytotoxic agents.** Tumours that **intrinsically express the MDR1 gene prior to chemotherapy** characteristically display **poor durable responses.** Chemotherapy agents subject to **MDR1- mediated resistance** include the **anthracyclines, vinca alkaloids, taxanes, and topoisomerase inhibitors. Targeted therapies** that **inhibit p-glycoprotein** are **under evaluation** in **combination** with **cytotoxic drugs.**

Liposomal formulations of chemotherapeutic drugs are a promising a **new approach** to **overcome** these **resistance mechanisms.** Liposomes are well-defined **lipid and lipoprotein vesicles** that offer immense **potential** for **targeting drugs** to **tumors.** FDA-approved **liposomal preparations** of **doxorubicin, daunorubicin, cytarabine**, and **amphotericin B** have proven to be attractive**, less toxic** alternatives to the conventional drug formulations.

Box 3.9:	Points regarding the causes for failure of chemotherapy

- Blood brain barrier - Reduced blood flow.
- Altered drug activation or inactivation.
- Decreased drug accumulation.
- Increased repair of damaged cells.
- Over expression of MDR1 gene.

Chemotherapeutic Agents Classified by Mechanism of Action

Alkylating Agents

The alkylating agents **impair cell function** by forming **covalent bonds** with the **amino, carboxyl, sulfhydryl, and phosphate groups** in biologically important molecules. The **most important sites** of **alkylation** are DNA, RNA, and proteins.

Alkylating agents depend on **cell proliferation** for activity but are **not cell-cycle phase–specific.** A **fixed percentage of cells** are **killed** at a **given dose. Tumour resistance** probably occurs through **efficient glutathione conjugation** or by **enhanced DNA repair** mechanisms. Alkylating agents are **classified** according to their **chemical structures** and **mechanisms of covalent bonding**; this drug class includes the nitrogen mustards, nitrosoureas, and platinum complexes, among other agents.

Nitrogen Mustards

The nitrogen mustards, which include such drugs as **cyclophosphamide, ifosfamide, and chlorambucil** are **powerful local vesicants;** as such, they can cause problems ranging from local **tissue necrosis**, to **pulmonary fibrosis, to haemorrhagic cystitis.** The metabolites of these compounds are **highly reactive in aqueous solution**, in which an active alkylating moiety, the **ethylene immonium ion**, **binds to DNA**. The **haematopoietic system** is especially **susceptible** to these compounds.

Nitrosoureas

The nitrosoureas including **Carmustine and Lomustine** are distinguished by their **high lipid solubility** and **chemical instability**. These agents rapidly and spontaneously **decompose** into two **highly reactive intermediates**: chloroethyldiazohydroxide and isocyanate. The **lipophilic nature** of the nitrosoureas enables **free passage** across **membranes;** therefore, they rapidly penetrate **the blood–brain barrier**, achieving **effective CNS concentrations**. As a consequence, these agents **are used** for a variety of **brain tumors**.

Platinum Agents

Cisplatin is an **inorganic heavy metal complex** that has activity typical of a **cell-cycle-phase–nonspecific alkylating agent**. The compound produces **intrastrand** and **interstrand DNA cross-links** and forms **DNA adducts**, thereby **inhibiting** the synthesis of **DNA, RNA**, and proteins.

Carboplatin has the **same active diamine platinum moiety** as cisplatin, but it is **bonded** to an **organic carboxylate group** that allows **increased water solubility** and **slower hydrolysis** to the alkylating aqueous platinum complex, thus **altering toxicity profiles**.

Oxaliplatin is **distinguished** from the other platinum compounds by a **di-amino-cyclohexane ring** bound to the platinum molecule, which interferes with **resistance mechanisms** to the drug.

Box 3.10:	Points regarding alkylating agents
• Non cell-cycle specific agents - Higher dose – Greater kill.	
• Nitrogen mustard group - Cyclophosphamide, ifosfamide and chlorambucil.	
• Nitrosourea - Carmustine and lomustine.	
• Platinum group – Cisplatin, carboplatin and oxaliplatin.	

Antimetabolites

Antimetabolites are **structural analogs** of the naturally occurring **metabolites involved in DNA and RNA synthesis**. As the **constituents** of these **metabolic pathways** have been **elucidated,** a large number of **structurally similar drugs** that **alter the critical pathways** of **nucleotide synthesis** have been developed.

Antimetabolites exert their **cytotoxic activity** either by **competing** with **normal metabolites** for the **catalytic or regulatory site** of a **key enzyme** or by **substituting** for a **metabolite** that is **normally incorporated into DNA** and **RNA**. Because of **this mechanism** of action, antimetabolites are **most active** when cells are in the **S phase** and have **little effect** on cells in the **G0 phase**. Consequently, these drugs are most **effective** against tumors that have a **high growth fraction**.

Antimetabolites have a **nonlinear dose-response curve**, so that **after a certain dose, no more cells** are **killed** despite **increasing doses** (5 fluorouracil [5-FU] is an exception). The antimetabolites include **Fluorouracil, Cytosine Arabinoside, Gemcitabine and Capecitabine.**

NATURAL PRODUCTS

A **wide variety of compounds** possessing **antitumor activity** have been isolated from **natural substances** such as **plants, fungi, and bacteria**. Likewise, selected compounds have **semisynthetic and synthetic** designs based on the **active chemical structure** of the **parent compounds**, and they, too, have **antitumour properties.**

Antitumor Antibiotics

Bleomycin preferentially **intercalates DNA** at **guanine-cytosine** and **guanine-thymine** sequences, resulting in **spontaneous oxidation** and formation of **free oxygen radicals** that cause **strand breakage**.

Anthracyclines The anthracycline antibiotics are products of the **fungus *Streptomyces peucetius var. caesius.*** They are **chemically similar**, with a basic **anthracycline structure** containing a **glycoside** bound to an **amino sugar, daunosamine**. The anthracyclines have **several modes of action**. Most notable are **intercalation between DNA base pairs** and **inhibition of DNA topoisomerases I and II. Oxygen free radical formation** from **reduced doxorubicin intermediates** is thought to be a **mechanism** associated with **cardiotoxicity.**

Epipodophyllotoxins Etoposide is a semisynthetic **epipodophyllotoxin** extracted from **the root of Podophyllum peltatum** (**mandrake**). It **inhibits topoisomerase II activity** by **stabilizing** the **DNA–topoisomerase II complex**; this process ultimately results in the **inability to synthesize DNA**, and the **cell cycle** is **stopped** in the **G1 phase.**

Vinca alkaloids: These are derived from the **periwinkle plant**

Vinca rosea: Upon **entering the cell,** vinca alkaloids **bind rapidly** to **tubulin.**

The **binding occurs** in the **S phase** at **a site different** from that associated with **paclitaxel and colchicine**. Thus, **polymerization of microtubules** is **blocked,** resulting **in impaired mitotic**

spindle formation in the **M phase**. The drugs include **vincristine and vinblastine.**

Taxanes: Paclitaxel and docetaxel (Taxotere) are **semisynthetic derivatives** of **extracted precursors** from the **needles of yew plants**. These drugs have a **novel 14-member ring**. **Unlike** the **vinca alkaloids**, which cause **microtubular disassembly**, the **taxanes promote microtubular assembly** and **stability**, therefore **blocking the cell cycle in mitosis. Docetaxel** is more **potent** than paclitaxel in **enhancing microtubular assembly** and **also induces apoptosis**.

Camptothecin analogs include irinotecan (CPT-11 [**Camptosar**]) and topotecan (**Hycamtin**). These **semisynthetic analogs** of the alkaloid **camptothecin** are derived from the **Chinese ornamental tree camphotheca** (happy tree). It **inhibits DNA synthesis** by its action on **topoisomerase 1.**

Box 3.11:	Points regarding other chemotherapeutic drugs

- Antimetabolites – 5 fluorouracil, gemcitabine and capecitabine.
- Antibiotics – Natural, semisynthetic and synthetic compounds.
- Bleomycin.
- Derived from fungus – Anthracyclins.
- Derived from vinca rosea – Vincristine and vinblastine.
- Derived from the root of podophyllum peltatum – Etoposide.
- Derived from the needles of yew plant – Taxanes.
- Derived from a Chinese ornamental tree – Camptosar and hycamtin.

■■■

Diseases of the Thyroid Gland

4

A CASE OF NODULAR GOITER

Setting

- Surgical outpatient department (OPD)

Chief Complaint

A 38-year-old lady presented at the OPD with a complaint of a **swelling** in the **front of the neck** of **10 years duration**.

History of Present Illness

The swelling was noted **10 years** ago in the **lower part** of the **front of the neck**. It was about **2 cm in size**. Since then it had been **gradually increasing** in size. There was no history of a **rapid increase** in size in the **recent past.**

- The patient did not complain of any **pain**.
- There was no history of **fever.**
- There was no history of **dyspnoea**, **dysphagia** or **hoarseness of voice**.
- The patient did not have any **symptoms** related to **altered hormonal status**.

Past and Personal History

- **Past and personal histories** were not significant.
- **None** of the relatives in the **family** had **similar complaints**.
- Her **menstrual history** was normal.
- She had not taken any **treatment** for this condition previously.

General Physical Examination

- It was normal. Her **pulse rate** was 76 per minute, **regular,** and the **BP** was 128 by 80 mm of Hg.
- There was no **pedal oedema**.

Local Examination

Inspection

There was a **swelling** occupying the **anterior aspect** of the neck extending from the **thyroid cartilage** to the **suprasternal notch**. Horizontally, it extended from the **posterior border** of the right **sternomastoid** to the same extent on the **opposite side.**

- The **size** was 12 cm by 10 cm. It was oval in **shape**.
- The **upper and lower borders** were well defined, but the **lateral borders** were indistinct.
- The **surface** was nodular.
- The **skin** over the swelling was stretched.
- The swelling was seen to **move upwards** when the patient was made to **swallow** a small quantity of **water**.
- The **surrounding areas** were normal.

Palpation

- The swelling was not **warm or tender**.
- The size was **larger** than on inspection, measuring 14 cm by 11 cm. The **lateral borders** were under **cover** of the **sternomastoid** on either side.
- The **lower border** became more **distinct** during **swallowing**.
- The **shape** was irregular.
- Both the **lateral lobes** as well as the **isthmus** were enlarged. The **right** lobe was **bigger** than the left.
- The **surface** was **nodular.** The **size** of the nodules varied from **2–4 cm**.

- The **consistency** of the nodules was **firm** and the **internodular** area was **soft**.
- The swelling **moved upwards** during **deglutition.**
- The swelling was **deep** to the **investing layer** of the cervical fascia. The **lateral lobes** were **deep** to the **sternomastoid** muscles.
- There was **transverse mobility**.
- The **trachea** was in the midline.
- On both sides, the **common carotid pulsations** were felt in the normal positions. The **external carotid pulsations** were felt on both sides.
- No **lymph nodes** were palpable in the neck.

Box 4.1:	Points regarding history
• Swelling – Front of the neck - Duration-site and size at onset	
• Rate of growth – Recent history of rapid increase	
• Pain – Absent in most cases - Fever	
• Dyspnoea, dysphagia and hoarseness of voice Symptoms due to altered hormonal status	

Box 4.2:	Points to be noted regarding inspection
• Swelling – Anterior aspect of neck	
• Extent – Margins Size and shape	
• Surface – Smooth – Nodular	
• Upward movement with deglutition	
• Skin over the swelling – Stretched	
• Visible pulsations - Rare	

Box 4.3:	Points to be noted on palpation

- Warmth and tenderness
- Enlargement of the portions of the gland – Lobes or isthmus or both
- Borders – Lower border-Retrosternal extension.
- Upward movement with deglutition
- Size – May be larger – Shape
- Surface – Smooth or nodular – Size – Location.
- Consistency – Soft or firm
- Mobility – Anatomical plane – Deep fascia – Lat. Lobes - Sternomastoid
- Trachea – Deviation
- Pulsations – Common carotid and external carotid arteries
- Palpable nodes in the neck

- Examination of the **oral cavity** was normal.
- There were no **eye signs**.
- Examination of cardiovascular system (**CVS**) was normal.
- All the **other systems** were normal.

Box 4.4:	Points to be noted on rest of the clinical examination

- Oral cavity – Lingual thyroid – Tremors of the tongue
- Eye signs – Proptosis – Other signs
- CVS – Pulse – Irregularities – Apex beat – Systolic hypertension
- Tremors of fingers
- Other systems

Q. 1. What was the clinical diagnosis?

(*a*) Single nodule thyroid.

(*b*) Multinodular goiter.

(*c*) Differentiated thyroid cancer.

(d) Medullary carcinoma.

The correct answer is (**b**). Single nodule thyroid arises from either **one lateral** lobe or **isthmus.** The **rest** of the gland is **not palpable**.

Differentiated thyroid **cancer** and nodular goiter can only be only be **distinguished** by fine needle aspiration cytology (**FNAC**).

Medullary carcinoma is an uncommon condition. The **suspicion is high** if it is a part of a multiple endocrine neoplasia (**MEN**) syndrome. **FNAC** is required for a diagnosis.

The clinical picture is typical of a multinodular goiter.

Q. 2. What were the investigations performed on this patient?

1. **Ultrasound (US)** study. It showed multiple nodules, some being cystic and the remaining solid, occupying both the lateral lobes and the isthmus. A large solid nodule measuring 4 cm was chosen for FNAC.

2. **FNAC** was done.

3. **Thyroid Function Test** were normal.

4. **Chest X-ray** was normal.

5. **ECG** was normal.

6. **Indirect laryngoscopy** was normal.

Setting: One week later the FNAC report showed a colloid goiter.

Q. 3. What was the treatment given to this patient?

She underwent a **total thyroidectomy**. She had a smooth postoperative period.

The histopathology report was a **colloid adenomatoid goiter.**

She was advised to take oral **thyroxine 100 mcg** daily for the rest of her **life.**

Q. 4. What is the incidence of nodular goiter?

It is an extremely common condition. Nodular changes in the thyroid are seen in **6% to 7%** of all **women** after the age of **30.**

Q. 5. What causes endemic goiter?

People living in **mountainous regions** had a high incidence of endemic **goiter** in the **past**. This was the result of usage of **rock salt** by these people, which led to **iodine deficiency**. **Sea salt** consumed by the rest of the **population** is enriched by **iodine** derived from decomposed **sea weeds**. Introduction of **iodized salt** has helped to overcome the **lack of iodine,** and hence endemic goiter is **hardly seen** in clinical practice. It is said to be **present** in some parts of South China. Still goiters are **more common** in **hilly** regions. This is the result of the **heavy rain**fall seen in these areas that **washes away** the **iodine** from the **soil,** leading to a **reduction** of the element in the **water** as well as in the **vegetables grown in that area.**

Q. 6. Why is family history important in these cases?

Dyshormonogenic goiter runs in **families,** and is the result of **lack of enzymes** needed for **uptake of iodine** by the gland or for the **coupling of** the **iodine** with the tyrosine molecules. Thus the **levels of T3 and T4** are **low** resulting in **elevated levels of TSH**. **TSH** induces both **hyperplasia** and **hypertrophy** in the gland resulting in a **goiter**. **Dominant genes** responsible for these **enzymes** are **absent** in these patients, and hence the condition is seen in all **siblings.** But when it occurs **sporadically,** it can lead to **difficulties** in diagnosis. In general, these goiters are seen at a **young age**, and are quite **large** and, most significantly, are also **vascular.** Administration of oral **thyroxine** gives good relief, and the treatment has to be continued **throughout life.**

Medullary carcinoma as a part of **MEN** or **familial** type is seen in all members of a **family.** The goiter appears at a **young age.** Serum calcitonin estimations are useful.

Fortunately both these conditions are **uncommon.**

Q. 7. How is a history taken in a case of nodular goiter?

This can be **quite confusing** unless a proper **stepwise** history is taken. The symptoms can be broadly divided into **three groups.**

Group I:

Symptoms due to the swelling.

(*a*) **Swelling:** This is the **primary** and may be the **only symptom.** The patient complains of a **swelling** in the **anterior aspect of the neck** of **many years** duration. In some instances, a **relative** might **detect** the **swelling** and the patient may be **totally unaware** of the same.

(*b*) **Site at onset:** If the patient has **noticed** the swelling, he or more often she may be able to **localise** the **site** where it was **noticed** at the **beginning.**

(*c*) **Size at onset: Only** if the **site** has been **detected**, the **size** at that stage will also be **remembered** by the patient. It may vary from the size of a **peanut** to that of a **lemon.**

(*d*) **Rate of growth:** Most goiters are **very slow** in their **growth.** A **rapid increase** in size occurring over a period of **few hours or days**, suggests a **bleed** into a nodule. But if the time span extends over a **few weeks** or **months,** a **malignant transformation** is likely.

(*e*) **Pain:** A **painful goiter** is seen in **subacute thyroiditis.** But this is a very **uncommon condition.** But most of the **nodular goiters** are **painless** and hence the patients **seek attention** only when the **swellings** reach a **large size. Pain** will be present if there is a **bleed** into a nodule or a **malignant** change has taken place.

(*f*) **Fever.** Not seen in most cases. Patients with **thyroiditis** have **fever** at **onset** of the disease.

Group II:

These are symptoms resulting from **pressure** on the structures in close relation to the gland, like the **trachea** and the **oesophagus.** In **malignant goiter, infiltration** of the **recurrent laryngeal nerve** will also produce symptoms.

(*a*) **Pressure** on the **trachea** will cause **dyspnea.** This is **inspiratory** in nature and can lead to **stridor** if there is a **sudden increase** in **size** due to a **bleed**. Also, lying in the **supine position** as well as the **mucosal oedema** from an upper **respiratory infection** worsens the **dyspnea.**

(*b*) **Pressure** on the **oesophagus** can cause **dysphagia.** Surprisingly, even in **large** swellings, it is **not seen frequently**. Again, in a patient with **dysphagia** in the **absence of dyspnoea**, the cause is very **unlikely** to be a **goiter.**

(*c*) **Hoarseness of voice** is due to **infiltration** of the **recurrent laryngeal nerve** by a **malignant tumour**, since **benign swellings** tend to only **displace** the **nerve.**

Group III:

These symptoms are the result of an **altered hormonal status. Hyperthyroidism** produces such **dramatic symptoms** that it is **identified** quite **easily.** But the clinical picture of **mild hypothyroidism** is often **subtle** and may be **missed easily.** Further, the **hormones** have **actions** on **various parts of the body.** Therefore it is safer to get the **information** with reference to **each system.**

(*a*) **Cardiovascular system: Palpitation (tachycardia)** and chest pain are suggestive of **excess of thyroxine.** Later,

symptoms of **congestive cardiac failure** may manifest. In **elderly patients,** the **cardiac element** may **predominate** and they are known as **thyrocardiacs. Patients** with **hypo status** may have **bradycardia.**

(*b*) **Gastrointestinal symptoms: Increased appetite, diarrhoea** and **weight loss** are seen in **hyperthyroidism. Hypothyroid** patients complain of **constipation** and **weight gain.** This clinical picture is so **often seen** in **middle-aged obese women** that unless investigated, the state of **hypothyroidism** may be **missed completely.**

(*c*) **Central nervous system: Anxiety, excitability** and an **easily disturbed emotional** state are manifestations of **hyperthyroidism.** Conversely, a **stoic state** and **depression** are so often seen in the **hypo state,** that this group may seek a **psychiatric consultation** before the **correct diagnosis** is **established.**

(*d*) **Musculoskeletal system: Proximal muscular weakness** is seen in **hyperthyroidism.** They may also complaint of **tremors** that may cause problems during **certain activities.**

(*e*) **Menstrual disturbances** like **oligo-** or **polymenorrhoea** and **menorrhagia** are common if there is **hormonal disturbance**.

Q. 8. Why is treatment history important in these cases?

This part of the history is quite often **neglected.** Essentially **three types** of **medications** are prescribed for thyroid diseases. If the patient says that she is taking a **liquid preparation** contained in a **coloured bottle**, it is likely to be an **iodine compound**. If a **small tablet** is advised to be taken in the **morning** on an **empty stomach**, **thyroxine** is a strong possibility. Lastly if the patient is consuming **tablets** at **eight hourly** intervals, or as a **single dose, antithyroid** medication has to be considered.

Q. 9. Why does the thyroid gland move upwards during deglutition?

The most **important clinical sign** of a **thyroid swelling** is **upward movement** of the swelling with **deglutition**. The reason is **anatomical**. The **thyroid gland** is **enclosed within** the **pretracheal fascia**. This is a **diamond-shaped** fascia, being **broad** in the **middle** to **accommodate the gland. Inferiorly,** it merges with the **fibrous pericardium** at the **root of the great vessels**.

This explains the **retrosternal extension** in some goiters. At the upper end it **condenses** to form the **ligament of Berry,** being **attached** to the **oblique line** of the **thyroid cartilage**. During **deglutition,** the **thyrohyoid apparatus** moves **upwards** due to the **contraction** of the **inferior constrictor** muscles. This **elevates** the **epiglottis, blocking the airway**. Thus the gland **within** the **pretracheal** fascia **moves upwards. Loss** of this **movement** signifies **malignancy**.

Q. 10. Describe the steps in palpation of the thyroid gland.

Most of the **palpation** is performed **standing** behind the patient. The **neck** is **flexed forwards** to **relax the cervical muscles. Lateral flexion** is added if the swelling is **unilateral**.

(*a*) **Warmth and tenderness: Vascular glands** as in hyperthyroidism feel **warm**. The most common cause for **tenderness** is a **recent haemorrhage. Thyroiditis** also produces a **tender swelling**.

(*b*) **Size and extent** are determined more **accurately** during palpation. In many instances, the swelling may be **larger on palpation**, particularly the **lateral**

lobes being covered by the **sternomastoid muscles.**

(c) **Borders:** This can be made out **more clearly** during palpation. The **lower border,** which was not detected during inspection, can be felt **clearly** during **deglutition** in several instances. The lateral borders are palpated **deep** to the **sternomastoids.**

(d) An important step in palpation is to **determine** the **portions** of the **gland** that are **enlarged**.The easiest method is to palpate the **thyroid cartilage** initially and then run the **fingers down** to **palpate the gland.** If **enlargement** is felt to the **left** of the **cartilage,** it implies an **enlarged left lobe** and **vice versa**. As the palpation is carried **downwards** in line with the **cartilage**, if the **rings of the trachea cannot be felt**, it suggests **enlargement of the isthmus**. In patients with **huge goiters**, this part of the **examination** may be **difficult.**

Having identified the **anatomical portion** of the enlargement, the **exact size** of **each lobe** and or **isthmus** can now be **determined.**

(e) **Surface** may be **smooth** as in a **colloid goiter.** Nodular

surface is much more **common.** The size of the **individual nodule** can be detected by careful **palpation**.

(f) **Consistency:** Thyroid poses **special problems** regarding the consistency. **Tensely cystic swellings** may be interpreted as **firm** and a **solid swelling** felt as **soft.** In general **nodules** are **identified** because they **feel firm** in comparison with the **remaining soft gland. Malignant and calcified** nodules are **hard.**

(g) **Mobility:** These swellings show **transverse mobility** along with the **trachea. Fixed thyroids** are often **malignant.** But **huge goiters** are **difficult** to **move** because of their **sheer size.**

(h) **Anatomical plane:** The thyroid gland lies **deep** to the **investing layer** of the **deep cervical fascia.** This can be demonstrated by asking the patient to **extend** his **neck** and tilt it **backwards.** The **fascia** now becomes **taut** and the **swelling** is seen to be **less prominent.** Since the **lateral lobes** are **deep** to **sternomastoid,** when the **muscles** are put into **contraction** against resistance, these become **less prominent** and **less mobile.**

(*i*) **Thrill:** The presence of a thrill indicates **increased vascularity**. The **superior thyroid artery** enters the gland at the **upper pole** from the **anterior aspect**. Thus **palpation** at the **upper pole** may reveal a **thrill.**

The next **stage** of palpation is done **standing in front** of the patient.

(*a*) **Position of the trachea: Unilateral enlargement** of the **thyroid** most often **displaces** the **trachea** to the **opposite side**. The **conventional** method of **palpating** the **trachea** at the **suprasternal notch** is often **difficult** with the **thyroid** almost **abutting** the **suprasternal notch**. Only if the **goiter is small** and the **lower border easily palpable is** it **possible to** feel the rings of the **trachea**. In other cases, **palpation** of the **thyroid cartilage** and then trying to **trace** the position of the **trachea** is more **practical**. **Gross deviations** of this structure will **shift** the **thyroid cartilage** also to **that side**. **Auscultation** of the **front of the neck** may reveal **breath sounds** of the **bronchial type** at the site, where the **trachea** is placed **deep** to the **enlarged thyroid**.

(*b*) **Carotid artery pulsations:** The **common carotid artery** is **palpated** at the **level of the swelling. Large goiters** tend to **displace the artery posteriorly**. The **external carotid** artery is felt **above the level** of the **upper pole**. In advanced malignancies of the gland, if the **carotid sheath** is **infiltrated, pulsations** at this level will be **absent (Berry's sign).**

(*c*) **Pemberton's test:** The **purpose** is to **detect** a **retrosternal goiter**. If it is **present, the neck veins** will get **engorged** due to **pressure** on the **brachiocephalic veins** and the superior vena cava in the **mediastinum,** when the patient is asked to **raise both upper limbs above the head.**

(*d*) **Lahey's test:** The **test** is performed in patients **presenting** with a **single nodule** occupying one **lateral lobe. Pressure** is applied with the **fingers on that** lobe **in an effort to rotate** the **whole gland. The posterior surface** of the **opposite lateral lobe** now becomes **posterolateral and is** palpated **with the fingers of the** other hand. **If** nodules **are now palpable,** the diagnosis is changed to a **multinodular goiter. The** advent of **ultrasonography (US)** has **reduced the significance** of this **test.**

Q. 11. What is the importance of percussion in a case of nodular goiter?

Percussion over the **manubrium sterni** is performed to detect a **retrosternal goiter** or massively **enlarged mediastinal lymph nodes.** But it is a very **poor clinical sign.**

Q. 12. What are the findings on auscultation?

A bruit heard at the **upper pole,** even in the absence of a thrill, indicates **increased vascularity** as is commonly seen in a **toxic goiter.**

Q. 13. Why lymph nodes should be examined in a case of nodular goiter.

Papillary carcinoma spreads along the **lymphatic route.** Hence it is necessary to palpate the **regional lymph nodes.**

Q. 14. What is the need to examine the oral cavity?

A lingual **thyroid,** an **uncommon entity,** is seen as a **cherry-shaped** swelling on the **dorsal surface of the tongue** at the **junction** of the **anterior two-thirds** and the **posterior one-third. Fine tremors** of the **tongue** are the manifestation of a **hyperthyroid state.**

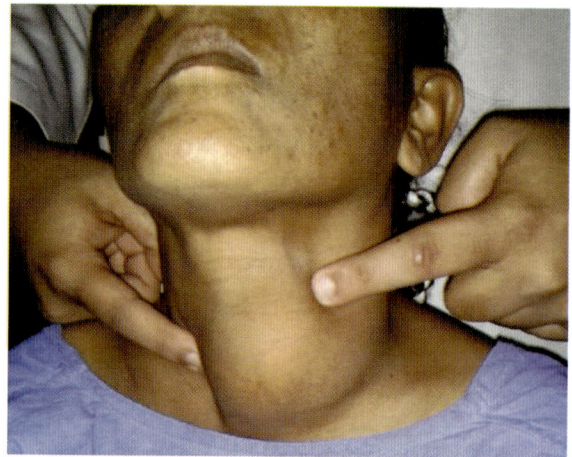

Fig. 4.1: Palpation of the thyroid cartilage to determine the parts of the thyroid gland that are enlarged.

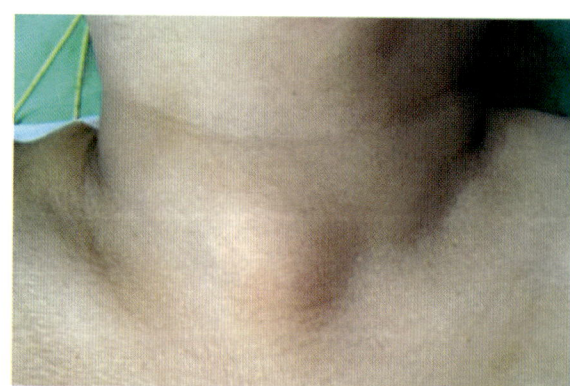

Fig. 4.2: Single nodule thyroid.

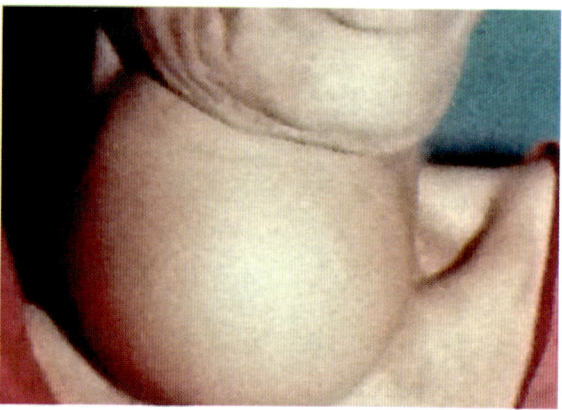

Fig. 4.3: Huge nodular goiter.

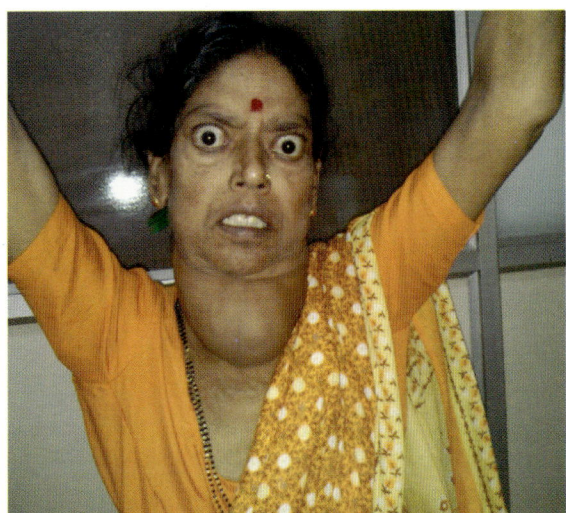

Fig. 4.4: Pemberton's sign in a case of toxic nodular goiter.

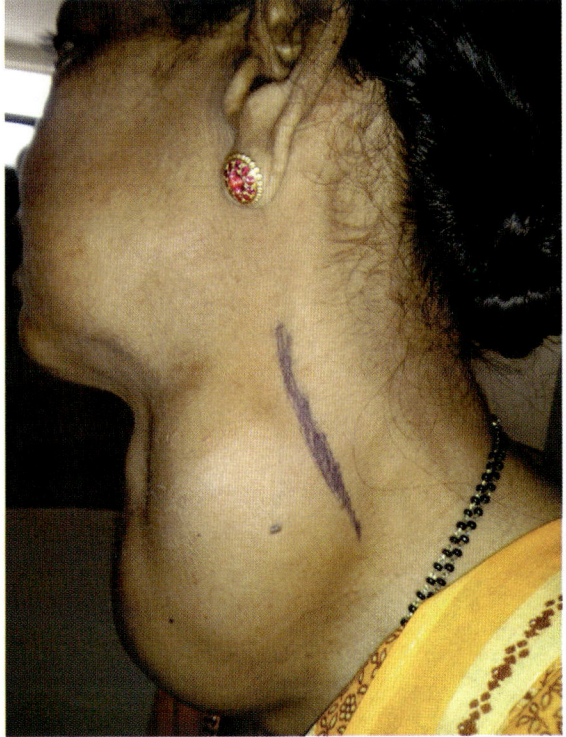

Fig. 4.5: Posterior displacement of the common carotid artery due to a huge goiter.

Q. 15. What are the investigations performed in a case of nodular goiter?

Well-differentiated malignancy of the thyroid gland is clinically indistinguishable from a nodular goiter. This is the **primary reason** for investigating this group of patients. Also, **subclinical alterations** in **thyroid function,** which have a bearing on the management, may not be detected by **clinical examination** alone. **US** examination has become such an **integral part** of the **investigation** that in the **developed countries,** it is taken as an **extension** of the **clinical examination** and the thyroid **surgeons** are the ones who **perform** this **test**.

US including the **Doppler examination**.

The clinical importance of the evaluation of a **nodular goiter** is primarily related to the need to **exclude thyroid cancer**, which is present in **4% to 6.5%** of these **nodules.**

1. The prevalence of cancer is **higher** in several groups:

   Children

   Males

   Adults less than 30 years or over 60 years old

   Patients with a history of previous **head and neck irradiation**

Patients with a **family history** of thyroid cancer.

2. The prevalence of cancer may be **lower** in **multinodular** goiters as compared to **single nodules.**

3. **Nonpalpable nodules** detected on imaging have the **same risk** of **malignancy** as **palpable nodules**.

Box 4.5:	Points regarding the role of US in nodular goiters

- Small, deeply located additional nodules are detected
- Cystic and solid nodules can be differentiated. Risk of malignancy is higher in a solid nodule
- Hypoechoic and vascular swellings (on Doppler study) have a higher risk of malignancy
- In multinodular goiter, a dominant solid nodule is chosen for FNAC
- US-guided FNACs are more reliable for deep-seated and small nodules

Computed tomography **(CT) and magnetic resonance imaging (MRI)** are **inferior** to US for characterizing **thyroid nodules,** and **small carcinomas** that are readily identified by US**,** may be **undetectable by CT and MRI.** The main role of **CT and MRI** is to demonstrate **extrathyroid tumour** extension into **major neck** structures, **nodal spread** and **distant metastases. CT** is always needed in **recurrent** **cancers** to detect the **extent** of **extrathyroid spread.**

Fine needle **aspiration cytology (FNAC)** of the thyroid gland.

FNAC has brought in a **remarkable change** in our understanding of the **nature** of various **diseases affecting** the **thyroid gland. Differentiated cancers** of the **thyroid gland** and **nodular goiters** are **clinically identical**. Hence **before FNAC** became popular, many a **patient** who underwent a **hemi- or a subtotal thyroidectomy** needed a **second operation** after the **histopathology** revealed **malignancy.** After the **advent** of **FNAC,** the **number** of such **completion thyroidectomies** has **come down** considerably.

The procedure is essentially **painless** and can be performed **with or without** local **anaesthesia,** preferably under **ultrasound guidance**. A small needle (**25–27 G**) is **inserted** into the periphery of the **nodule,** and the sample obtained by an **up-and-down** movement. As soon as **blood** appears, the needle is **rotated and removed**. The patient is told **not to swallow** during the **aspiration.** Complications are **minimal** because of the use of a **fine**

needle, and **rarely** a **haematoma** formation has been described. The **assessment** of the results of fine needle aspiration is **complex** and the **interpretation** of the results is listed below. The commonly followed **THY diagnostic system** is described in detail. The report ranges from **THY1,** which is non-diagnostic, to **THY5,** which is diagnostic of thyroid malignancy. The **success** of this investigation is directly related to the **competency** of the **cytopathologist**. The smears could be interpreted in the following manner.

THY1 Non-diagnostic

The smear does not provide **enough evidence** for a definitive **diagnosis**. The smear may show only a **blood clot**. This smear may also be reported as having **inadequate cellularity**. If the **number of follicles** or the **cluster of cells** in a given smear is **less than six,** the **cytopathologist** is **unlikely** to give a report. Under these circumstances, the FNA must be **repeated.**

THY2 Non-neoplastic (non-malignant)

This is the **most common report** and is seen in most patients with either a **single** or a **multinodular goiter**. **Colloid goitre** is the most frequently reported one. The smear shows **abundant colloid** and **scanty cells**. A diagnosis of **Hashimoto's** and **subacute thyroiditis** can also be made by FNA. If **conservative treatment** is adopted for patients with **colloid goiter**, FNA needs to be **repeated** at **six months** or **yearly** intervals, since **malignancy** can develop at a **later stage** in a **small percentage** of this group of patients.

THY3 Follicular neoplasm.

The cytopathology report is a **follicular neoplasm**. Follicular **adenoma** and **carcinoma** can be **distinguished** by the presence **capsular or vascular** invasion, **detected** only on **histopathology**. If the F.N.A.C report is a follicular neoplasm the lesion should be **removed** and subjected to formal **histology (5%–30% are malignant**). The **percentage** of **THY3** lesions **varies** from **centre to centre**.

THY4

The cells in this group may show many **atypical follicular cells** with a high degree of **suspicion** of **cancer. Hurthle cell tumours** also belong to this **group.** If the smear is unable to **exclude medullary thyroid** cancer or lymphoma, then a **core needle biopsy** must be performed and the tissue subjected to appropriate tests like **immunocytochemistry (medullary thyroid cancer)** or **flow cytometry (lymphoma)**, though both these conditions are **uncommon**. In all other cases, a **THY4** report indicates the need for an **immediate thyroid exploration**.

THY5

Papillary carcinoma is the type of malignancy identified by **FNAC** with a success rate of **97%–99%. Anaplastic and medullary carcinomas** are also diagnosed by this method. In a patient with **Hashimoto's thyroiditis**, a **malignant transformation** is **difficult to prove** and may demand **further investigations** as mentioned above.

Box 4.6:	Points regarding FNAC in nodular goiters

- Thy 1 Non-diagnostic
- Thy 2 Non-malignant – Colloid goiter, Hashimoto's and subacute thyroiditis
- Thy 3 Follicular adenoma
- Thy 4 Highly suspicious of malignancy – Atypical follicular cells
- Hurthle cell tumours – Rarely medullary carcinoma and lymphoma
- Thy 5 Malignant – Papillary carcinoma – Anaplastic and medullary carcinoma

Thyroid Function **Tests.**

Though the patient appears to be euthyroid clinically, these studies are always needed. Subclinical changes (10% to 15%) are significant, especially while planning the treatment. Surgery in a patient who is marginally hyperthyroid may precipitate a life-threatening thyroid storm. The main biochemical tests are as follows:

Serum free T3 and free T4 and TSH levels.

Free T3 **3-8 ng/dl**

Free T4 **4-11 ng/dl**

TSH **0.5-5 ng/dl**

TSH levels are the most sensitive tests of thyroid function. Lowered levels of TSH suggest a hyperthyroid state even in the presence of normal or slightly elevated levels of T3 and T4.

Additional tests like thyroid antibodies (Hashimoto's Thyroidits) and Thyroglobulin levels (Thyroid cancer) are needed in specific circumstances.

Q. 16. What are the other investigations needed in a case of nodular goiter?

X-rays of **the neck,** both anteroposterior and lateral views, are needed when **deviation** and **narrowing of the**

tracheal lumen is suspected.

If surgery is being planned, an **indirect laryngoscopy** to visualise the vocal cords is mandatory. It is done primarily for avoiding **postoperative medico-legal** problems.

Q. 17. What is the treatment of a nodular goiter?

There has been a **paradigm shift** in the **management** of this condition. This is the result of a **better understanding** of the **genesis** of these **nodules** and several **long-term studies** on their **behavior.** In the past, the **presence** of a **nodular goiter** was a clear **indication for surgery** because of the complications that might develop, some of which were considered to be **life threatening**.

The **list of complications** includes the following:

(*a*) **Haemorrhage** into a nodule. This will cause a **sudden increase** in the size of the **nodule**, leading to **compression** of the **trachea**, resulting in **inspiratory stridor,** and occasionally **asphyxia** and even **death.**

(*b*) **Secondary toxicosis:** The **internodular** tissue may undergo **hyperplasia** and produce symptoms of **toxicosis.** A **single nodule** may become **toxic** at a **later date. Toxic patients** are liable for many **complications**.

(*c*) **Malignancy:** **Follicular carcinoma** has been described in patients with **nodular goiter** when they are **followed up** for a **long time**.

(*d*) **Calcification:** Goiters lasting for **several years** are likely to develop **calcification.** The nodule will feel **hard** and may be **mistaken** for **malignancy.** A plain X-ray will show a dense **circular rim** of **calcification** at the **periphery** of the **nodule.**

(*e*) **Pressure effects:** As the **swelling enlarges** in size over a **period of time,** it is liable to press upon the **trachea** and the oesophagus.

(*f*) **Cosmetic disfigurement:** Although not a complication, a **swelling** in the **anterior aspect** of the neck can be quite **embarrassing,** especially in **women.**

But many **long-term studies** involving a **very large number of patients** have shown that all the **complications** mentioned above are **uncommon,** if not **rare.** Again a **better understanding** of the **aetiopathology** has made the **surgeon more reluctant** to **operate** on **nodular goiters**. The **common** indications for **surgery today** are **cosmesis,** followed by **pressure effects** of a large goiter.

Box 4.7:	Points regarding complications

- Haemorrhage
- Secondary toxicosis
- Follicular carcinoma
- Calcification
- Pressure effects
- Cosmetic disfigurement

Q. 18. What is the aetiopathology of a nodular goiter?

Although the condition is **very common,** the **exact mechanism** of nodule formation has **not been understood**. The main causative factor is likely to be **fluctuating levels of thyroid stimulating hormone (TSH)**. Since this **hormone** is regulated by the thyroid regulating hormone (**TRH),** the **hypothalamus** has also been **implicated** in the aetiology of nodular goiter. In the **thyroid gland, all** the **acini** are **not active** at a **given time**. As a result of **increased** levels of **TSH** a **group of acini** become **hyperplastic**. But the **response** of these **acini** is **not uniform**. Some remain in a **stage of hyperplasia**. Some **others** may undergo **necrosis**

due to **paucity of blood supply**. **Haemorrhage** is also seen in **some acini**. As the **levels of TSH decrease, hyperplasia** is replaced by **involution**. These **acini** are **distended with colloid** and lined by a **layer** of **flattened cells**. So the **natural history** of these nodules is one of **hyperplasia** and **involution,** induced by **fluctuating levels of TSH**. Thus the fact that all the **complications** described above are **very uncommon** can be **easily explained**. In addition, the **term** used to describe the **histopathology** of a **nodular goiter** has **changed** from **colloid goiter** as it was reported earlier to a **colloid adenomatoid goiter**.

Box 4.8:	Points regarding aetiopathology

- Fluctuating levels of TSH - Related to TRH
- Hypothalamus
- Changing response by a group of acini
- Hyperplasia, haemorrhage, necrosis and involution
- HP – Colloid adenomatoid goiter

Q. 19. What is the surgical treatment for a nodular goiter?

Total thyroidectomy is the **operation of choice**. It has the **following advantages**:

1. The rate of **recurrence is zero**. If **recurrences** were to **develop** following a **subtotal**

thyroidectomy, the patient needs a **second operation**. A **second operation** on the gland **increases** the incidence of **injuries** to the **recurrent laryngeal nerves** and the **parathyroids,** even in **experienced hands**. Both are **serious complications** leading to **poor quality of life** and are **difficult** to **treat**.

2. The belief that **injuries** to the **recurrent laryngeal nerves** and the **parathyroids** are **more frequen**tly seen following **this operation,** as compared to a **subtotal thyroidectomy, has now been** proved to be false.

3. If a **subtotal thyroidectomy** is done, the **quality** of the **remaining thyroid tissue** may be so **poor** and the **patient** may need **thyroxine** postoperatively to maintain a **euthyroid** status.

4. If the **histopathology report** shows **malignancy,** there is no need to perform a **completion thyroidectomy** with its **inherent increased morbidity**.

Following a total thyroidectomy, these patients are given **thyroxine** for the rest of their **life**.

The usual dose is **100 mcg** daily. But it is **titrated** to maintain a **normal TSH** level. **Long-term** thyroxine has been found to have certain **undesirable side effects**.in a small group of patients. It is said to **increase** the **risk of hypocalcaemia** in **young patients**. In **elderly patients**, the incidence of **cardiac disease increases** following **thyroxine** therapy.

Patients having a **single nodule** occupying one **lateral lobe** are treated by a **hemithyroidectomy.** The **lateral lobe** and the **isthmus** are removed in this **operation**. Following the surgery, these patients need to be under **surveillance** for the **development of nodules** in the **opposite lobe**.

Box 4.9:	Points regarding the surgical treatment

- M.N.G – Total thyroidectomy – No recurrence
- Risk of injury to recurrent laryngeal nerves and parathyroids – Low
- Subtotal thyroidectomy – If recurrence develops, risk of injuring recurrent laryngeal nerves and parathyroids high – Significant morbidity
- Following subtotal excision – Quality of remaining tissue – Poor – Thyroxine
- HP – Malignancy – No further surgery
- Single nodule – Hemi-thyroidectomy

Q. 20. What are the indications for conservative treatment in nodular goiters?

Older patients with **small goiters** and who are available for **regular surveillance** are **suitable candidates** for this line of treatment.

Q. 21. What is the role of thyroxine as the sole method of treatment in nodular goiters?

Obese women who present **primarily with a swelling** in the neck may be found to have **small nodules** in the thyroid gland. These are **more often detected** on **US.** Such patients show **improvement with thyroxine therapy**. Some of the **nodules** (in the stage of **hyperplasia**) may **regress in size**. But the **internodular tissue** undergoes **atrophy.** The **swelling** gets **reduced in size** due to these **two reasons.** The **cosmetic effect** is very **satisfying** to the patient. These patients also need **regular surveillance**.

A CASE OF SECONDARY THYROTOXICOSIS

Setting

- Surgery OPD.

Chief Complaint

- A **55-year**-old **lady** presented with the complaint of a **swelling in** the front of the neck of **10 years** duration.
- She also had **palpitation, sleeplessness** and **anxiety** for the last 6 months.
- She said her relatives told her that her **eye** appeared to be **bulging** and **prominent** recently.

History of Present Illness

The patient had noticed a **swelling** in the front of the **neck** about **ten years** ago. It was noted in the **lower part** of the **front of the neck**. It was the size of a small **lemon**. It was gradually **increasing in size.** Since it was totally **asymptomat**ic, she had not consulted a doctor regarding this problem. For the **last six months** she had developed a series of symptoms. She had **palpitatio**n, which worsened with **anxiety,** and **insomnia**. She had **lost weight** despite eating more. There was no history of diarrhoea.

There was no history of **rapid increase** in the size of the swelling or **pain.** She did not have **dyspnoea, dysphagia or hoarseness of voice**.

Personal history was insignificant.

Family History

No other **membe**r of the family had **similar** complaints.

Menstrual History

The patient had attained menopause five years earlier.

Treatment History

She had **not taken** any treatment for this condition.

General Physical Examination

The patient was moderately built and well nourished. She appeared anxious. Her pulse rate was 96 per minute, respiratory rate was 18, and the B.P. was 148 by 90 mm of Hg. There was no pallor, jaundice or clubbing of fingers.

Local Examination

Inspection

A s**welling** was seen in the **anterior aspect of the neck**.

It was extending from above the **thyroid cartilage** to the **suprasternal**

notch, vertically. The horizontal extension was beyond the **posterior borders** of the **sternomastoid muscles** on both sides.

The upper and **lower margins** were distinct, but the lateral margins could not be made out clearly.

The **shape** was irregular.

It was about 12 cm by 8 cm in **size**.

The **skin** over the swelling appeared to be **stretched** and a few **dilated veins** were visible over the swelling.

The **surface** was **nodular**.

The swelling was seen to move **upwards during deglutition**.

Palpation

The swelling was **warm,** but not tender.

It was **larger** in size than made out during inspection, extending from above the **thyroid cartilage** to the **suprasternal notch**. Horizontally, it extended 1 cm beyond the **posterior border of the sternomastoid** on both sides.

All the borders could be felt and the **lower border** became more **distinct** when the patient was asked to **swallow**.

The **size** was 14 cm by 10 cm.

Both the **lateral lobes** and the **isthmus** were found to be **enlarged.**

The right lobe was slightly larger than the left lobe.

The surface was **nodular**. Nodules could be palpated in both the **lobes** and the **isthmus**. Their size varied from 2 cm to 4 cm.

The nodules were **firm in consistency**. The remaining part of the thyroid was **soft.**

Upward movement of the swelling with **deglutition** was clearly demonstrated.

It was **deep t**o the **investing layer** of the deep fascia. Major parts of the lateral lobes were **deep** to the **sternomastoid**s.

There was limited **horizontal mobility**.

A **thrill** could be felt near the **upper pole** of both lateral lobes.

Position of the **trachea** was central.

Carotid pulsations. Left **common carotid** was found to be **displaced** posteriorly.

Both **external carotid** pulsations were **felt** above the level of the swelling.

Lymph Node Examination

No enlarged lymph nodes were palpable in the neck.

Box 4.10:	Points to be noted in the history

- Goiter – Duration - Site of onset – Size at onset
- Rate of growth. Symptoms due to toxicity
- CVS – Palpitation, precordial pain – Nocturnal dyspnoea
- GIS. Increased appetite, diarrhoea - Weight loss
- CNS – Anxiety, irritability – Emotional disturbances, insomnia
- Musculoskeletal system – Tremors and proximal muscular weakness
- Pain over the swelling
- History of pressure symptoms

Auscultation

A **bruit** was heard on both sides at the **upper pole**.

Box 4.11:	Points to be noted during inspection

- Swelling – Site and extent – Anatomical landmarks
- Thyroid cartilage, suprasternal notch and sternomastoids
- Borders – Lower – most important
- Size and shape
- Surface – Nodular or smooth
- Skin over the swelling – Stretched – Dilated veins
- Movement with deglutition – Present
- Surrounding area

Box 4.12:	Points to be noted during palpation

- Warmth and tenderness.
- Site, size and extent.
- Borders - Inferior border during deglutition.
- Surface and consistency - Nodular and firm.
- Parts of the gland which are enlarged.
- Mobility - Transverse.
- Anatomical plane - Deep fascia and sternomastoid muscles.
- Tracheal position.
- Displacement of the common carotid artery.
- Berry's sign.
- Palpable thrill at upper pole.

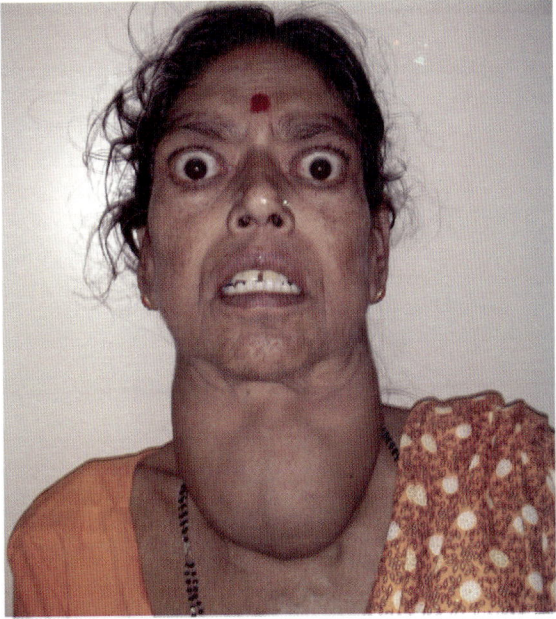

Fig. 4.6: Secondary thyrotoxicosis with proptosis.

Eye Signs

There was marked proptosis.

The following eye signs were present.

1. **Dalrymple's sign:** A **ring of sclera** was visible around the **cornea** when the patient looked straight forward.

2. **Naffziger's test:** In this test the examiner stands behind the patient and tilts the **neck backwards** till the eyes of the examiner fall in **line with the upper eye lid** of the patient. A **portion of the eye ball** was seen **protruding** beyond the eye lid in this patient.

3. **Rosenbach's sign: Fine tremors of the upper eye lid** on slight closure of the eye were present.

4. **Joffroy's sign:** There was **lack of wrinkling** of the **forehead** when a patient was asked to look upwards.

5. **Moebius' sign: Lack of convergence** was present when the patient was asked to **look** at a **close object.**

6. **Von Graefe's sign:** The **upper eye lid was lagging** behind when the patient was made to **look downwards** without **moving the head** (**lid lag sign**).

7. **Stellwag's sign: Infrequent blinking** was noticed in this patient.

Pretibial myxoedema: The patient had bilateral **pretibial myxoedema.**

Examination of other systems did not show any abnormality.

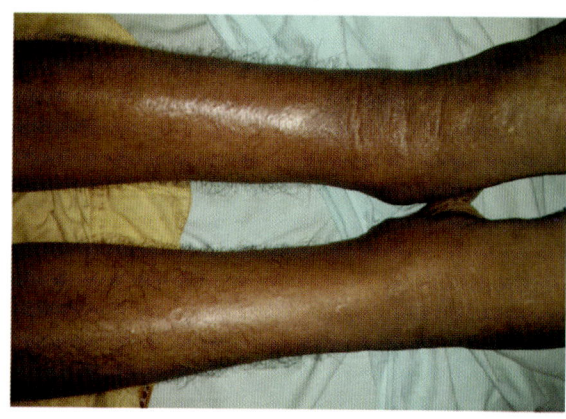

Fig. 4.7: Bilateral pretibial myxoedema.

Q. 1. What is the clinical diagnosis?

(*a*) Multinodular goiter.

(*b*) Primary thyrotoxicosis.

(*c*) Secondary thyrotoxicosis.

(*d*) Follicular carcinoma of the thyroid.

The right answer is (c). The patient had a **nodular goiter** for several **years.** But for the last **six months** she had symptoms of **toxicity**. In addition toxic signs are also present. In **primary toxicity**, the **goiter** and **toxicity** appear at the **same time**. **Functioning follicular carcinoma** is a **rare** condition. The diagnosis needs **histopathology** for confirmation. Hence the clinical diagnosis was **secondary thyrotoxicosis**. In this condition the **toxicity** was **superimposed** on a pre-existing **nodular goiter**.

Q. 2. **What was unusual about this patient?**

Eye signs and pretibial myxoedema are features commonly seen in the **primary variety**. Again **neurological symptoms** predominate in **primary** toxicosis. **Cardiovascular** involvement is seen more frequently in **secondary** toxicity. This patient had all the **eye signs** as well **pretibial myxoedema**. The CVS showed only **tachycardia.**

Q. 3. **What is the pathophysiology of exophthalmos in toxic thyroid?**

Symptoms referable to the **eye** are seen in **5% to 15%** of patients with moderate and **severe thyrotoxicosis**. The **antibodies** liberated by **T lymphocytes** present in the **thyroid** gland are responsible for the **ophthalmopathy**. But they are probably **different from TSAb** and are usually referred to as exophthalmos producing factors (EPF). The proptosis is produced by the following factors.

(*a*) **Enlargement** of the **extra-ocular muscles**.

(*b*) **T lymphocyte** infiltration of the **retro-orbital space**.

(*c*) Accumulation of **glycosamino-glycan** in the **retro-orbital tissue** due to **overproduction** by the fibroblasts.

Q. 4. **What are the complications following exophthalmos?**

Conjunctival irritation, congestion, diplopia, and exposure keratitis are all **due to exophthalmos**. In severe cases, there may be **corneal ulceration, external ophthalmoplegia** and even **panophthalmitis**, with **loss of vision**.

Q. 5. **What causes pretibial myxoedema?**

Dermopathy is seen in **1% to 2%** of patients only. The patients complain of **swelling** in the **anterior aspect of the leg** (**Pretibial myxoedema**). The swelling is due to the **accumulation** of **glycosaminoglycan** in the **subcutaneous plane** on the anterior aspect of the leg. **The aetiopathological factors** are probably the **same** as those responsible for **exophthalmos.**

Box 4.13:	Points regarding history of present illness in primary toxicosis

- Age 20 to 40 years
- More common in females (10:1)
- Goiter and toxic symptoms appear at the same time
- Exophthalmos is a prominent feature
- CNS symptoms are frequently seen
- May be associated with CVS, GIS and musculoskeletal system symptoms
- Dermopathy seen in some patients

Primary toxicosis differs in many respects from the **secondary** variety. The **aetiopathology,** **clinical features** and to a certain extent the **management** strategies are **different**. The **clinical features** are given in **Boxes 4.13, 4.14 and 4.15.**

Box 4.14:	Points regarding inspection in primary toxicity
• Swelling in the anterior aspect of the neck
• Uniform enlargement of the whole gland
• Shape of the thyroid retained
• Moves up with deglutition
• Surface appears smooth
• Skin over the swelling normal or shows dilated veins
• Uncommonly visible pulsations

Box 4.15:	Points regarding palpation in primary toxicity
• The gland is warm but not tender
• There is uniform enlargement of both the lateral lobes and the isthmus
• The consistency is soft
• The surface is smooth
• It is deep to the investing layer of the cervical fascia
• Enlarged lateral lobes are deep to sternomastoid.
• There is horizontal mobility
• A thrill may be palpable at the upper pole
• Bruit may be heard over the upper pole and in some cases over the entire gland
• Trachea is central
• Carotids are felt on both sides
• No palpable lymph nodes

Q. 6. What is the aetiopathology of Grave's disease?

Primary thyrotoxicosis (Grave's disease) is considered to be an **autoimmune disease**. But there is an **important difference** between this **condition** and all **other autoimmune diseases**. In **most autoimmune diseases**, the **antibodies** are **cell destructive**, but in **this condition** they are **cell stimulating**. As a result, **excess of thyroxine** is formed, leading to **hyperthyroidism.** The causative antibody is known as **Thyroid Stimulating Antibody (TSAb).** For reasons not clear yet, **T lymphocytes** infiltrate the **thyroid gland**. These **T lymphocytes** are responsible for the **production** of the **antibody**. When the **cells** of the **gland** are exposed to these **lymphocytes,** a process of **autoimmunization** takes place, resulting in the **release** of the **antibodies** by the **T lymphocytes. TSAb** thus formed, **binds** with the **T**hyrotropin receptors on the **thyroid cells,** resulting in **hyperplasia** and **increased production of the hormones. Activated lymphocytes** also release **growth** factors, causing **further hyperplasia.** This **degree of hyperplasia,** in turn, causes **increased vascularity.** All these factors **contribute** to the **formation** of a **goiter** in these patients. The presence of **T lymphocytes** is also responsible for a **reactive inflammation** resulting in **destruction** of the **thyroid cells** and **fibrosis** in the gland. Over a period of time, due to the **massive lymphocyte** infiltration and **fibrosis,** the number of **functioning** thyroid **acini** is markedly **reduced.** At this stage, the patient may develop **hypothyroidism.** This fact is significant, since **hypothyroidism** once detected is **easily treatable**. Hence if the **same result** is obtained as a result of **treatment,** it is **not** to be considered as a **disadvantage**.

Box 4.16:	Points regarding aetiopathology of Grave's disease

- Autoimmune disease: The unique feature is that the antibodies are cell stimulatory unlike other autoimmune diseases wherein they are cell destructive
- The presence of T lymphocytes in the gland sets off the reaction. When they come in contact with the thyroid cells, they liberate the antibody TSAb (thyroid stimulating antibody)
- This competes with the TSH at the cellular level. The result is hyperplasia of the thyroid acini. In addition, the lymphocytes also produce growth factors making the condition worse
- These changes are associated with increased vascularity of the gland
- Thus the increased secretions from the gland result in a state of hyperthyroidism

Q. 7. What is the aetiopathology of secondary thyrotoxicosis?

The **aetiopathology** of **secondary toxicity** is not as clear as that of primary thyrotoxicosis. The patient usually has a **nodular goiter** of several **years** duration. The nodule could be **single** or the gland may have **several nodules. Toxicity** develops as a complication at a **later date.** In a case of a **single nodule,** the nodule itself may become **toxic**. In the remaining cases, the **internodular tissue** becomes **toxic.** Most of these nodules are **colloid** in nature and are **nonfunctioning.** In addition, the role of **autoimmunity** is also **not** so clearly **established** in these cases. The factors responsible for inducing toxicity are not yet known. But the nature of the **pathology** is important in the **treatment**. These can only be i**dentified** with the help of **investigations.**

Box 4.17:	Aetiopathology of secondary toxicosis

- Toxicity develops on a pre-existing nodular goiter
- A single toxic nodule or in the internodular tissue
- Autoimmunity not significant
- Older age group. Hence CVS. more vulnerable.
- Cardiac damage severe - Thyrocardiacs

Q. 8. **What are the investigations for patients with toxicosis?**

Thyroid Function Tests.

1. The levels of free **T3 and T4** are **elevated.** It is necessary to estimate the levels of both these hormones because a **small number** of patients show raised levels of only free **T3. Low levels of TSH.** This test is more **reliable** than raised T3 or T4.

   In some patients with toxicosis, these may be within the normal limits.

2. **Raised** levels of **TSAb** confirm the diagnosis of Grave's disease.

   F.N.A.C. This test is **not needed** for the following reasons.

   (*a*) The **clinical features** and the **biochemical tests** are adequate as far as the **diagnosis** is concerned.

   (*b*) If the gland is **vascular**, the risk of a **bleed** following the procedure is real.

   (*c*) **Functioning follicular carcinoma** of the thyroid gland, though described, is extremely **rare.** This **cannot** be detected by FNAC.

Radioiodine (RI) Studies.

The test is indicated in patients with **toxicity** presenting with a **single nodule** in the thyroid. A **tracer dose** of **4 to 10 microcurie** is given orally and a **scintiscan** of the neck is performed. If the **nodule** is the seat of **hyperplasia**, the **RI uptake** by the nodule will be **high** (**hot nodule**), and the rest of the gland will show minimal uptake. On the other hand, if the **internodular tissue** is **hyperplastic**, those areas will take up **more of RI** and the nodule is referred to as a **cold** nodule. The **surgical treatment** will be **different** in these two groups. It is important to remember that this is the **only indication** for **RI uptake** studies in the management of **nonmalignant goiters.**

Box 4.18: Points regarding investigations

1. Thyroid function tests – Low levels of TSH diagnostic
   - T3 and T4 may be elevated
   - TSAb raised in primary toxicosis
2. FNAC NOT DONE – Risk of bleed due to vascularity
   - Clinical and biochemical tests adequate for diagnosis
   - Functioning carcinomas are of follicular variety
   - These not diagnosed on FNAC
3. RI studies. Single nodule – More uptake - Toxic nodule
   - Uptake more in the rest of the gland - Cold nodule

Q. 9. What is the treatment strategy for this patient?

(*a*) Antithyroid medication

(*b*) Total thyroidectomy

(*c*) Radioiodine treatment

(*d*) All of the above

The correct answer is (*b*). Presence of a **toxic nodular goiter** is an indication for **surgical treatment**. Long-term results following either **medical or RI** therapy are **inferior** to surgery. The advantages of surgery are the **short duration** of treatment coupled with a **success rate** of more than **95%**. The primary **disadvantages** are the need to take **lifelong thyroxine**, the **risk of damaging** the **recurrent laryngeal nerves** and the development of **permanent hypoparathyroidism**. The latter two are **serious** problems and are **difficult** to manage. The **quality of life** is also **compromised** to a great extent. But with the **expertise now available**, the **incidence** of these **complications** is very **low**.

Setting: **The operation theatre,** after the **patient** had reached a **euthyroid** state with **antithyroid drugs for six weeks** and had been given **Lugol's iodine** for **ten days.**

The patient was posted for a **total thyroidectomy**. The advantages of this operation are as follows. The **risk** of **recurrence is zero**. Even if **histopathology** shows **malignancy,** the operation is the **right choice**. But there are some **disadvantages** also. The chances of developing the major **complications** mentioned above are **higher** in the hands of an **inexperienced surgeon. Lifelong thyroxine** therapy increases the risk of **hypocalcaemia** in **young patients, whereas** in **elderly** patients, **thyroxine increases** the incidence of **cardiac disease.**

Subtotal thyroidectomy, which involves the removal of a major portion of both the lateral lobes and the entire isthmus, may be an alternative that can avoid the above mentioned side effects. **Here,** a **small** part of the **lateral lobe** on each **side** in relation with the **recurrent laryngeal nerves** and the **parathyroids** is **left behind.** But in case of **recurrence,** the risk of **damaging** the **vital structures** is **much higher** during the **second operation.**

Dunhills' **modification** of **subtotal thyroidectomy.**

In this operation, **one lateral lobe** along with the **isthmus** is **removed** and a **small part** of the **opposite lobe** is **retained.** The **advantage** is that if a **completion thyroidectomy** were to become necessary at a later date, only the **recurrent laryngeal nerve** and the **parathyroids** on **that side** are at **risk**.

If the patient has **a single nodule** proved to be **toxic** on RI studies, only a **hemithyroidectomy** is needed. The **lateral lobe** containing the **nodule** along with the **isthmus is** excised.

Q. 10. How is the patient prepared for surgery?

Operating on a patient who is **toxic** invites the **life threatening complication** of a **thyroid crisis.** The gland is also **very vascular,** which makes the **surgery hazardous**. Hence it is essential that the **patient** must be brought to a **euthyroid state** prior to **surgery**. The patient is started on **antithyroid medication**. It usually takes about **6 to 8 weeks** for the patient to reach this **state. Sleeping pulse** rate is a **rough guide** towards response. Estimations of **T3, T4, and TSH** are more **reliable**.

If the patient is receiving **beta blockers** in addition to antithyroid drugs, it is necessary to **continue** the same for **one week** after the **surgery**, since the **half-life** of **thyroxin**e is about **7 days**. The dosage is to be **tapered off** over the **nex**t **week**.

Even after the toxicity has been controlled, the thyroid remains very **vascula**r and **friable,** making the **operation** a **difficult one. Lugol's iodine** in a dose of **10 minims three times** a day in milk **controls these two problems** making the **surgery safer**. But there is a **caveat** regarding **iodine therapy**: if the **drug is continued** beyond **two weeks**, the gland **escapes** from the **effect of the drug,** resulting in a **rebound phenomenon**. The ideal time **to operate** is about **8 to 10 da**ys after **starting iodine treatment.**

Q. 11. What are the guidelines for treating primary thyrotoxicosis?

The **rationale** for **treatment** depends on the **natural history** of the disease. The following are the possible outcomes for patients with toxicosis.

(*a*) A **small percentage** of patients are known to undergo a **spontaneous remission** for reasons that are not clear, reaching a **euthyroid state.**

(*b*) **Cardiac complications** can lead to **congestive cardiac failure,** which can be fatal, especially in elderly patients. The **cardiac condition** may be **worse** than the original **thyroid disease**. These patients are known as **thyrocardiacs.**

(*c*) **Thyroid** storm or **crisis** is a dramatic and **serious complication** associated with significant **morbidity** and **mortality. Sepsis, stress, surgery** (other than on the thyroid gland also) and **trauma** are the common precipitating factors.

(*b*) **Treated** or sometimes **untreated** patients will reach **a hypothyroid state** over a period of time. The reasons for this change have been explained earlier. But this is **not** a **serious complication** as long as it is **recognised early** and treated adequately.

The following are the **main guidelines** of **treatment.**

All patients with **mild-to-moderate primary toxicity** respond to the **medica**l line of treatment. It is only for those in the **severe** group that different **options** are considered regarding the treatment. To a large extent the **treatment** depends upon the **preferences** of the **patien**t or the **clinician**. The question of **availability** may also influence the treatment, especially of **RI**. **Medical, surgical and RI**—all the **three modalities** are **used** for treatment. The details regarding **medical and RI treatment** are described, **before the indications** are mentioned.

Medical line of treatment.

Antithyroid drugs are used to reduce the **hormonal secretion** by the gland. **Carbimazole** (neomercazole) is the drug of choice. It is available in tablet form of **10 m**g each. It acts by **reducing the uptake** of iodine by the gland. Neomercazole is given in a dose of **10 mg three times** a day and the dose is **gradually increased** over a period of **several weeks** till the **patient reaches** a **euthyroid** state. The drug can be given as a **single daily dose**. This **regime** is continued for a period of **six to nine months**. The dose can then be gradually **tapered** to a low **maintenance** dose. It may vary between **10 and 15 mg** per day. This has to be continued for a **total period** of **18 to 24 months**. Neomercazole is also used as an **adjunct for surgery** as mentioned earlier, as well as the **Radioactive Iodine (RI) treatment** that will be described later.

Propylthiouracil was used in the past in a dosage of **300 to 450 mg daily**. In addition to **agranulocytosi**s, this drug can cause **fatal liver damage,** and hence is no longer in use.

Advantages of medical treatment:

(*a*) **Major surgery** on the thyroid gland is avoided owing to its inherent **morbidity** (though low). The incidence of **hypothyroidism** is less as compared to **Radioactive Iodine** (RI) treatment

Disadvantages:

(*a*) The **duration** of treatment extends over a period of **years** and in this country, **patient compliance** in the **absence of symptoms** is **rather poor.**

(*b*) The **success rate** at the **end of treatment** ranges between **60% to 65**%. These patients tend to have **recurrences in a few months**

(*c*) **Drug sensitivity:** Patients **allergic** to neomercazole tend to develop severe **skin rashes** and **arthralgia.** The treatment may have to be **stopped** for this reason.

(*d*) **Drug toxicity: Agranulocytosis** is the most **dreaded** life-threatening **complication** associated with **neomercazole.** It is likely to occur within the first **six months** of treatment. This complication is **not dose related**. The patient complains of **fever** and **sore throat.** A **simple blood examination** will clinch the **diagnosis**. **Hospitalisation** is always required. **Granulocyte infusion** along with **antimicrobial therapy** is the treatment of choice, but this complication is still associated with significant **morbidity and mortality**. So it is necessary to **warn** the **patient** of this possible complication at the **initiation** of treatment. **Weekly blood counts** are usually ordered, but do **not guarantee** that agranulocytosis **will not develop.**

(*e*) **Drug Resistance:** A small percentage of patients do **not respond** to medical treatment **despite increasing** the **dosage.**

Potassium Perchlorate is another **antithyroid drug** used in clinical practice. It is useful in patients where **neomercazole** is **contraindicated** as well as in **children and pregnant women**. The usual dosage is **400 mg three times a day.**

Q. 12. What is the role of beta blockers?

These are **not antithyroid drugs** in the **true sense** of the word. The thyroid **hormone** acts on the **target cells** via the **catecholamines. Beta blockers** act **against** these **drugs** and prevent the **actions** of the **hormone** at the **cellular level.** Thus **adverse actions** of the hormone on **various systems** of the body are **negated**. Hence **symptomatic relief** is obtained **soon** after the **administration of these drugs**. This is **significant** because **reduction** in the **circulating levels of the**

hormones occurs only after a **few weeks** after starting **antithyroid medication. Propranalol** is the commonest drug used in a dosage of **40 mg three times** a day. It is primarily indicated in patients with **severe toxicity,** and is administered **along with neomercazole.** It is also used in the **preoperative preparation** of patients undergoing **surgery** as well as **along** with **RI therapy. Bronchospasm** is a known side effect of propranalol and hence the drug is **contraindicated** in patients with bronchial **asthma. Newer beta blockers** are now available without the undesirable **side effects.**

Box 4.19:	Points regarding medical treatment

- Antithyroid medication – Carbimazole
- Action – Prevention of uptake of iodine from the blood
- Dosage initial small dose 10 mg tid or 30 mg od
- Gradual increase in dosage till euthyroid status is reached (6 to 8 weeks)
- Maintain high dosage for 6 to 9 months
- Gradual decrease till a maintenance dose of 10 to 15 mg is reached
- Total duration – 18 to 24 months
- Potassium perchlorate – Preferred in children and during pregnancy
- Beta Blockers – No direct effect on the gland
- Prevents the action of the hormone on the target cells by blocking the catecholamines
- Immediate symptomatic relief.
- Needed in severe cases

Q. 13. What are the principles of radio iodine treatment?

The treatment is based on the physiological fact that **iodine** is **selectively taken up** by the **thyroid cells. Radioactive iodine131** is the isotope chosen for this purpose. The drug is given **orally** either in **liquid or capsular** form. The **dosage** depends on the **size** of the gland and varies between **10 to 15 millicuries.** Once it is **absorbed** into the **blood stream** it is **trapped** by the **thyroid cells.** These **cells** are **destroyed** by the effect of **ionizing radiation.** In some cases, to **reduce** the risk of **hypothyroidism** the drug can be given in **two split** doses.

Advantages:

(*a*) **Simplicity** of treatment. The patient has to swallow the required **dose orally** and stay in the hospital for a **couple of days**.

(*b*) **Risks** associated with **major surgery** and the **complications** of **thyroidectomy** are **completely avoided.**

(*c*) The need for **long-term medication** with **antithyroid drugs** and the associated **problems** are eliminated.

Disadvantages:

(*a*) The drug acts on the **rapidly multiplying cells**

of the **gonads,** which could cause **sterility**. Hence it is used only in **patients** who have **completed** their **reproductive activity**. Ideally RI treatment is given to **patients** who are more than **40 years** of age.

(*b*) All **radioactive isotopes** have **teratogenic** potential. Hence this mode of treatment is absolutely **contraindicated** in **children** and during **pregnancy**.

(*c*) When this treatment was **first introduced**, there was a **fear** of **increased incidence** of **haematological cancers** and **carcinom**a of the **thyroid**. Both of these have now been proved to be **not true.**

(*d*) **Action** of the drug on the cells is rather **slow,** and **symptomatic relief** may become manifest only after about **six months**. During this period many of the patients will need additional **antithyroid drugs** and **beta blockers**.

(*e*) Risk of **hypothyroidism**. Since the drug acts on **every thyroid cell, hyperplastic or otherwise**, this complication is **doome**d to occur in patients **following RI therapy**. The **risk increases** over a period of **time.** It is suggested that

after **10 years** of **treatment** the risk increases by **10% every year**. But as mentioned earlier, **early recognition** and treatment makes this complication **less dangerous**.

Box 4.20:	Guidelines for treatment:

Advantages:
- Simplicity of treatment
- Avoidance of long-term medical treatment
- Avoidance of morbidity associated with major thyroid surgery

Disadvantages:
- Teratogenicity
- Carcinogenesis
- Sterility
- Slow action
- Hypothyroidism

It is important to decide what the mode of treatment will be for a particular patient. **Personal preferences** of the **patient** as well as the **treating physician** play a **major role** in this regard. Again the **availability of a mode of treatment** like **RI** may modify the decision. The **following guidelines** will be useful in planning the **treatment.**

(*a*) All **patients** with **mild-to-moderate Grave's disease** will respond to **medical treatment.**

(*b*) The **role of either surgery or RI treatment** involves only the group with **severe primary toxicosis.**

(c) **Failure of medical treatment** due to reasons mentioned above demands either **surgery or RI treatment.**

(d) All patients with **toxic nodular goiter** need **surgery**. Even if **nodularity** develops **following administration** of **antithyroid drugs**, **surgery** is preferred.

(e) Patients with **large goiters** and or with **pressure symptoms** are treated by surgery.

(f) In the presence of a **nodule suspicious of malignancy**, **surgery** again is the choice of treatment.

Box 4.21:	Points regarding advantages and disadvantages of RI treatment

- Personal preference of the patient and clinician.
- Availability – Especially RI treatment
- Mild-to-moderate primary toxicosis – Medical treatment
- Secondary toxicosis (nodular toxicosis) – Surgery
- Large goiters with pressure symptoms – Malignancy suspicion - Surgery
- Small goiters in patients above 40 years – RI therapy

A CASE OF PAPILLARY CARCINOMA OF THE THYROID GLAND

Setting

- Surgical OPD

Chief Complaint

- **Swelling** in the **front of the neck**.

History of Present Illness

- This **28**-year-old **lady** had noticed a **swelling** in the front of the **neck** about **one year** ago.
- It was the **size** of a gooseberry and was **located** in the middle of the neck.
- The **rate** of growth was **gradual**.
- There was **no pain**.
- She did not complain of **dyspnoea, dysphagia** or **hoarseness of voice**.
- She did not have any **symptoms** referable to **altered hormonal** status.
- Her **past a**nd personal **histories** were **insignificant.**
- **No** other member of the **family** had similar swellings.
- She had a six-year-old son. Her **menstrual** history was **normal**. Her last LMP was 22 days ago.
- She had **not** taken any t**reatment** for this swelling.

General Physical Examination

General physical examination revealed a **healthy** lady. There was no pallor, jaundice, pedal oedema or clubbing of fingers.

Local Examination

Inspection

- A **swelling** was noted in the **anterior** aspect of the **neck.**
- It extended from one centimetre below the **thyroid cartilage** to one centimetre above the **suprasternal notch**. In the horizontal axis it extended from the **midline** to the **posterior** border of the right **sternomastoid.**
- It was **oval in shape** measuring 8 cm by 5 cm in **size.**
- Except for the right lateral border, all other **borders** were **distinc**t.
- The **surface** was **smooth.**
- The **skin** over the swelling was **normal.**
- The **swelling** was moving **upwards** on **deglutition.**

Palpation

The swelling was not warm or tender.

- It was arising from the **right lateral lobe** of the thyroid gland. The **isthmus** and the **left lateral** lobe were **not enlarged**.
- It measured 9 cm by 5 cm in **size** and was **oval in shape.**

- All the **border**s could be **felt** and the **right lateral border** was behind the **sternomastoid**. The **lower border** was **clearly** made out.
- The **surface** was **smooth.**
- It was **firm** in **consistency.**
- It was **mobile** in the **transverse** direction along with the **trachea.** There was **no vertical mobility.**
- The swelling was **deep** to the **investing layer** of the deep cervical fascia. **Part** of the swelling was **deep** to the right **sternomastoid** muscle.
- **No** palpable **thrill** could be made out at the **upper pole** of the right lateral lobe.
- The **trachea** was shifted to the **left** side.
- The carotid pulsations were felt **above** the swelling.

Examination of Lymph Nodes in the Neck

- A level **III node** was found to be **enlarged** on the **right side** of the neck measuring **2 by 2** cm in size, **soft, mobile and not tender**.
- **Multiple** nodes were palpable at **level IV**. They were **1.5–2.0 cm in size**. All were **soft, nontender and discrete**.
- **No** other group of **lymph nodes** was palpable in the **neck.**
- Examination of the **oral cavity** was normal.

- There were **no signs** of **altered hormonal status**.
- **Examination** of other **systems** did not reveal any abnormality.

Box 4.22:	Points regarding history of present illness
• Swelling – Duration - Site and size at onset	
• Rate of growth	
• Associated pain	
• Symptoms due to involvement of adjacent structures	
• Symptoms resulting from altered hormonal status	

Box 4.23:	Points regarding inspection
• Site and extent of the swelling	
• Size and shape	
• Borders – Lower border most important	
• Surface	
• Skin over the swelling	
• Upward movement with deglutition	

Box 4.24:	Points regarding palpation
• Warmth and tenderness	
• Site and extent – Borders	
• Upward movement with deglutition	
• Part of the thyroid that is enlarged	
• Whole gland or restricted to one lateral lobe or isthmus	
• Size and shape	
• Surface	
• Consistency	
• Mobility – Transverse	
• Anatomical plane – Deep to fascia and sternomastoid	
• Trachea – Displacement	
• Carotid pulsations	
• Palpable thrill at upper pole	

Box 4.25:	Points to be noted in examination of regional nodes

- Level III and IV. Level V.
- Nodes soft (Cystic in papillary cystadenocarcinoma). Mobile and discrete.
- Both sides to be palpated.
- Level VI nodes not clinically detected. Soft nodes embedded in pretracheal fat.

Q. 1. **What is the clinical diagnosis?**

(*a*) Nodular goiter with tuberculous lymph nodes.

(*b*) Papillary carcinoma of the thyroid.

(*c*) Medullary carcinoma of the thyroid.

(*d*) Anaplastic carcinoma of the thyroid.

The right answer is (*b*). Though nodular goiter and tuberculous nodes are both **common conditions**, nodes in **tuberculosis** are **matted**. Soft nodes indicate cold abscess formation. **Skin changes** are likely to occur in the presence of a **cold abscess**. **Medullary** carcinoma is a **pathological** diagnosis unless it belongs to the **familial** variety. **Anaplastic** cancers grow very rapidly. They usually occur in **elderly** people. The duration is measured in **weeks and months**. The **consistency** of the **primary tumour** and the **nodes** is **hard.** Early **fixity** is seen in anaplastic carcinoma.

Hence the **clinical picture** fits with a diagnosis of **papillary carcinoma**. The **age, sex** and the clinical features fit in with this diagnosis.

Q. 2. **What are the other modes of clinical presentation of papillary carcinoma of the thyroid gland?**

(*a*) **Single nodule** thyroid. **Differentiated thyroid cancers** and **nodular goiters** are clinically **indistinguishable**. The risk of **malignancy** is **higher** if the patient is a **male a**nd the age **over 45** years. **FNAC** is helpful to diagnose malignancy.

(*b*) The patient presents with **enlarged lymph nodes** in the neck of several **months** duration. The nodes are **soft, mobile** and **discret**e. There is **no** evidence of **enlargement** of the **thyroid. FNAC** of the **lymph node** shows **papillary carcinoma**. The **primary** is said to be **occult**, since it is **not detected** by a **clinical examination**.

(*c*) Patient has undergone a **subtotal** or a **hemithyroidectomy** earlier for a **nodular goiter**. The FNAC done prior to surgery was reported as a **colloid goiter**. The **histopathology** of the **resected specimen** has been reported as **papillary carcinoma**. The patient did not have any lymphadenopathy**.**

Box 4.26:	Points to be noted regarding the common characteristics of papillary carcinoma

- 60% of all thyroid cancers
- Age – 20 to 40 years. Can be seen in children.
- More common in females
- Slow growing tumour
- Spreads primarily by the lymphatic route
- Intraglandular lymphatic spread common
- Spread outside the capsule (extrathyroidal) - Poor prognosis
- Can be multicentric in origin
- TSH-dependent tumour
- Anaplastic change after a long duration

Q. 3. What were the investigations done?

FNAC was diagnostic: Both the **primary** tumour and the enlarged **node** were biopsied. The presence of **psammoma bodies** and multinucleated tumour giant cells with **orphan eye nuclei** were characteristic of papillary carcinoma.

US study of the neck: The **thyroid** did not reveal **additional nodules,** not detected clinically. Additional **lymph nodes** were not identified by the ultrasonologist.

Chest X-ray: Chest X-ray was normal. Papillary carcinoma spreads primarily by the lymphatic route. Hence **secondary** deposits in the lung are **uncommon**. But **long-standing** cancers may change into an **anaplastic type** and haematological **spread** can occur to the lungs.

MRI chest: This investigation was not done in this patient. If there is a suspicion of **enlargement** of **mediastinal nodes level VII** (**lymphatics** accompanying the **inferior thyroid veins** drain into this group), **MRI** of the chest is needed. Their presence as well as **infiltration** into the **vital structures** is made out by this investigation.

Thyroid function tests: T3, T4 and TSH. The patient was **euthyroid**. But **TSH** levels act as a **baseline** for **postoperative management**.

Box 4.27:	Points regarding investigations

- FNAC - Psammoma bodies and cells with orphan eye nuclei
- US study of the neck - Additional nodules in thyroid
- Additional nodes in the neck
- Chest X-ray - Normal
- Thyroid function tests - Usually euthyroid
- TSH - Baseline for later treatment

Q. 4. What are the prognostic factors in cancers of the thyroid gland?

Various **classifications** are available that take into consideration a **number** of

prognostic factors. This is termed as **tumour stratification.** The **MACIS** classification is a **popular one.**

M – Presence of **metastases.** Unlike many other cancers, the presence of lymph node metastases **does not make** the **prognosis** much **worse.** As mentioned earlier, **spread** beyond the **regional nodes** is **uncommon.** Since the nodes are **amenable** for **surgical extirpation** or RI treatment, the patient has a fairly **good outcome.**

A – **Age** of the patient. The **common age group** where this cancer is seen is between **20 and 40** years. Any patient **above 45** years has a **poorer prognosis. Men** do **worse** as compared to **women.**

C – **Completeness** of the operation. The **first** operation gives the **best** chance of **survival.** A **R0 resection,** wherein the **margins** show **no evidence** of the **tumour** on **microscopy,** ensures a **better** outcome. The **main cause** of **postoperative morbidity and mortality** is **local recurrence.** The **recurrent tumour** is invariably **fixed** to **vital structures** like the **trachea** and the **oesophagus.**

I – This indicates an in**trathyroidal** cancer. It would mean that the **tumour** is still **within the capsule.** Extracapsular spread (**extrathyroidal** cancer) has a **worse** prognosis.

S – **Size** of the tumour. Tumours less than **1 cm** in size have the **best** outcome. Once the tumour is **more than 2 cm** in size, the outlook becomes **poor.** With the advent of newer **imaging studies, smaller cancers** are being **detected.** These are termed as **microcarcinomas** and have an **excellent** prognosis.

Setting: One week later. FNAC reported a **papillary carcinoma. Thyroid function** tests were **normal. Chest X-ray** was **normal. US study** showed that the **rest** of the gland was **normal,** and there were **no nodes** on the **left side** of the neck.

Q. 5. **What are the treatment options for the primary tumour for this patient?**

(*a*) Right hemithyroidectomy.

(*b*) Subtotal thyroidectomy.

(*c*) Total thyroidectomy.

(*d*) Oral thyroxine therapy.

The correct answer is (*c*). Irrespective of the **location** and the **size** of the tumour, the **treatment of choice** for a papillary carcinoma is a **total thyroidectomy.** This **patient** underwent a **total thyroidectomy,** because this cancer could be **multicentric** and **intraglandular lymphatics** tend to carry the tumour cells **within the gland** far and wide.

Even if the **thyroid is not enlarged** and the **diagnosis is** made on **FNA** of a lymph **node,** the **same schedule** is followed. In the group where a **previous surgery** has been performed, a **completion thyroidectomy** is the answer. This is a more **difficult** operation and the risk of **damaging** the **recurrent laryngeal nerves** and **parathyroids increases** to a **great extent**. Obviously performing any **other operation** would lead to **local recurrence,** which most often is **fatal**. Oral **thyroxine** has a place in the **postoperative** management.

Q. 6. How were the lymph nodes treated in this case?

This patient needed a **functional** or **modified radical lymphadenectomy** of the neck on the **right side**. The structures removed included **fat, fascia** and **lymph nodes** on the right side of the neck. The fascia included the **investing layer** and the **carotid sheath**. The **lymph nodes** removed included levels **II, III, IV, V and VI**. Since the **nodes** were **discrete and mobile**, a **modified** procedure was carried out. The

structures that were **retained** included **the internal jugular vein, the spinal accessory** nerve and the right **sternomastoid** muscle. Retaining these structures helped to **reduce the postoperative morbidity**.

Q. 7. What are the advantages of a modified radical neck dissection?

If the **internal jugular vein** is removed, the **venous flow from the brain** is **impaired**. If the vein is removed on **both sides**, there is a risk of **raised intracranial pressure**. **Division** of the spinal **accessory nerve** leads to **paralysis** of the **trapezius**. This causes **drooping of the shoulder**. The resulting **traction** on the **brachial plexus** causes **severe pain** radiating down **the limb**. The patient tends **to restrict the movements** of the shoulder in an effort to **reduce the pain**. The result is a **painful frozen shoulder**.

Since the patient was **fit** this procedure was **combined** with a **total thyroidectomy**. In other circumstances the **lymphadenectomy** would have been done after an interval of **three weeks**.

Q. 8. What was the postoperative management of this patient?

Differentiated thyroid cancers like the **papillary** variety have the **capacity** to **imbibe iodine**. Following surgery, the patient was asked to **return** after six weeks to the **hospital**. During this period the patient's **thyroxine** levels would have become **nonrecordable**. In response, the **TSH** levels would be **very high.** If there were any **secondary deposits** (**level VI nodes**), or a small **remnant** of the **gland** was **retained** during the **operation**, they would be **sensitized** by the **high levels** of TSH **t**o take up **iodine.** During the second admission, the patient was given a **tracer dose of RI** and a **scintiscan** of the body was performed. The **scintiscan** was reported as **normal**. If any **deposits** were detected he would have been given a **curative dose of RI.**

Q. 9. **What is the role of thyroxine in the management of this patient?**

Papillary carcinoma is a **TSH-dependent** tumour. Due to the **feedback** mechanism, administration of **thyroxine** will bring **down** the levels of **TSH.** But the **dose** needed is a **high suppressive** one to **reduce** the levels of **TSH** to **nonrecordable levels**. The usual dose is between **200 and 300 mcg** per day. At this stage the patient may develop **symptoms** of mild **toxicity**. These are to be **controlled** by **beta blockers**, rather than reducing the dose of thyroxine. **Thyroxine treatment** is to be continued **lifelong**.

Q. 10. What would be the surveillance pattern in this patient?

The patient would be asked to come to the hospital **once a year** for examination. The suppressive dose of **thyroxine** would be stopped **six weeks** before this visit. This is to increase the levels of TSH. In addition to a **complete physical examination** and a **chest X-ray**, a **RI scintiscan** would also be performed. If all the findings were normal, the **thyroxine therapy** would be continued.

Q. 11. How are patients without lymph node involvement managed?

A **negative clinical examination** is **not adequate.** An **US study** of the neck should be done to **confirm** this status. Such patients are put on **suppressive doses** of **thyroxine** and kept under **observation**. If **metastase**s into **lymph nodes** were to be detected at a **later stage**, a **modified block dissection** is performed. The **surveillance** continues as mentioned above.

Q. 12. In general what is the prognosis of papillary carcinoma?

Women **below 40 years** of age with a **single focus** of **tumour,** less than **2 cm** in size and **no** enlarged **nodes,** and who undergo a **proper total thyroidectomy** have an **excellent** prognosis. They have a **normal life span**.

Q. 13. How are cancers of the thyroid gland classified?

The classification of all thyroid cancers is mentioned in Box 4.28.

Box 4.28:	Points to be noted regarding classification of thyroid cancers

- Arising from the thyroid cells-
- Differentiated
  - Papillary carcinoma
  - Follicular carcinoma
- Undifferentiated
  - Anaplastic carcinoma
- Arising from cells in the thyroid gland – Medullary carcinoma.
- Arising from lymphocytes
  - NHL
- Direct extension from adjacent cancers – Laryngeal cancers.
- Metastatic cancers – Renal, bronchogenic (rare).

Q. 14. Describe the common characteristics of a follicular carcinoma.

1. **20% to 25%** of malignancies belong to this type.
2. Occurs at a **later age group** as compared to the papillary type.

3. It is also more common in **women**.

4. Unlike a papillary carcinoma, **FNAC** is **not useful** in this malignancy. The **cellular characteristics** are **not adequate** to identify the malignancy in many instances. The presence of **capsular** and **angio invasion** is needed for diagnosis. These findings are noted only on **histopathological** examination. This assumes significance when the **management strategies** are considered.

5. The tumour **spreads** essentially by the **blood stream**. Hence **secondaries** are likely to occur in the **bones, lungs and brain**. The tumour is **biologically** more **aggressive,** and **secondaries** are more **common.**

6. The **prognosis** is **worse** than the papillary type because the occurrence of **metastases** in **vital organs is** often **fatal.**

Box 4.29:	The points to be noted about the characteristics of follicular carcinoma

- 20% to 25% of thyroid cancers
- Disease of the middle age
- Common in women
- FNAC not useful – Capsular and angio invasion on histopathology
- Spread along the blood stream - Secondaries in lung, bones etc
- More aggressive tumour
- Hence poorer prognosis

Q. 15. What are the clinical features of follicular carcinoma?

The following modes of presentation are described.

(*a*) The picture is one of a **single nodule** of the thyroid or less commonly a **multinodular goiter** of several **months** or even **years** duration. If there may a history of **recent increase** in **size** over a **short period** of time, the **suspicion** of malignancy is **higher. Pain** as a symptom is **uncommon. US** examination will show either a **single** or multiple nodules that are **solid** in nature. **Doppler** studies will show **increased vascularity. FNAC** is reported as a **follicular neoplasm**. This group may **present** as a **histological surprise.** Following the FNAC report of a follicular adenoma, the patient might have had a **hemi- or a subtotal thyroidectomy.** If the histopathology report is a **follicular adenoma, no further treatment** is needed. But the **histological report** may show a **follicular carcinoma. Frozen section** reports are **unreliable** in this situation.

(*b*) **Follicular carcinoma** with **metastatic** disease. This is the **easiest** group as far as diagnosis is concerned. They present with a **nodular goiter** with **secondaries. Bones** are the **commonest seat** of **secondary** deposits. The **bones involved** are those with **red marrow,** such as the **vertebral bodies**, the **skull,** the **flat bones** of **the pelvis** and the **upper ends** of the **humeri** and **femora.** When the **skull** is infiltrated, the **swelling** is unusually **soft** and **pulsatile** due to the increased vascularity. **Secondaries** may also be seen in the **lungs** or the **brain.**

(*c*) The patient presents with a **secondary deposit** in the **bone, lung** or **brain.** The **thyroid gland** may **not palpable (occult primary).** Investigations like a **FNAC or a CT-guided biopsy** of the **secondary** lesion will reveal the nature of the **primary tumour.** The **cytological** features may **not** suggest malignancy. But the **presence** of **thyroid follicles** or **cells** at these sites is adequate for a **diagnosis** of **follicular carcinoma.**

(*d*) This **group** presents with a **histological surprise.** Following **FNAC** report of a **colloid goiter**, the patient has had **a hemi- or a subtotal thyroidectomy.** But the **histological report** shows **follicular carcinoma.** In addition, a **small number** of patients are even **more unfortunate.** They present with **symptoms of secondaries** in the **organs** mentioned above, **months** or **years** after the **operation.** Even the **histological report** at that stage would have been a **follicular adenoma.** Investigations like **X-ray and biopsy** point out the **diagnosis.**

Box 4.30:	The points to be noted regarding the various types of presentation of follicular carcinoma

- Nodular goiter with blood-spread metastases
- Skull secondaries: Soft and sometimes pulsatile
- FNAC of secondaries – Diagnostic. May need CT guidance
- Presentation with a nodular goiter – Single nodule – More common
- FNAC – Follicular neoplasm or colloid goiter (uncommon)
- Hemi – or subtotal thyroidectomy
- H.P. report – Follicular carcinoma
- Thyroid surgery earlier – Presentation with metastases-FNAC - Follicular carcinoma

Q. 16. Describe the treatment modalities for follicular carcinoma.

All patients with a diagnosis of follicular carcinoma need a total thyroidectomy. A patient having undergone a **hemithyroidectomy, {FNAC report follicular adenoma}** may return to the hospital with a **histopathology report** of a **follicular carcinoma.** This patient needs a **completion total thyroidectomy.** The **same routine** is followed for patients who have undergone a **subtotal thyroidectomy** for a **multinodular goiter** (less common) and present with a **histological** report of **follicular carcinoma.** The **reasons f**or performing this operation are **different** from that of **papillary carcinoma.** **RI** plays an **important part** in the **diagnosis** and **treatment** of **metastases** from **follicular carcinoma.** If one **lateral lobe** or **parts of the thyroid** (following subtotal resection) are **retained,** all the **dose** of **RI** given for **diagnostic purpose** is **taken up** by **the thyroid tissue** and even if **secondarie**s are present, they will **not be detected.** Following a total thyroidectomy, the secondaries if present are sensitized to take up RI.

Q. 17. Discuss the role of RI in the treatment of follicular carcinoma.

Since **follicular carcinomas** are **differentiated cancers,** they still retain the **capacity t**o take up

iodine. The **RI test is delayed** for **six weeks** following the **total thyroidectomy.** During this period, the patient will become **athyroid**, and hence the levels of **TSH** will be very **high.** Thus if **secondary deposits** are present they will be **sensitised** to take up **iodine.** At this stage, a **tracer dose** of **RI i**s given and a **scintiscan** is performed. If **metastases** are **detected,** they are destroyed by a **curative dose of RI.** The curative dose is between **100 to 150 millicuries.** If the investigation needs to be performed **earlier** due to **time constraints**, the **scintiscan** can be performed **immediately** following an injection of **recombinant TSH..** If **no secondary** metastases are detected, the patient is kept under **observation.**

Q. 18. What is the role of oral thyroxine in this group of patients?

The patients are put on permanent **replacement thyroxine** therapy. The dose is to maintain the **TSH** levels within **normal** limits, and usually it is about **100 mcg p**er day. Every **year** the patient needs a repeat **RI scan. Thyroxine** is **withheld f**or **six weeks** before the **test.** If **metastases** are **detected,** a **curative dose** of **RI** is administered. The usual dose ranges between **100 to 150 millicuries.** Because of **severe** **side effects,** efforts have been made to **reduce** the dose without **compromising** its **efficacy. Thyroglobulin levels** in the blood can be used as a **tumour marker.** It is nearly **zero** after a **total thyroidectomy. Raised levels** of **TG** are an indication of **metastatic** disease and are detected before symptomatic secondaries make their appearance.

Q. 19. What is the role of external beam radiotherapy (EBRT)?

Unfortunately, many **recurrences** that **appear** at a **later date** are **undifferentiated.** They **lose** their capacity to **take up iodine. Hence** they are **not detected** by **RI** studies. They become **manifest** much **later** with **symptoms and signs.** Though **isolated** single **deposits** in **bones** have been **excised**, more often they are **multiple** and **palliative EBRT** is the only possible remedy. As mentioned earlier, they are invariably **fatal.**

Q. 20. Describe the treatment of patients presenting with synchronous or metachronous secondaries.

For the group of **patients** who present with a **goiter** and **metastases,** the principles of **management** are **easy** to **comprehend.** The **diagnosis** is confirmed by **FNAC** of the **metastatic** lesion. These patients undergo a **total thyroidectomy** for reasons mentioned earlier. The **rest** of the **management** is the **same** as mentioned above.

For patients who had undergone various types of **thyroid surgery** earlier and present with **metastatic disease months** or **years** later, a **completion thyroidectomy** followed by **RI treatment** described earlier is the treatment. But in general this **group** has a **poor prognosis.**

Box 4.31:	Points to be noted in the management of follicular carcinoma

- Total thyroidectomy. Even in the presence of secondaries.
- Need for removal of the entire gland-
- Reasons – Different from papillary carcinoma.
- Metastases are treated by RI.
- If major portions of the gland are retained, all the tracer dose of RI is absorbed by this remnant
- Secondaries are not detected.
- Hence completion thyroidectomy following either a hemi- or subtotal thyroidectomy.
- Curative dose of RI for detected secondaries.
- Replacement therapy with thyroxine to maintain euthyroid state.
- Thyroglobulin – Tumour marker.
- Undifferentiated secondaries. Palliative EBRT.

Q. 21. What are the clinical features of anaplastic carcinoma?

Anaplastic carcinoma fits into the **classical description** of a **malignant tumour** completely. It represents only **about 5%** of patients with thyroid cancers. The tumour may arise in a normal thyroid. But it may also occur as a **transformatio**n of a pre-existing **papillary** carcinoma. These patients give a history of a **rapid increase** in **size** along with **pain** of a **few weeks** duration.

The **clinical features** are as follows:

(*a*) It affects **elderly** patients.

(*b*) It is seen equally in both the sexes.

(*c*) The **goiter** is of a **short duration**, being present for some weeks or a few months.

(*d*) **Pain** is a prominent symptom.

(*e*) **Dyspnoea** and **dysphagia** occur frequently.

(*f*) Presence of **hoarseness of voice** due to **infiltration of the recurrent laryngeal nerves** is almost **diagnostic**.

(*g*) Movement **upwards** with **deglutition** may be absent if the **tumour** has become **extrathyroidal.**

(*h*) On palpation, the **consistency** is **hard,** and **mobility** either **restricted** or **absent.**

(*i*) There may be evidence of **tracheal** deviation or **compression.**

(*j*) **Carotid pulsations** may be **absent** on one or both sides. (Positive Berry's sign)

(*k*) The cancer is known to **infiltrate** the adjacent structures like **trachea** and **oesophagus**.

(*l*) The tumour spreads both via the **lymphatics** and the **blood stream**.

(*m*) **Lymph nodes** when present are **hard**. In early stages they are **mobile**, but once extracapsular spread occurs, they are **fixed**.

(*n*) **Haematogenous** spread will produce **secondaries** in **bones, lung** and **brain.**

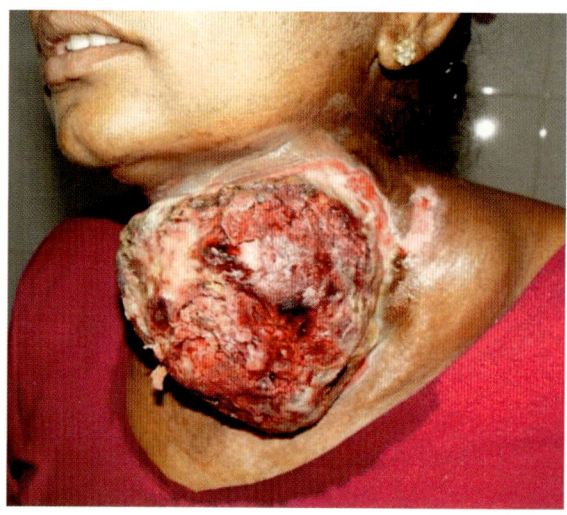

Fig. 4.9: Fungating anaplastic carcinoma thyroid.

Box 4.32:	Points to be noted about the clinical features of anaplastic carcinoma

- Elderly patients – Rapidly growing goiter
- Pain present. Dyspnoea, dysphagia and hoarseness of voice
- Hard in consistency. Upward movement with deglutition
- May be absent. Restricted or no mobility
- Regional nodes may be enlarged
- Late stages – Blood-spread secondaries

Q. 22. Describe the investigations for anaplastic carcinoma.

FNAC shows **spindle cells** as well as **multinucleated giant cells.** Signs of **anaplastic changes** are seen in the cells.

Chest X-ray may show evidence of metastases.

Plain X-ray or CT scans will depend on the site of the secondaries. **Bony secondaries** are **osteolytic** in nature.

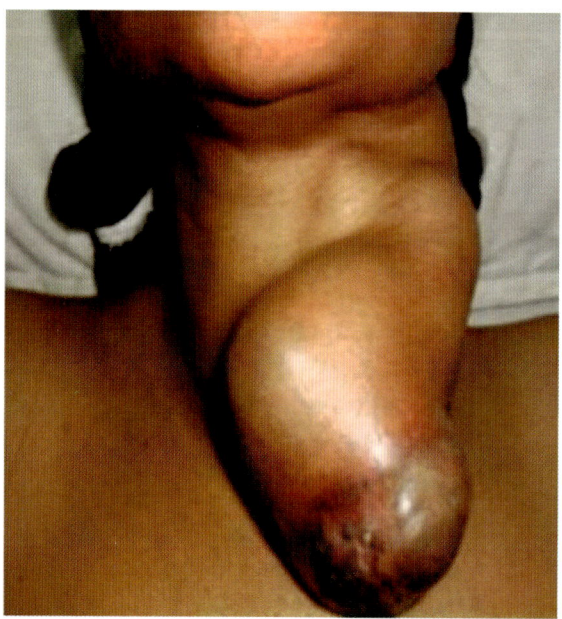

Fig. 4.8: Anaplastic carcinoma extending in front of the sternum with skin necrosis at the lower end.

CT scan of the neck is indicated only if **curative surgery** is being planned.

Box 4.33:	Points regarding investigations for anaplastic carcinoma

- FNAC – Spindle cells with multinucleated giant cells
- Chest X-ray – To detect secondaries
- CT neck – If curative surgery is feasible

Q 23. What are the principles of treatment?

Most of our **patients** by the time they reach the hospital have **advanced inoperable** disease.

If detected early with a **mobile tumour,** a **CT** is done to confirm **operability.** Such patients undergo a **total thyroidectomy** followed by **radiotherapy. Extended radical surgery** is performed in advanced **oncology centres** by removing involved **adjacent structures** and **plastic surgical reconstruction.** If the patient has **mobile** secondary lymph **nodes, radical lymphadenectomy** is performed.

But this **scenario** is **rare** in our **country. Inoperable** cancers are treated by **palliative EBRT.**

Patients presenting with **inspiratory stridor** pose special problems. An **urgent CT** followed by a **bronchoscopy** is needed to rule out **intraluminal extension.** If it is **absent,** a **wedge resection**

of the portion of the tumour present **in front** of the trachea, followed by a **tracheostomy** is advised. But this can be **technically** a very **challenging procedure.**

Prognosis is very **poor** and most patients survive only for a **few months. Death** is the result of **asphyxia** or **lung** and **bony** metastases.

Box 4.34:	Points regarding treatment

- Operable cases – Total thyroidectomy followed by EBRT.
- Extended radical surgery if feasible-
- Reconstruction of trachea
- Post. op EBRT
- Mobile nodes – Radical lymphadenectomy
- Most of our patients – Advanced stage
- Palliative EBRT
- Lifespan – Weeks or months only.

Q. 24. Describe the clinical features and management of medullary carcinoma of the thyroid gland.

Medullary carcinoma is an **uncommon thyroid malignancy,** accounting for about **3% to 4%** of all thyroid cancers. It is a tumour arising from the **parafollicular** or **C cells** present **in** the **thyroid** gland. These **C cells arise** from the **ultimobranchial body**, derived from the **IVth pharyngeal pouch,** and secrete **calcitonin.**

Its importance lies in the fact that it may be a part of **familial cancer** or **MEN type 2A or 2B** wherein, **pheochromocytoma** and **parathyroid tumours** are also seen. These tumours are the result of a **dominant gene mutation** and are responsible for **20% of medullary carcinoma cases**. They are seen at a **younger age** and have a **poor prognosis.** The remaining **80% are sporadic** in nature and occur in persons above **45 years** and have a **better outlook**.

Box 4.35:	Points regarding general characteristics of medullary carcinoma

- 3% to 4% of all cancers
- Arising from C cells – Secreting calcitonin
- 20% – Familial. Part of MEN type IIA or IIB
- Young age – More aggressive
- 80% sporadic – Older age
- Spread – Both by lymphatic and haematogenous routes

Q. 25. Describe the clinical features of medullary carcinoma.

The patient may present with an **asymptomatic nodular goiter.** More often in the **familial variety both the lobes** are **enlarge**d. **Unilateral** lobe may be enlarged in **sporadic** cases. The tumour **spreads** by the **lymphatic** as well as the **haematological** routes. Nearly **50%** of the **patients** have **palpable nodes in** the neck at the time of **presentation.** These nodes are **hard** and **mobile** initially and become **fixed** at a later stage. **Clinically,** there are no **specific features** to arrive at a **diagnosis.** Hence it is a **cytological** or **histological** diagnosis. The degree of **suspicion** is **high** in the **familial** variety.

Box 4.36:	Points regarding clinical features

- Asymptomatic nodular goiter.
- High degree of suspicion in MEN syndromes.
- 50% have enlarged nodes at presentation.
- Nodes are hard, nontender, mobile in early stages.
- No specific features in the sporadic variety.

Q. 26. What are the investigations to be done in a case of medullary carcinoma?

1. **FNAC** is **diagnostic**. The cells may be **round** or **spindle** shaped with **eosinophilic** cytoplasm. These cells are separated by a **homogenous eosinophilic amyloid** {diagnostic}.

2. **Calcitonin**. It is a **tumour marker** for **medullary carcinoma**. Serum **calcitonin levels** are usually **raised**. If the level **comes down** after **t**reatment, it indicates a **good response. Raised** levels after the **operation** are significant because they occur **before symptomatic secondaries** appear. Again **calcitonin** is

important as a **screening** procedure in the **familial type** of cases.

3. But **genetic studies** have been found to be **more reliable** than calcitonin levels in **predicting** the development of the **cancer** in other members of the **family** at a **later date.**

4. Investigations to rule out **phaeochromocytoma** and **hyperparathyroidism .**

5. **Chest X-ray and CT chest and neck** (if **major ablative surgery** is being planned).

Box 4.37:	Points regarding investigations

- FNAC – Diagnostic. Round or spindle shaped cells,
- with eosinophilic cytoplasm – Presence of amyloid.
- Serum calcitonin - Usually raised.
- With treatment calcitonin levels reach normal.
- Increase occurs before symptomatic secondaries appear.
- Necessary to identify susceptible members of family.
- Genetic studies more reliable.
- Investigations specific to MEN.
- CT chest and neck prior to radical surgery.

Q. 27. Describe the treatment of medullary carcinoma.

Operable cases need a **total thyroidectomy** followed by **EBRT**. When indicated, a **radical neck dissection** is also performed. **Inoperable** cancers are treated by **palliative** **radiotherapy**. Following a **total thyroidectomy**, these patients need **replacement therapy** with **thyroxine**. Annual **calcitonin estimations** are done to detect **metastatic** disease. Once **metastases appear**, the outlook is **poor**. A **monoclonal antibody,** which is a **tyrosine kinase inhibitor,** called **vandetanib** is being tried as a palliative treatment.

Q. 28. What are the indications for prophylactic total thyroidectomy?

Prophylactic total thyroidectomy is indicated in **relatives** if the levels of **calcitonin** are **high** or **genetic studies** are **positive.** This operation is to be done at a **very young age**, since the risk of developing the cancer is **100%.**

Box 4.38:	Points regarding the treatment

- Operable cases – Total thyroidectomy followed by EBRT
- Thyroxine replacement
- Positive nodes – Radical neck dissection
- Inoperable cancers – Palliative EBRT
- Regular calcitonin estimation
- Familial type
- Calcitonin and genetic studies
- Risk of medullary carcinoma – 100%
- Prophylactic total thyroidectomy at a very young age

■■■

Diseases of the Salivary Glands

5

A CASE OF PLEOMORPHIC ADENOMA OF THE PAROTID GLAND

Setting

- Surgical outpatient department (OPD).

Chief Complaint

A **swelling** in the **left parotid** region for a duration of **10 years.**

History of Present Illness

A **42-year-old man** presented to the OPD with the complaint of a **swelling** in the **left parotid** region of **10 years** duration. The swelling was first noticed in front of the **tragus** of the ear. Since then it had been **gradually increasing** in size. The patient had noticed that the swelling had been **extending** to the **adjacent regions**. There was no history of **rapid increase** in size. The patient did not complain of any **pain**. He had not noticed any **change** in the **size** during **eating**. There was no history of **excessive salivation**. There was no history of **fever**.

Past, personal and family histories were **insignificant.**

He had **not** taken any **treatment** for this condition.

General physical examination showed a well-built and well-nourished 42-year-old man who had no abnormalities on general examination.

Local Examination

Inspection

A **single** swelling was seen in the **left parotid** region. It was extending from the **zygomatic arch** to 1 cm below the **lower border of the mandible** vertically. The horizontal extent was from the **mastoid process** to about 4 cm behind the **angle** of the **mouth**. The **groove** between the **mandible** and the mastoid process was **obliterated**.

It was present **in front, below and behind** the **lobule** of the left ear. The lobule appeared **elevated** in a **forward** direction.

- All the **margins** were well defined.
- It measured 8 cm by 5 cm in **size** and the **shape** was irregular.
- The **surface** was **lobular**.
- The **skin** over the swelling was **stretched.**
- The **surrounding area** appeared normal.

Palpation

- The swelling was not **warm** or **tender.**
- The **site** and **extent** were the same as noted on inspection.
- The **size** was 8 cm by 5 cm and the **shape** was irregular. All the **borders** could be easily palpated.
- The surface was nodular.
- The consistency was basically firm. Few soft areas were felt at the summit of some nodules.
- The overlying **skin** was **free** from the swelling.
- There was minimal **vertical** and **transverse mobility**.
- The **swelling** could not be **pushed upwards beyond** the **zygomatic arch**.
- There was no **change in** the mobility on putting the **masseter** on contraction against resistance.

Examination of the VII Nerve

- There was no evidence of nerve deficit.

Examination of the Regional Lymph Nodes

- No enlarged nodes were palpable in the left side of the neck.

Examination of the Oral Cavity

- The **orifice** of the **Stensen's duct** was normal. There was no **medial deviation** of the **left tonsil**, indicating an absence of **deep lobar** enlargement.

Examination of the other Major Salivary Glands

- None of the other major salivary glands were enlarged.

Box 5.1:	Points to be noted in history
• Swelling – duration – site and size at onset	
• Rate of growth	
• Pain- change in size during eating	
• Salivary symptoms – excessive salivation – dryness of the mouth	
• Fever	

Box 5.2:	Points to be noted during inspection
• Swelling – site and extent – parotid region	
• Present in front, below and behind the lobule	
• If the whole gland is enlarged – lobule of the ear – elevated	
• Not seen if only a part of the gland is enlarged	
• Shape and size	
• Surface – smooth or nodular	
• Skin over the swelling	
• Surrounding area	

Other systems were clinically normal.

Q. 1. What was the clinical diagnosis?

(*a*) Pleomorphic adenoma of the parotid.

(*b*) Chronic sialadenitis.

(*c*) Monomorphic adenoma.

(*d*) Carcinoma of the parotid.

The right answer is (a). **Chronic sialadenitis** is usually **secondary** to a **stone** blocking the **duct.** The **submandibular** salivary gland is the one most **frequently** involved. The typical history is that of a **painful swelling** that **enlarges** during **eating.** The **orifice,** being the **narrowest part** of the **duct,** is the site for the **stone** to be **lodged. Monomorphic adenomas** are **rare** and are diagnosed by **cytological examination.** The duration in a case of **carcinoma** is measured in **months.** The **rate of growth** is **rapid.** There may be associated **pain.** The swelling is **hard** and most often **fixed.** Evidence of **VII nerve palsy** and palpable **nodes** strengthen the diagnosis.

The **history** and the **clinical features** in this patient were **typical** of a pleomorphic adenoma. It happens to be the **commonest** tumour arising from the **parotid** gland. The swelling was of a **long duration** with a gradual increase in size. It was **asymptomatic.** Hence it was **cosmetic** embarrassment that brought the patient to the hospital.

Q. 2. What was the investigation done in this patient?

Fine needle aspiration cytology (FNAC) of the swelling was done. The report showed **pleomorphic adenoma.**

Q. 3. What is the incidence of a pleomorphic adenoma of the parotid?

80% of all **salivary gland** tumours occur in the **parotid gland. 80%** of these are **pleomorphic adenomas.** The **superficial lobe** of the parotid is involved in **80%** of these cases**.**

Q. 4. What are the clinical signs that help to identify the anatomical nature of these swellings?

If the **entire parotid gland** is enlarged, it is present **in front, below** and **behind** the **lobule** of the ear. Under these circumstances, the **lobule** of the ear is **elevated.** But a tumour may be seen only **in front** of the **tragus** of the ear or **in front** of the **mastoid process.** The **groove** between the **mandible** and the **mastoid** may be **obliterated.** A tumour arising from the **lower pole** can easily be **mistaken** for an enlarged **lymph node.**

The **"curtain sign"** helps to distinguish between a

subcutaneous swelling and a swelling of the **parotid gland**. The **parotid fascia,** which is an extension of the **investing layer** of the **cervical fascia,** is **attached** to the **zygomatic arch**. Hence a parotid swelling **cannot be pushed upwards beyond** this **arch,** similar to an **object** placed **within the curtain**. A **subcutaneous** swelling can easily be pushed **beyond this point**.

This clinical sign assumes **significance** since a pleomorphic adenoma present **in front** of the **tragus** may be so **freely mobile,** as to be mistaken for a **subcutaneous** swelling. This may end up with an **enucleation** of the lesion. It would mean a **100 % recurrence**.

Q. 5. Why should other major salivary glands be examined in a case of a parotid swelling?

Warthin's tumour is **bilateral in 10% to 15 %** of cases. **Congenital sialectasis** of the **parotid** glands are also **bilateral.** Certain **autoimmune diseases** like **Mickulicz** syndrome and **Sjogren's** disease produce **enlargement** of all the **major salivary glands**.

Q. 6. What was the investigation done to prove the diagnosis?

FNAC The **smear** showed **ductal cells** along with a **chondromyxoid stroma** and **myoepithelial cells** confirming the diagnosis.

Q. 7. Does FNAC carry any risk to the patient?

Pleomorphic adenomas **recur frequently**. Hence it was thought that the **needle track** could provide an **access** for the tumour **cells** to spread and increase the **incidence** of **recurrence**. But that has **not** been proved to be **true**. In addition, a **low**-grade **mucoepidermoid carcinoma** behaves like a **pleomorphic adenoma**. Hence **all patients** with a pleomorphic adenoma need an **FNAC**.

Q. 8. What is the natural history of pleomorphic adenoma of the parotid gland?

Pleomorphic adenoma **commonly recurs** and it also has a potential to turn **malignant.** The **risk** of malignancy **increases** with the **number of recurrences**. When a **malignant transformation** occurs, the outlook is **very poor**.

Q. 9. What were the treatment options for this patient?

(*a*) Total parotidectomy.

(*b*) Partial parotidectomy.

(*c*) Superficial parotidectomy.

(*d*) Extracapsular excision.

The correct answer is (*c*). The tumour is confined to the **superfiicial lobe**. Hence a superficial **parotidectomy** is the correct answer. The term **partial parotidectomy** is no longer **used** since it is a **nonspecific** term. **Extracapsular excision** would mean removal of the **tumour** along with a **rim** of **normal parotid** tissue. This operation also carries the **risk** of **injuring** the branches of the VIIth **nerve**. The **only indication** for this operation is a **pleomorphic adenoma** arising from the **lower pole** of the parotid in relation to the **cervical branch of the VIIth nerve.** This branch supplies the **platysma** and hence can be **sacrificed.**

A **superficial parotidectomy** means removal of the **superficial lobe** of the gland, which has the tumour. This operation has the **least incidence** of **recurrence**.

Q. 10. Describe the relation of the VIIth cranial nerve to the parotid gland.

The VIIth **nerve** exits the skull via the **stylomastoid foramen**. Then it enters the **substance** of the parotid **gland**. Within the gland it **divides** usually into **five branches** before exiting **along** the **anterior border** of the gland to supply the **muscles of the face.** Thus the facial nerve divides the gland into a **superficial** and a **deep lobe.** Since the **veins** are also present in the **same plane,**

this has been termed as the **faciovenous** plane of **Patey.**

Q. 11. What are the macroscopic features of the tumour?

They appear as well-**encapsulated solid** tumours. The **thickness** of the **capsule** may be **variable** and can be **extremely thin** in some areas. The cut **surface** is **homogenous** and **whitish tan to gray** in colour. It also has a **glistening** appearance. **Haemorrhage and necrosis** are often seen with areas of **cystic degeneration.**

Q. 12. Explain the terminology "pleomorphism" used to describe the tumour.

Pleomorphic adenoma shows a remarkable degree of morphological diversity (**pleomorphism** on microscopic examination means **histological variations**). The essential **components** of the **tumour** are the **capsule,** the **epithelial** and **myoepithelial cells** as well as the **stroma.** The **epithelial** cells are **secretory wedge-shaped cells** surrounding a **lumen, which** becomes the **origin** of the **intercalated ducts.** The **cytoplasm** of these cells contains strongly **basophilic granules.**

Myoepithelial cells are **contractile** and are present **between** the **acinar cells.** They contain **actin**, **myosin** and **intermediate filaments**.

The **stroma** is composed of **modified myoepithelial cells** and may contain **mucoid, hyaline, chondroid** or even **osseous tissue**. Thus **metaplastic changes** in the **myoepithelial cells** can result in the **formation** of various tissues, including **cartilage.** In the **past,** these tumours were named as **mixed salivary tumours**. It was presumed that the **ectodermal** elements gave rise to the **adenoma** and the **embryological remnants** of the **mesoderm trapped within**, produced **cartilage**. This term is no longer in use.

The most **significant part** of microscopy is the **study** of the **capsule.** If **serial sections** of the tumour are taken, **capsular deficiency** is seen in almost **all cases. Finger-like projections** can be demonstrated **extending beyond** the **capsule** into the **adjacent glandular tissue.** Sometimes the tumour **bulges through the capsule** and forms **satellite nodules** in the **peritumoural** region. These are **invariably attached** to the main **tumou**r by a **narrow isthmus**.

Q. 13. Explain the causes for recurrence of a pleomorphic adenoma though it is a benign tumour.

An **operation** on the **parotid** gland is basically an operation on the **facial nerve**. As mentioned earlier, the **facial nerve and its branches** pass through the **substance** of the **gland,** dividing it into a **superficial** and a **deep lobe. Pleomorphic adenoma** being a **benign** tumour has a **capsule**. But the **capsular deficiency** can give rise to **finger-like projections** of the tumour into the **adjacent glandular** tissue. In addition, the tumour **bulges through the capsule,** being **attached** to the main body by a narrow **isthmus.** Pleomorphic adenoma being a benign tumour, the **facial nerve** needs to be **preserved** under all **circumstances.** Thus the problem is to be **as far away** as possible from the **capsule** of the tumour to ensure a **complete resection** without **sacrificing** any branch of the **facial nerve.** If a **branch of the nerve** is found in **close proximity** to the **capsule,** chances are that a **finger-like projection** of the tumour has **not been removed,** leading to a **recurrence.** In addition, **operative manipulation** may cause a number of **tumour cells** to **spill over** on to the **operative field. Rupture** of the **capsule** during **surgery** increases this **risk.** These **cells** have a tendency to get **implanted** in the **operative area,** giving rise to **recurrence** at a **later date**. Thus **surgery** for pleomorphic adenoma carries a **definite risk** of **recurrence**. The **recurrences** may be in the **remnant of the gland,** in the **subcutaneous tissue,** or in the **skin flaps**. The **standard statement** for pleomorphic adenoma runs as follows. They **commonly recur** but **uncommonly become malignant**. To confound matters further, the **risk of malignancy increases** with each **recurrence.**

Setting: A week later the patient was posted for a superficial parotidectomy.

Q. 14. Describe the main steps of a superficial parotidectomy.

An **incision** was made starting at the **zygoma,** running in front of the **tragus** vertically downwards. The incision then was extended in a broad curve **around** the **lobule** of the ear. The last part of the incision turned **round at the mastoid** and continued downwards along the **anterior border** of the **sternomastoid.** The **skin flaps were raised.** The **sternomastoid** and the **posterior belly of the digastric** were **retracted,** exposing the **trunk of the facial nerve** at the **posterior border** of the **gland.** The **nerve and its branches** were then traced through the **substance** of the gland **exiting**

at its **anterior border**, thus forming the **fasciovenous plane.** The **portion** of the **parotid gland superficial** to this plane was **removed**. Care was taken not to **injure** any of the branches of the **nerve** as well as not to **rupture** the **capsule** during the operation. The entire operative field was irrigated with **sterile water** to **destroy** the tumour **cells** that might have **spilled** on to the **tissues.** This step has been found to **reduce** the chances of **recurrence.** The incision was **closed** with a suction **drain.**

Q. 15. What are the clinical features that suggest a deep lobar tumour?

Restricted mobility even when the **size** of the tumour is **small** should raise the suspicion of a **deep lobe** tumour. The **deep lobe** is intimately related to the **lateral wall of the pharynx. Enlargement** of the deep lobe causes a **medial displacement** of the **pharyngeal wall.** Hence an **intraoral examination** shows a **medial displacement** of the **tonsil.** The **space** between the **uvula** and the **tonsil** on the affected **side appears to be reduced when compared to** the **opposite** side. A **MRI** scan may be needed to **localise** the tumour **accurately**.

Q. 16. How are deep lobe tumours treated?

Tumours of the **deep lobe** and those tumours **extending** from the **superficial** to the **deep** are treated by a **total conservative parotidectomy.** It would mean **the removal** of the **entire gland** with **conservation of the VII**[th] **nerve** and its branches**.**

Q. 17. **How are recurrent tumours managed?**

A **recurrent adenoma** poses **special problems**. The **time interval** may range from **months to years. Recurrence** can arise from the remaining **deep lobe** or in the **subcutaneous fat** overlying the gland, in the **skin flaps,** or even at slightly **distant sites**. The **risk** of recurrence is **higher** in **men,** especially **over 40** years of age, and if the tumour is **more than 2 cm** in size. A **FNAC** is performed to confirm its **benign nature.** It is pertinent to note that in **many other** clinical **situations,** a **recurrence** is equated with **malignancy**. The salivary glands are an **exception** to this rule. A **MRI scan** is always needed since recurrences are **multifocal** and the **extent** of recurrence can be **accurately** defined by **an MRI scan. Imaging** also helps in identifying the **location** of the facial nerve.

The operation consists of a **total parotidectomy** **preserving** the **facial nerve**. The involved **skin** and **subcutaneous fat** are **excised**. The surgery is technically **difficult**. Because

of **previous surgery,** there is extensive **fibrosis** and the **tissue planes** are **difficult** to **dissect**. Identification of the **nerve** and its branches is also **problematic**. A **nerve stimulator** is used by some surgeons for this purpose. It is **safer** to explain the **nature of the operation** and the possible **complications** to **the patient** in detail **before the operation** to avoid **medicolegal** problems later. It is unfortunate that even a **second** operation does not bring **down** the incidence of **recurrence** to **zero.** The role of **postoperative radiation** is **controversial**. As a principle, benign tumours are not treated by radiation. But if the capsule is ruptured during the operation, or after **2 or 3 recurrences,** some surgeons employ **superficial radiation** to the operated area. It does bring **down** the rate of **recurrence.**

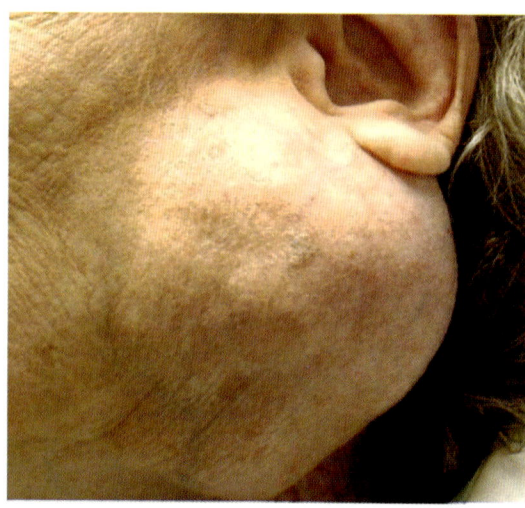

Fig. 5.1: Pleomorphic adenoma of the parotid gland with elevation of the ear lobule.

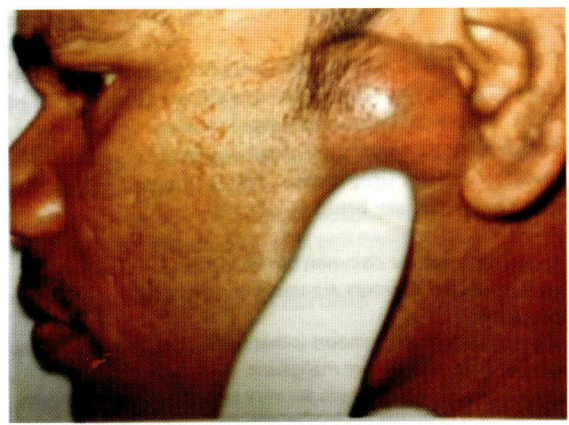

Fig. 5.2: Demonstration of the "curtain sign."

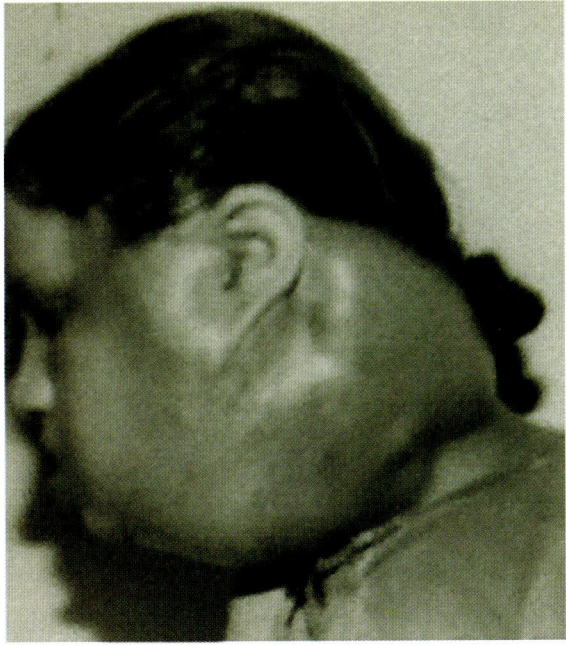

Fig. 5.3: Recurrent pleomorphic adenoma of the parotid gland.

Q. 18. Describe the clinical features of a malignant tumour of the parotid gland.

Malignant salivary gland tumours are **rare** and are responsible only for about **0.3%** of all cancers. The incidence among **head and neck cancers** is about **6%.** Of these **60% to 80%** occur in the parotid gland, mostly located in the **superficial lobe**. Though more than **40** histological **varieties** have been described, only the **common types** are important for the **clinician.**

Clinical Features

1. **Age:** The **fifth decade** has the highest incidence. But when a **malignant** transformation occurs in a **pleomorphic adenoma**, it occurs at a **later age** group.

2. **Gender:** It is seen **equally** in both the sexes.

3. The chief **complaint** is a swelling in the **parotid** region. The duration is of a **few months**. But the **pleomorphic group** may give a history of several **years.** The **rate** of growth is **rapid. A sudden spurt** in the growth of a pleomorphic adenoma raises a suspicion of **malignancy.**

4. **Pain** is a significant symptom. When the **nerves** are involved, the pain is **severe. Infiltration** of the mandible or the **base of the skull** leads to **intense pain.**

5. Patients may present with **enlarged lymph nodes** in the neck in **addition** to the primary tumour.

6. **Facial nerve paralysis** may bring the patient to the hospital.

7. **Blood-borne metastases** occur only at **a late stage**, mostly after the **primary** has been **treated.**

Box 5.3:	Points to be noted in the clinical features of a malignant tumour of the parotid

- Age – Fifth decade. Malignant change in a pleomorphic adenoma occurs in elderly patients
- Swelling in the parotid region of a short duration
- Rate of growth – Rapid
- Pain present. Involvement of nerve, mandible and base of the skull – Pain becomes very severe. Facial nerve palsy
- Presentation with metastatic disease

Local Examination

1. **Swelling** in the parotid region.

   (*a*) The **size** may vary from a few centimetres to a huge swelling.

   (*b*) The **shape** is usually irregular.

   (*c*) The **consistency** is **hard**. But it is variable if there are areas of **necrosis.**

   (*d*) **Mobilty:** Restricted mobility is an important sign due to involvement of the **adjacent structures**. If the tumour is adherent to the **masseter** muscle, the mobility is **lost** when this muscle is put on **contraction** against resistance. When the **mandible** or the

base of skull is infiltrated by the tumour, there is **total fixity. Skin involvement** occurs **late** in the course of the disease except for the group of patients who have undergone **previous surgery** on the gland.

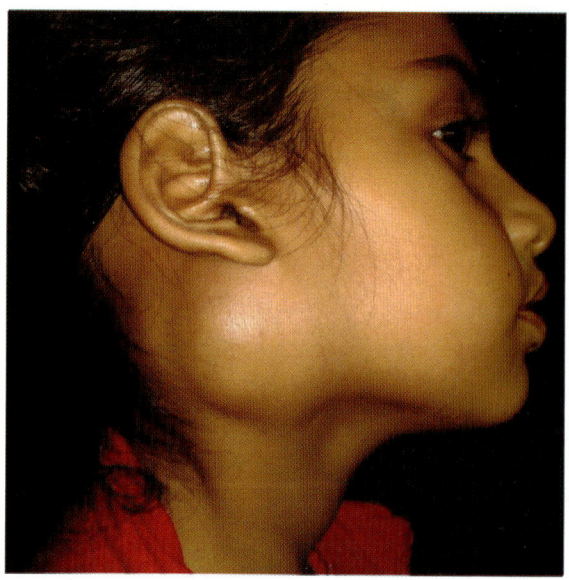

Fig. 5.4: Adenocarcinoma of the parotid gland.

2. **Lymph node examination:** The lymph nodes that could be the site for **secondaries** include the **preauricular** and **level IB,** II and **V groups. Skip** lesions are also **known** to occur. The lymph nodes are **hard.**

3. **Facial nerve examination:** At admission, most of our patients have evidence of **VIIth nerve palsy** due to infiltration by the tumour. To some extent, it is related to the **pathological type** of malignancy.

An **adenoid cystic** carcinoma produces **early** nerve involvement due to **perineural spread.** Many patients with **mucoepidermoid carcinoma** may not have nerve paralysis till a very **late stage**.

Box 5.4:	Points to be noted regarding the clinical features

- Swelling in the parotid region.
- Hard in consistency .May also be variable.
- Fixed to masseter, mandible and base of skull as the disease progresses.
- Facial nerve palsy.
- Enlarged lymph nodes – Preauricular, level II and V

Q. 19. What are the investigations?

1. **FNAC** helps to diagnose **malignancy**. In many instances, the **pathological type** can also be determined. Core needle biopsy (**CNB**) is needed if **FNAC** is **inconclusive**. The prognosis differs depending on the type of tumour. But the **finer details** like the tumour grade can only be determined by **histopathology.**

2. An **ultrasound-guided FNAC** is necessary for **small** and **deeply** located lesions.

3. **Chest X-ray**. Blood-borne metastases can occur in the **lung,** in late or **recurrent** malignancy.

4. **CT scan** provides informa-tion on the exact **location of** the tumour in the gland and **infiltration** of the **neighbor-ing structures**.

5. **MRI** scan will demonstrate the extent of infiltration of the **adjacent soft tissue and bone**. CT and MRI will help to decide whether **extensive radical surgery** with **intent to cure** can be undertaken or not.

Box 5.5:	Points to be noted for investigating a malignant parotid swelling

- FNAC – Confirms malignancy and the type.
- CNB – if inconclusive
- Tumour grade – only on histopathology
- Chest X-ray
- CT scan – Involvement of mandible and base of skull
- MRI better for soft tissue infiltration

Q. 20. Describe the common patho-logical varieties of carcinomas of the parotid gland.

Mucoepidermoid Carcinoma

This is the **most common** type of malignancy of the salivary glands. The parotid gland is the most frequently affected than the other major glands.

Macroscopy

These tumours are **firm and smooth** with a **whitish** or **pink** colour. **Cystic areas** are often present. The **edges** may be **well-** or **ill-defined**.

Histopathology

Mucoepidermoid carcinoma is characterised by **epidermoid** and **mucus secreting** cells as well as cells of the **intermediate type**. It is to be noted that **embryologically,** the salivary glands develop from the **ectoderm.** These tumours are **multicystic** with some **solid** areas. The **epidermoid** cells are **cuboidal or polygonal,** but **keratinisation** is **not seen**. The **mucus secreting cells** are **large** with **pale cytoplasm** and **peripherally placed nuclei. Neural invasion** is **uncommon.** Depending on the histopathology, they are classified as **low, intermediate- and high**-grade tumours. The treatment as well as the **outlook** is determined by the **grade** of the tumour. A **low**-grade tumour has a very **good prognosis**.

Adenoid Cystic Carcinoma

This is a more **aggressive** tumour. It is responsible for about **10%** of malignant tumours and the **parotid** is again the most **common** site. **Pain** is a predominant symptom due to early **perineural invasion**.

Macroscopy

These are **solid** tumours with a **whitish tan** appearance .They appear to be **circumscribed,** but are **not encapsulated**. The tumour invariably has **infiltrative edges.**

Microscopy

The tumour consists of **two cell types,** namely, the **ductal** and the modified **myoepithelial cells**, having **hyperchromatic angular nuclei** and **clear cytoplasm**. Three well-defined patterns have been described. They **are tubular, cribriform and solid**. **Perineural** and **intraneural** invasion is a **specific feature** of this tumour. The tumor may **extend** along the **nerve** for a considerable **distance** beyond its **macroscopic edges**.

Adenoid cystic carcinoma has a **poor prognosis**. Involvement of the **base of the skull** occurs early in the course of the disease making the tumour **inoperable.** Again histologically, the **solid** type has the **worst** outcome.

Carcinoma Arising in a Pleomorphic Adenoma

As mentioned earlier, a **malignant transformation** can develop in a **pleomorphic adenoma**. It is seen in **elderly patients** who have had a **benign** tumour of a **long duration**. The **risk** of this complication is low, being about **6%. Rapid increase** in size and associated **pain** are the common symptoms. **Histopathology** reveals a **poorly differentiated adenocarcinoma.** These are **aggressive** tumours. In addition, the **patients** tend to come for **treatment** rather **late,** since they had the **swelling** for **several years.** Thus in general the outlook is **poor**.

Adenocarcinoma

The **clinical picture** fits the earlier description of a **malignant parotid** tumour **completely.** The **duration** is **short. Pain** is always present. On examination, the swelling is **hard,** with **restricted mobility** or is **fixed** to the deeper structures. **VIIᵗʰ nerve palsy** is commonly seen. In late stages, the regional **lymph nodes** are **enlarged**.

The tumour arises from the **epithelial** or ductal cells. Depending on the degree of differentiation, they are classified as **low, intermediate** and **high grades**. But **local infiltration** occurs **early,** and again the prognosis is **poor. Blood**-borne **metastase**s can occur at a **later stage.** The **lungs** are the common site of **secondaries.**

Box 5.6:	Points regarding the pathological types
<ul><li>Mucoepidermoid carcinoma – Low, intermediate and high grade</li><li>Low grade – Good prognosis</li><li>Adenoid cystic carcinoma – Perineural invasion early</li><li>VIIth nerve palsy present. Poor prognosis</li><li>Malignancy in a pre-existing pleomorphic adenoma</li><li>Aggressive tumour – Poor prognosis</li><li>Adenocarcinoma de novo – Low, intermediate and high grades</li><li>Clinical features easily identified</li><li>Poor prognosis.</li></ul>	

Q. 21. What is the treatment for cancer of the parotid gland?

In **operable** cases, **radical parotidectomy** offers the **best outcome.** The operation consists of **removal** of the **entire gland,** including the **fascial coverings** and the **facial nerve.** In properly selected patients an **extended radical surgery** is performed. It includes, depending on the extent of involvement, the **masseter**, the **temporal bone**, the involved portion of the **mandible** and the **overlying skin** and **subcutaneous fat**. **The mastoid** is **drilled** to get an **access** to the **healthy facial nerve**. These patients need plastic surgical reconstruction, with **myocutaneous** or **osteomyocutaneous flaps**. The **only indication** for **conserving the facial nerve** in malignancy of the parotid is in patients with a **low-grade mucoepidermoid carcinoma**. Postoperative external beam radiotherapy (**EBRT**) **improves** the **prognosis**. **Palliative radiotherapy** is advised in **advanced cases** but the results are **poor. Relief of pain** is vital when the cancer invades the **base of the skull**.

Excision of the **facial nerve** leads to considerable **morbidity**. It includes **facial asymmetry** and **exposure keratitis,** with the risk of developing **corneal ulcers** and its **complications. Drooling of saliva** makes the patient **miserable.** If immediate reconstruction is planned, the **greater auricular** or the **sural nerve** is used as a **cable graft**. To protect the cornea, a **lateral tarsorraphy** is performed. The **temporalis muscle** can be used to replace the **paralysed orbicularis oculi. Facial asymmetry** can be managed by properly placed **slings.** Sophisticated **reconstructive procedures** are now available to reduce the morbidity.

Box 5.7:	Points regarding treatment

- Radical parotidectomy – Excision of the gland with the fascia
- VIIth nerve excised. Exception – Low grade mucoepidermoid carcinoma
- Extended resections – Masseter, mandible and base of skull
- Drilling of mastoid to remove involved VIIth nerve in adenoid cystic carcinoma
- Plastic surgical reconstruction – Myocutaneous flaps
- Reconstructive surgery for VIIth nerve palsy
- Postoperative EBRT
- Inoperable cases – Palliative radiotherapy

A CASE OF WARTHIN'S TUMOUR

Setting

- Surgical OPD.

Chief Complaint

- Swelling in the right parotid region.

History of Present Illness

A **65-year**-old **man** came to the OPD with the complaint of a **swelling** in the right **parotid** region of **5 years** duration. The swelling was **small** initially and had been **gradually increasing** in size. There was no history of **pain.** The patient did not have any **symptoms** referable to the **salivary system**.

Past history and family history were nonsignificant.

Personal History

The patient was a **smoker** for the last **30 years**.

General physical examination did not reveal any abnormality.

Local Examination

Inspection

A **swelling** was present in the **right parotid** region. It was present **in front** of the **tragus** of the ear. Vertically, it was extending from 1 cm below the **zygoma** to 1 cm below the **angle of the mandible**. The horizontal extension was from the **tragus** 4 cm **anteriorly**. There was **no deviation** of the ear **lobule**.

- The **size** was 6 cm by 4 cm. The shape was a vertical oval.
- All the **margins** were **distinct.**
- The **surface** was **smooth.**
- The **skin** over the swelling was **normal**.
- The **surrounding area** looked normal.

Palpation

- The swelling was **not warm or tender**.
- It was confirmed to be a **swelling** from the **parotid** by the "**curtain sign**".
- It was **soft** in consistency. The lower part was **cystic and transilluminant**.
- There was **mobility** in both vertical and horizontal directions.
- The **skin** could be **lifted off** the swelling. It was **not fixed** to the **masseter.**
- VIIth **nerve functions** were **normal.**
- **Regional nodes** were not palpable.
- **Intra-oral** examination was normal.
- Examination of other **major salivary glands** did not reveal any abnormality.

Box 5.8: Points to be noted in history
- Swelling – Site – Duration
- Size and site at onset
- Rate of growth
- Pain
- Salivary symptoms

Box 5.9: Points to be noted on inspection
- Swelling – Site – Extent – Margins. Deviation of the ear lobule
- Size and shape
- Surface – Smooth or nodular
- Skin over the swelling – Normal, stretched
- Surrounding area

Box 5.10: Points to be noted during palpation
- Warmth and tenderness
- Site – Extent – Borders
- Curtain sign – Confirmation of a parotid swelling
- Consistency – Soft – Cystic – Transilluminant
- Skin and masseter – Free
- VIIth nerve – Not involved
- Lymph nodes – Not palpable
- Intra-oral examination – Normal
- Other major salivary glands – Not involved – 10% to 15% bilateral

Q. 1. What is the clinical diagnosis?

(a) Pleomorphic adenoma.

(b) Warthin's tumour.

(c) Lymph cyst.

(d) Tuberculous cold abscess arising from intraparotid lymph nodes.

The right answer is (b). **Pleomorphic adenoma is the** **commonest** tumour arising from the **parotid.** But the **consistency** is basically **firm. Few soft** and **cystic areas** may be present due to **cystic degeneration. Transillumination** will be **negative**.

Lymph cysts are **rare** in **adults**. The **common** site is the **neck**. They are **cystic** and **brilliantly transilluminant**.

Tuberculosis involving **lymph nodes** is a disease of **childhood**. The **cervical** nodes are **most often** involved. But **intraparotid** node involvement is seen in **poor children** in **our country** .Once **cold abscess** develops, the **mobility** gets **restricted** and the **skin** may be **fixed** to the swelling. **FNAC** confirms the diagnosis.

An **elderly male** who was a **smoker,** had presented with an **asymptomatic** swelling arising from the **parotid** of a **long duration**. The swelling was **soft,** and some areas were **cystic and transilluminant**. The clinical picture was very suggestive of a **Warthin's tumour**.

Q. 2. What are the common characteristics of Warthin's tumour?

The disease was once considered to be seen **exclusively** in Caucasians. But now it is also **seen** in **other sections** of people as well.

Majority of the patients are **men**.

Smoking is considered to be an important **aetiological factor**. Most patients give a **history of smoking**. Since the number of **women smokers** is **increasing,** the incidence of the disease in **this group** has also shown an **increase.**

Parotid is the **commonest** of the salivary glands to be affected by this disease. In **10% to 15%** of patients, the condition is **bilateral.**

The patients present with an **asymptomatic swelling** of a **long duration**.

The swelling is **soft** often **cystic** and **transilluminant.**

It is well **encapsulated. Excision** results in a **cure.** Unlike with a pleomorphic adenoma, **recurrences are not known.**

Box 5.11:	Points to be noted regarding the common characteristics
• Disease of elderly men – Smokers • Asymptomatic swelling – Long duration • Soft – Cystic – Transilluminant • Encapsulated – Excision – Zero recurrence	

Q. 3. **What is the aetiology of Warthin's tumour?**

The **exact aetiological** factors are **not known**. Since most patients are **smokers, tobacco** has been implicated in the **aetiology.** A **retrograde flow** of tobacco **smoke** or certain **noxious elements** derived from **tobacco**, into the **salivary ducts** is said to be the **main cause**. These factors are likely to induce **inflammatory changes** in the salivary **ducts** leading to a partial **block of the ductal system,** resulting in a **collection of the fluid** inside the gland. The **fluid** has plenty of **oncocytes.**

Embryonic origin. This hypothesis states that **Warthin's tumour** is due to **salivary gland heterotopia** in **periparotid** and **intraparotid lymph nodes**. The epithelial **cells trapped** within the **lymphoid tissue** during **embryological development** are said to give rise to the **tumour** at a **later date.**

Box 5.12:	Points regarding the aetiology of Warthin's tumour
• Related to tobacco smoking. Blockage of the ducts leading to retention of contents inside the gland, and fluid collection with oncocytes. • Embryological origin. Heterotopia of the salivary tissue, trapped within the periparotid and intraparotid lymphoid tissue leading to development of the tumour later.	

Q. 4. **What were the investigations performed?**

Ultrasound study. It showed **multiple anechoic areas** in the superficial part of the gland.

FNAC smear showed **oncocytic epithelial cells** (acidophilic and granular) in a **lymphoid stroma**.

MRI scan was done. It demonstrated **multifocal** areas with **cystic changes**.

Q. 5. **What are the treatment options for this patient?**

(a) Total parotidectomy.

(b) Aspiration.

(c) Superficial parotidectomy.

(d) Enucleation.

The correct answer is **(c)**. **Total parotidectomy** with sacrifice of the VIIth nerve is done only for **malignancy.** **Aspiration** does not solve the **aetiological problem**. **Enucleation** is **indicated** for a **tumour** occupying the **deep lobe** as detected by a **MRI scan**. If **enucleation** is **attempted** for a tumour in the **superficial lobe**, there is a **risk** of **damaging** the branches of the **VIIth nerve**.

Hence **superficial parotidectomy** was the **best option** for this patient.

Setting – A week later. **FNAC report** showed **Warthin's tumour**. A **superficial parotidectomy** was performed.

The **histopathology** report confirmed the diagnosis of **Warthin's tumour**.

Q. 6. **What is the treatment for a Warthin's tumour in the deep lobe of the parotid?**

Deep lobe tumours are **uncommon**. **MRI scan** is needed for proper **localisation.** The **fasciovenous plane** is initially identified, and the **nerve** branches along with the superficial lobe are **retracted** to expose the **deep lobe**. The tumor is then **enucleated** from within the **capsule**.

A CASE OF SUBMANDIBULAR SALIVARY GLAND CALCULUS

Setting

- Surgical OPD.

Chief Complaint

Swelling in the **submandibular region** of **3 months** duration.

History of Present Illness

A **38-year-old man** presented to the OPD with the complaint of **a swelling** in the **right submandibular** region of **3 months** duration. Initially, the swelling was **small,** but had **gradually increased** in size. It was noted that the swelling used to become **bigger** during **eating**. It was also associated with **pain** during these **episodes**. There was no history of **excessive salivation**. There was no history of **fever.**

- **Past, family and personal histories** were noncontributory.
- **General physical examination** showed a healthy individual.

Local Examination

Inspection

A **swelling** was present in the **right submandibular** region. It was extending from the **anterior border** of the right **sternomastoid** to about 2 cm **behind** the **midline. Vertically,** the extent was from the lower border of the **mandible 3 cm downwards**. Except for the upper, the other borders were well defined.

- The **size** was 5 cm by 3 cm. The **shape** was a horizontal **oval.**
- The **surface** appeared **smooth**. The **skin** over the swelling was normal.
- The **surrounding area** was normal.

Palpation

The swelling was **not warm,** but was slightly **tender.**

- The **site, size and shape** were **confirmed.**
- All the borders were palpable. The **upper border** was close to the lower border of the **mandible.**
- The **surface** was **smooth.**
- The **consistency** was **firm**.
- The overlying **skin** was **free** from the swelling.
- There was minimal **transverse mobility.**
- The swelling was **bidigitally palpable** indicating its anatomical origin from the **salivary gland**.
- Regional lymph **nodes** were **not palpable**.
- **Intra-orally**, a stone could be palpated at the **orifice** of the **Wharton's duct** in the floor of the mouth. It measured about **0.75 cm** in size.

Box 5.13:	Points to be noted in the history

- Swelling in the submandibular region – duration – Few months
- Enlarges during eating – Pain present
- Fever – Usually absent
- No episodes of excessive salivation

Box 5.14:	Points to be noted during clinical examination

- Swelling in the submandibular region
- All borders made out clearly
- Size variable. Shape oval
- Surface smooth
- Consistency firm
- Restricted transverse mobility
- Skin – Free
- Bidigitally palpable
- Intra-oral - Stone felt at orifice of Wharton's duct

Q. 1. What is the clinical diagnosis?

The clinical diagnosis is a **stone** in the **orifice** of the submandibular duct with chronic **sialadenitis**. The clinical findings are **so typical** that no other condition can be thought of.

Q. 2. What was the investigation performed?

An **intra-oral X-ray** was done. It showed a **radio opaque calculus** in the floor of the mouth, confirming the **diagnosis**.

Setting: A couple of days later, the patient was posted for treatment.

Q. 3. How was this patient treated?

Under **local anaesthesia,** an incision was made on the duct at the site of the stone. The **mucosa** of the floor of the mouth and the **duct wall** were incised, exposing the **stone**. The **stone** was easily **extracted**. A large amount of **saliva** was seen flowing out of the **duct**. The **incision** was **kept open**. The patient made an uneventful recovery.

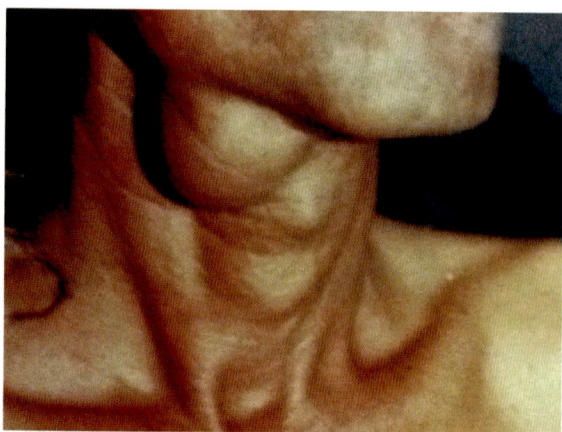

Fig. 5.5: Submandibular salivary gland swelling due to a calculus blocking the duct.

Q. 4. Describe the borders of the submandibular triangle.

The **upper border** is formed by the **lower border of the mandible**. The anterior and **posterior bellies** of the **digastric** muscle form the **lateral and medial borders**.

Q. 5. Why are stones common in the submandibular salivary gland?

The **secretion** of the **submandibular** gland is more **viscous** as compared with the **parotid** secretion, which is **serous** in nature. The **thicker**

saliva makes it prone for **stone formation.**

The **gland** is at a **lower level** in relation to the **duct**. Hence the **flow** of saliva is **against gravity**. This induces **stasis**. Stasis leads to **stone formation**. The stone is comprised of **calcium carbonate** or phosphate. Hence it is **radio opaque**.

Q. 6. What causes enlargement of the gland?

Due to a **block** by the *stone,* the ductal system dilates (**sialectasis**). **Sepsis** always follows **stasis**. Hence there is **chronic sialadenitis** resulting in enlargement of the gland.

Box 5.15:	Points to be noted in the aetiopathology

- The submandibular salivary gland is the most common site for stone formation.
- The saliva secreted by these glands is more viscous as compared to parotid secretions.
- The flow of saliva is against gravity since the gland lies at a lower level, leading to stasis.
- The calculus is made of either calcium carbonate or calcium phosphate.
- Due to obstruction caused by the stone there is sialectasis.
- Stasis is followed by sepsis, resulting in sialadenitis.

Q. 7. How is the bidigital examination performed and what is the significance?

The test is performed by **palpating** the swelling in the neck and trying to feel the same **swelling** at the **floor of the mouth**. If it is palpable **bidigitally**, it indicates that the swelling is arising from the **salivary gland,** because the **deep lobe** of the salivary gland lies above the **myelohyoid** muscle and is in relation to the **floor of** the **mouth**. Conversely, an **enlarged submandibular lymph node** is **not palpable bidigitally.**

Q. 8. How are stones located in the intraglandular portion of the ductal system diagnosed?

A **CT sialogram** will detect the presence of these **stones**. It also gives a clear picture of the **morphological changes** in the gland, including **sialectasis**.

Q. 9. What is the treatment for these stones?

The treatment is excision of the salivary **gland** along with the **duct** containing the **stone.**

Q. 10. Name the important structures in relation to the submandibular salivary gland.

The **marginal mandibular** branch of the VIIth cranial nerve, the **lingual** and the **hypoglossal nerves** and the **facial artery** are the vital structures in relation to the gland.

A CASE OF RANULA

Setting

- Surgical OPD.

Chief Complaint

- **Swelling** in the **floor of the mouth.**

History of Present Illness

- A **5-year-old girl** was brought to the surgical OPD by the mother with the complaint of a **swelling** in the **floor of the mouth** of **one year duration**. The swelling was **noted below the tongue** on the right side.
- The **size** at onset was that of a **grape**. Since then it had been **gradually increasing** in **size**.
- The child did not complain of **pain.**
- The child did **not** have any **difficulty in talking or intake of food**.
- **Past, personal and family** histories were insignificant.
- **General physical examination** showed a healthy child.

Local Examination

Inspection

- Swelling was present in the **floor of the mouth** to the **right** of the **frenulum** of the **tongue.**

- It appeared like a **bluish dome**. Margins were well **defined**.
- The swelling had a diameter of 2 cm. It was **globular** in **shape**.
- The **mucosa** over the swelling appeared **translucent**.
- Rest of the **oral cavity** was **normal.**

Palpation

- The swelling was not **warm or tender**.
- The **site, size and shape** were **confirmed** by palpation.
- The **consistency** was **tensely cystic.**
- **Fluctuation and transillumination** were both **positive.**
- The swelling was **mobile.**
- The overlying **mucosa** was **not free** of the swelling.
- **Movements** of the **tongue** were **normal.**
- Rest of the **oral cavity** was **normal.**
- Regional lymph **nodes** were **not palpable.**

Box 5.16: Points to be noted in the history

- Site – Floor of the mouth – Duration
- Size at onset – Rate of growth
- Pain
- Difficulty in talking, chewing and swallowing

Box 5.17:	Points to be noted on clinical examination

- Swelling – Site, extent and margins – Floor of the mouth – Lateral to frenulum
- Size and shape, surface – Appears like a bluish dome
- Consistency – Tensely cystic – Brilliantly transilluminant
- Mobility present
- Movements of the tongue – Not restricted
- Lymph nodes – Not palpable

Q. 1. What was the clinical diagnosis?

The diagnosis was a **ranula.** The clinical picture was **typical** of this condition. The only **other cystic** swelling that is seen in the floor of the mouth is a **sublingual dermoid.** The **dermoid cyst** occurs in the **midline** and is **not transilluminant**.

Q. 2. What is the etymology of the term ranula?

Rana is the term used in **Latin** for a **frog.** Since the **bluish surface** of the swelling **resembles** the **belly of a frog**, it is called as a **ranula**.

Q. 3. What is the present concept regarding the aetiopathology of a ranula?

Traditionally, ranula was described as a **retention cyst** arising from **minor salivary glands** present in the **floor of the mouth**. It is now believed that the **cyst arises** in relation to the **sublingual salivary gland**. This gland is **unique** in that it is a **spontaneous secretor** of mucus even in the **absence** of any **stimulus**. There are **two theories** regarding the formation of a ranula. **Partial congenital occlusion** of the **duct** may lead to the formation of an **epithelial-lined retention cyst.** But this is **uncommon**

More often it is considered to be an **extravasation mucocoele** arising from the **sublingual gland**. The cyst probably results from a **tear in the duct** following **minor trauma** during **mastication.** The **extravasated** mucus induces an **inflammatory reaction** leading to the formation of a thin fibrous wall. A **better term** to describe this condition therefore would be a **"mucus escape reaction".**

Q. 4. What is a plunging ranula?

Anatomical **dissections** have demonstrated that in some cases, **part** of the **sublingual gland** descends into the **neck** through a **hiatus** in the fibres of the **myelohyoid** muscle. If a **ranula** occurs **under** these **circumstances,** it can **descend**

down into the **neck**. Thus the **cyst** has **two components**, one in the **floor of the mouth** and the other in the **submandibular region**. **Cross fluctuation** can be demonstrated between the two parts. This is known as a **plunging ranula.**

Box 5.18:	Points to be noted regarding the aetiopathology

- Considered to be a retention cyst of a minor salivary gland in the past.
- Present concept – Related to the sublingual salivary gland and duct.
- Unique feature – Continuous secretion even without stimuli.
- Minor trauma to the duct from food particles.
- Extravasation of mucus – Fluid collection jn the floor of the mouth.
- Mucus evoked reaction results in a very thin fibrous wall.
- Thus ranula is an extravasation mucocoele due to a mucus escape reaction.
- Congenital cause – Uncommon. Blockage of the duct leads to increased pressure. Further changes same as above.
- Plunging ranula – Hiatus in the myelohyoid muscle.
- Gland – Descent into the neck – Ranula with 2 components.
- Floor of the mouth and neck – Cross fluctuation.

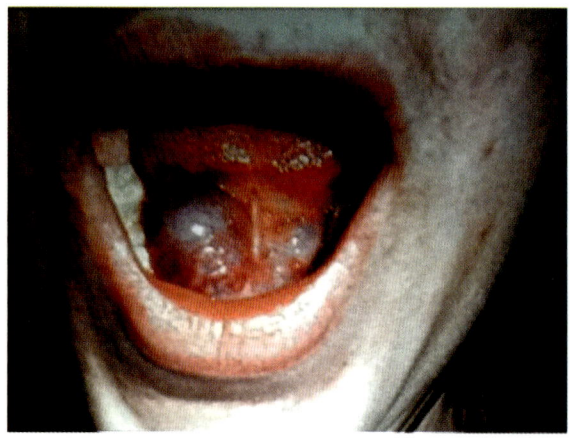

Fig. 5.6: Ranula on either side of the frenulum of the tongue.

Q. 5. **What was the treatment adopted for this patient?**

Excision of the sublingual gland along with the **cyst** by an incision in the floor of the mouth **was performed**. The **rationale** behind this operation was the removal of the **source of mucus**. The **excision** was made **easy** by **aspirating the contents before** the **incision** was made. This step helped in **reducing the risk** of **rupture** during **surgery**. The **extremely thin wall** made the operation a **delicate** and an **intricate** one. **If a portion** of the **cyst wall** was to be **retained, recurrence** would be a strong **possibility.**

Q. 6. **What are the other options available for the management of ranula?**

Marsupialisation can be performed, but the **rates** of **recurrence** are **high**. It involves **deroofing** the cyst and **suturing the remaining cyst wall** to the **mucous membrane** lining the **floor of the mouth.** The **purpose** is to allow **free drainage** of the mucus **secreted** by the **sublingual salivary gland.** **Inflammatory fibrosis** leading to **retention of secretions** is the cause for **recurrence. Injection of silver nitrate** to induce **fibrosis,** aiming to **seal the leak** in the **duct** after **aspirating the** **contents** has been tried. But **recurrence rates** are **high**. It also makes **future surgery** if needed, **more difficult**.

Box 5.19:	Points regarding treatment

- Excision of the ranula along with the sublingual salivary gland
- Marsupialisation – Still practiced – Recurrence not uncommon
- Injection of silver nitrate – To seal the defect in the duct
- Recurrence rates high
- Future surgery more difficult

■■■

Oral Cancer

6

A CASE OF CARCINOMA OF THE TONGUE

Setting

- Surgical outpatient department (OPD).

Chief Complaint

- **Ulcer** in the **tongue** of **6 months** duration.

History of Present Illness

- A **52-year-old man** presented to the OPD with the complaint of an **ulcer in** the **tongue** of **six months** duration. He had noticed a **small ulcer** on the **left side** of the **tongue six months** ago. It had **gradually increased** to the **present size.**

- He was complaining of **pain** for the previous **three weeks**. The pain was **pricking** in nature. It was **worse** during intake of **hot and spicy food**. The pain was **not disturbing** his **sleep**. The **pain** was **radiating** to the **left ear.**

- He gave a history of **excessive salivation.**

- The patient also complained of **halitosis.**

- There was **no** history of **bleeding** from the **ulcer.**

- He had some **difficulty** while **talking** and **chewing food.**

- The patient did not have **chronic cough** or **fever**.

- **Past and family histories** were insignificant.

Personal History

- He was a **smoker** and **tobacco chewer** for **30 years**. He used to consume **alcohol** regularly.

- **General physical examination** did not reveal any abnormality.

Local Examination of Oral Cavity

Inspection

- The **mouth opening** was normal.
- A **proliferative type** of **ulcer** was seen along the **lateral margin** of the **anterior two-thirds** of the **tongue** on the left side. It **extended** from about **2 cm behind the tip** for a **length of about 3 cm.** Vertically, it extended for about **1cm** both on the **dorsal and ventral surfaces** of the tongue. The **floor of the mouth** was **not involved.**
- The **margins** were distinct.
- The **size** was 3 cm by 2 cm. The **shape** was oval.
- The **floor** of the ulcer was **raised** in relation to the **surrounding area**. It comprised of **slough** and **reddish nodular tissue.**
- The remaining part of the tongue appeared **normal.**
- There was **no restriction** regarding **movements** of the tongue.
- The **oral and dental** hygiene was **poor.** The **teeth** showed **tobacco staining**. There were **no** patches of **leucoplakia.**

Palpation

- There was **no tenderness**.
- A **proliferative ulcer** was present along the **lateral border** of the **left side** of the tongue. The **size** and **shape** were confirmed.
- The **edges** were **raised** and **everted**.

- There was **induration** at the **base** formed by the **muscles** of the tongue. The induration did **not extend** beyond the **margins** of the lesion.
- The **remaining part of the tongue** was normal on palpation.
- The **movements** of the tongue were **normal.**
- There was **no thickening** of **the horizontal ramus** of the left side of the **mandible.**
- The **rest of the oral cavity** was normal on palpation.

Examination of Regional Lymph Nodes

- Level **IA, IB and III group** of lymph **nodes** were enlarged and **palpable** on the **left side** of the neck. Their size varied from **1 cm to 2 cm,** and the nodes were **hard** and **nontender.** They were **mobile**.
- **No nodes** were palpable on the **opposite side** of the neck.
- The **chest** was clinically **normal.**
- **Other systems** were normal.

Box 6.1:	Points regarding history

- Ulcer tongue – Site – Duration - Rate of growth
- Pain – Late – Nature – Intensity – Aggravating factors – Radiation
- Halitosis
- Excessive salivation
- Bleeding from the ulcer
- Difficulty in talking and chewing
- Chronic cough and fever

Box 6.2:	Points regarding inspection

- Extent of mouth opening – 4 fingers normal
- Ulcer – Site and extent
- Size and shape
- Margins – Distinct
- Floor – Slough with reddish granular or nodular tissue
- Remaining part of the tongue
- Movements of the tongue
- Oral cavity – Dental status – Leucoplakia

Box 6.3:	Points regarding palpation

- Site – Extent - Size and shape - Confirmed
- Edge – Raised and everted
- Base – Muscles of the tongue – Induration – Extension
- Remaining part of the tongue
- Movements of the tongue
- Mandible – Bidigital examination – Tenderness – Thickening
- Regional nodes – Levels I to IV – Skip lesions
- Opposite side – Nodes

Q. 1. What was the clinical diagnosis?

(*a*) **Carcinoma** of the tongue.

(*b*) **Chronic dental ulcer.**

(*c*) **Tuberculous** ulcer.

The answer is **(a).Tuberculous ulcers** of the tongue are **rare** at the present time. They are associated with **pulmonary tuberculosis**. The ulcer is seen at the **tip** of the **tongue.** It is very **painful and tender**. The **edges** are **undermined.** There is no **induration.**

Chronic dental ulcers are common. They occur along the **lateral margin** of the **anterior** two-thirds of the **tongue**. They are the result of **repeated minor trauma** caused by a **sharp tooth**. They are **painful** and **slightly tender**. They have **sloping edges** and are **not indurated**. These **ulcers** heal when the **causative factor** has been **controlled.** But over a **period of time** a **chronic dental ulcer** can become **malignant.**

The **symptoms and signs** in this **patient** support a **diagnosis of malignancy**. The raised edges and induration present in the ulcer are important findings. In addition, the patient had **multiple hard nodes** in the neck.

Q. 2. What was the clinical stage of the cancer?

The stage was **Stage III (T2, N2B and MX)**

Q. 3. What were the investigations carried out in this patient?

Multiple edge biopsies.

Ultrasound (US) examination of the **neck.**

Chest X-ray.

Setting: A week passes.

Biopsy report showed a **well-differentiated squamous cell carcinoma.**

US neck did not reveal any **additional lymph nodes** in the neck.

Chest X-ray was normal.

Q. 4. How was this patient treated?

The patient underwent a hemiglossectomy followed by a pectoralis major flap for the primary tumour. The secondary nodes were treated by a functional neck resection After the incisions had healed completely he had External Beam Radiotherapy (EBRT) to the left side of the neck

Q. 5. What is the incidence of oral cancer?

It is the **most common** cancer seen in **our country** with several studies showing an incidence of **30%** of **all malignancies**. Further its occurrence at a **younger age** is **quite alarming.**

Q. 6. What are the aetiological factors?

1. The universal habit of **chewing of tobacco** is the primary cause, but a combination of **paan leaf, arecanut and lime** without tobacco is **equally culpable.**

2. **A sharp tooth** in relation to the **lateral border** of the **anterior two-thirds** of the **tongue** produces an **ulcer** that can later turn **malignant.** Chronic **mucosal irritation** is probably the underlying factor in all these cases, though **chemical carcinogens** have been isolated from **tobacco** as well as **arecanut.**

3. Smoking of **beedi** and **cigarette** along with consumption of **alcohol** and **poor oral hygiene** are additional **aetiological factors.** Combination of **smoking** with **alcohol** consumption **increases the incidence** considerably.

When the **mucous membrane** of the oral cavity is exposed to the action of the **physical or chemical factors** mentioned above, it is likely to become **malignant.** This effect is known as **field cancerization.**

4. A **genetic susceptibility** explains the prevalence in **young patients** who **neither chew tobacco nor consume alcohol.**

Q. 7. What are the premalignant conditions?

Leucoplakia. It presents as a **whitish** or **discoloured** patch in the **mucosa** of the oral cavity. The **tongue** and the **cheek** are the **common** sites. The patch usually has well-**defined edges**. There is **no induration.** A **biopsy** is needed to rule out **malignancy.** The treatment is **essentially conservative.** The patient must **abstain** from **smoking and**

chewing of tobacco products as well as use of **alcohol.** The patient is kept under **regular surveillance.** Since the **patient compliance** is rather **poor** in **our country, localised patches** are best treated by **excision.** The **risk** of **malignancy** is said to vary from **3% to 17%.**

Erythroplakia: The lesion presents as a **raised velvety reddish patch** in the mucous lining of the oral cavity. The patch tends to **bleed** even after **minor trauma.** It is **less common** when compared to leucoplakia. But the risk of **malignancy** is as high as **50%. Biopsy** is always performed. **Localised** lesions are best **excised.**

Submucous fibrosis: It is a condition almost **exclusively seen** in the **Indian subcontinent.** It is directly related to the habit of **chewing paan or Ghutka,** resulting in **chronic inflammation.** The inflammation leads to **fibrosis.** The patient may have **limitation** in **opening the mouth.** The oral **mucosa** appears **pale** and **white. Transverse fibrous bands** are felt along **the submucous layer** of the **cheek. Treatment** is **conservativ**e. **Abstinence** is most important to **prevent further progression. Intralesional steroid** injections have been tried to **reduce** the **fibrous reaction. Excision** may need **plastic surgical reconstruction** to **restore function.** The risk of **malignancy** is between **7% and 15%.**

Box 6.4:	Points regarding aetiology and premalignant conditions

- Most common cancer in our country – 30%
- Tobacco chewing – Paan with arecanut – Smoking – Alcohol
- Chemical carcinogens – Chronic irritation
- Premalignant – Leucoplakia, erythroplakia, submucous fibrosis

Q. 8. What are the important points in history in oral cancers?

1. The primary symptom is always a **nonhealing ulcer** in the oral cavity. The duration is of **several months.** The **cardinal rule** is that any **ulcer** in the **oral cavity** that **does not heal** within **three weeks of adequate treatment** is to be considered **malignant** until **proved otherwise.**

2. The **four symptoms** that are **frequently complained** of, **irrespective of** the **location** of the tumour are the following.

   (*a*) **Excessive salivation,** since the lesion acts as a **foreign body.**

   (*b*) **Halitosis:** The bad smell is due to the presence of **infection.**

Necrosis occurs when the **blood supply** is **not adequate** to sustain the growth of the tumour. This tissue is **invaded by bacteria**, producing **sepsis.**

(*c*) **Bleeding: Increased vascularity** makes these tumours **bleed** even after **minor trauma. Severe bleeding** can be a challenging problem in **cancers** of the **tongue.**

(*d*) **Pain** is a **late symptom**. Initially the patient may complain of **discomfort** after **consumption** of **hot liquids** or spicy **food**. But later, when the **deeper nerves** are involved, the patient has **severe pain. In tongue cancer,** the pain **radiates to the ear**, since the **lingual** and **auriculotemporal** nerves are **branches** of the **mandibular division** of the **trigeminal nerve.**

(*e*) A **cancer** arising from the **mucoperiosteum** of the **jaw** may present with **loosening of the teeth** as a prominent symptom.

3. The next **group of symptoms** depends on the **site of malignancy**.

(*a*) **Lip:** Local symptoms are **minimal,** and in **late stages** there may be **difficulty** in **eating and talking**.

(*b*) **Cheek: Progressive difficulty** in **opening** the **mouth** is the cardinal symptom. As a result there is **inanition** leading to **loss of weight**. If the tumour extends **outward**, an **external swelling** may be the **chief complaint**. Further infiltration leads to the **development** of an **orocutaneous fistula** at this site. Such patients usually come from areas of **poor education** and **health** facilities.

(*c*) **Tongue:** A **frequent site** for malignancy, the main symptoms of which are **difficulty in talking, chewing and swallowing**. Lesions in the **posterior one-third** of the tongue are notorious in presenting **late** with hardly **any local symptoms**. Interestingly, **macroglossia** is an **uncommon manifestation** of a cancer at this site due to **lymphatic obstruction** of the **anterior two-thirds of the tongue.**

4. Systemic symptoms: Loss of appetite and **weight** are common. **Chronic cough** with **expectoration** is due to **spread of infection** into the **respiratory tract.**

Q. 9. What are the clinical findings in oral cancers?

The **clinical findings** depend on the **site** of the tumour. The **initial step** in **all cases** is to **determine** any **limitation in opening the mouth. Normal**ly mouth opening is **four fingers width**. Since **submucous fibrosis i**s seen in a vast majority of patients, there may be **mild-to-severe restriction** leading to **trismus.** It makes **clinical examination** more **difficult**.

Lip: A **proliferative type** of ulcer is most often seen in the **lip.** The **margins** are **well defined** and the **floor** is **comprised** of **granulation-like tumour tissue. Extensions** on to the **inner surface of the lip** and the **gingivolabial sulcus** are **not uncommon.** On **palpation**, the edges are **everted** and the **base** is **indurated. Induration** is a **specific feature** of **squamous cell cancers,** and is the result of a **desmoplastic reaction (fibrosis)** on the part of the **body (host)** towards the **tumour.** This could also be a result of **infiltration of malignant cells** into the

soft tissue. It is the **extent of induration** that decides the true **size of the tumour** and not that of the **ulcer.**

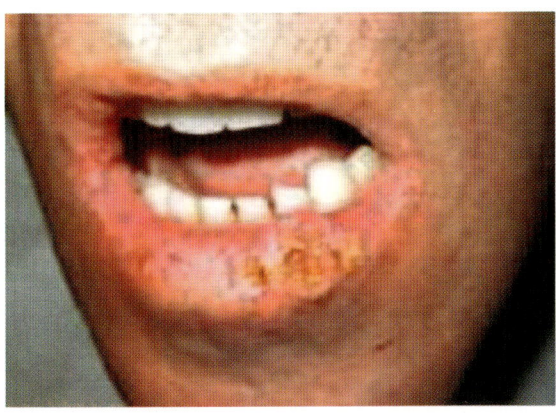

Fig. 6.1: Carcinoma of the lip.

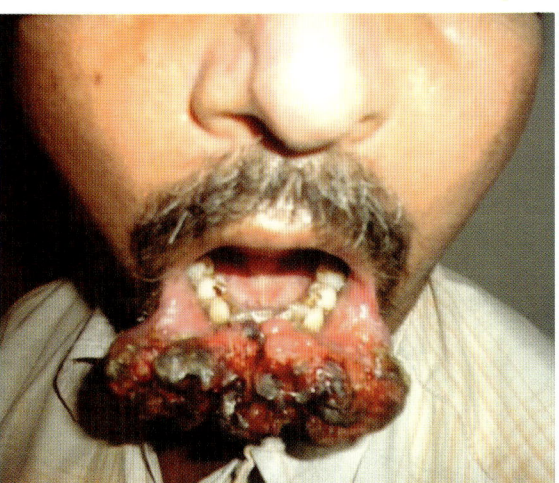

Fig. 6.2: Advanced carcinoma of the lower lip.

Cheek (buccal mucosa): A very **common site** in **tobacco chewers**, it usually presents as a **proliferative ulcer** with **raised edges** and **induration. Spread** of the tumour can occur **anteriorly** to the **angle of the mouth** and **posteriorly** to the

retromolar trigone. Infiltration of the **overlying skin** results in **erythema** and **induration** initially, and later a **fistula** lined by a **malignant ulcer. Infiltration** of the adjacent bone, **mandible** more often than the maxilla, produces **bony thickening**. The **horizontal ramus** of the **mandible** is **commonly involved**, which can be made out by a **bidigital examination**. Since this **part of the bone** is **developed from membrane**, there is **no new-bone** formation. Hence the clinical finding is **not due to any periosteal reaction** but the **growth** of the **tumour between** the **two tables** spreading them **apart**. The **inner table** is **primarily involved** by the malignancy. **Advanced** tumours infiltrate the **buccinator and** the **masseter** muscle as well, resulting in **progressive trismus**.

A **tumour** arising in the **gingivobuccal sulcus** has the **notorious reputation** of being **labelled** as "**The Indian Oral Cancer**". This is the result of the **vicarious habit** of our people keeping the **tobacco quid** in the **sulcus** over a **period of several hours**. The lesion presents as an **excavating type** of **ulcer**. It has raised and **everted edges,** but the **floor** is at a **deeper level** indicating a **greater degree of infiltration** than the **proliferative type.** Therefore these carry a **poorer prognosis**. The cancer **spreads** to the **mandible** very **early** and hence the **base** is formed by the bone. A small number of **tumours** develop from the **mucoperiosteum** of the **jaw**. Since they are **fixed** to the **bone, induration** as a sign **loses its significance**. These tumours may involve the **cortex** of the mandible **minimally** or spread to the **medullary canal**. There is also a possibility of a spread along the **inferior dental nerve** producing **severe pain.**

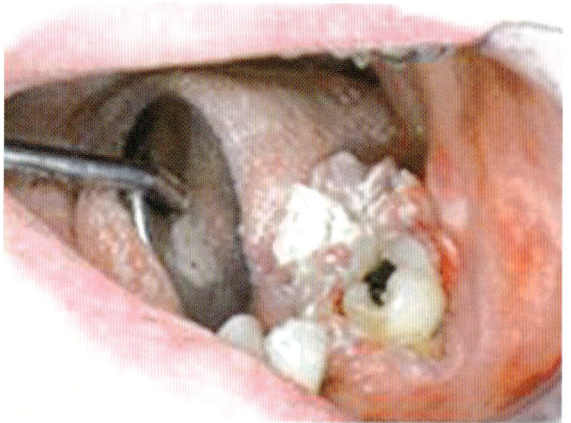

Fig. 6.3: Verrucous carcinoma at the gigivolabial sulcus.

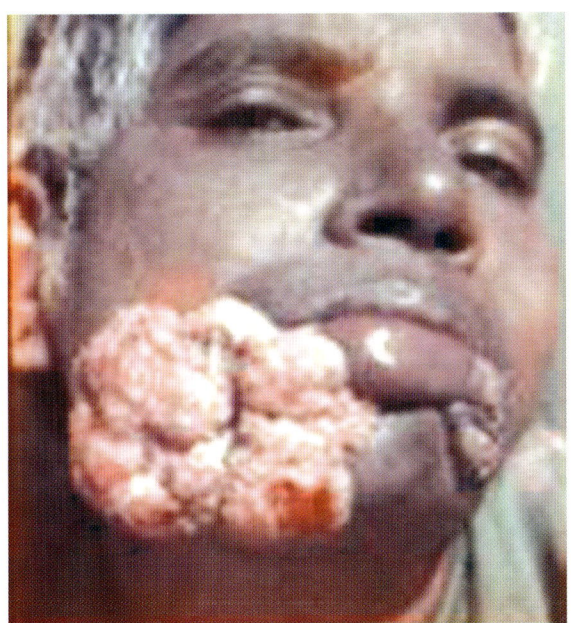

Fig. 6.4: Carcinoma of the cheek producing a fungating growth externally.

Tongue: Compared to cancers of the **lip and cheek**, these tumours are **biologically more aggressive**. The **lateral margin** of the **anterior two-thirds** of the tongue is the **most common** site. But **the dorsum** of the tongue could also be a **seat of the disease**. These tumours can **spread** to the **posterior one-third,** or the latter site may be the **focus** of the **primary tumour**.

Proliferative ulcers are the most **frequent type** of **presentation**. In many of these patients, the **induration tends to extend well beyond** the margins of the **ulcer**. **Examination for induration** is always done with the **tongue kept well inside the mouth**, since a **false sense** of **induration** may be felt due to **contractions** of the **intrinsic muscles** when the tongue is protruded out. A **cancer** of the tongue may also manifest as an **indurated plaque** with **minimal ulceration,** and in a **small number** of cases as a **fissure** with markedly **indurated edges**.

Infiltration of the **extrinsic muscles** leads to **limitation of movements** of the tongue. **Inability** to **protrude the tongue forwards** is known as **ankyloglossia.** Tumours at the **lateral margin** are prone to **spread** to the **floor** of the **mouth.**

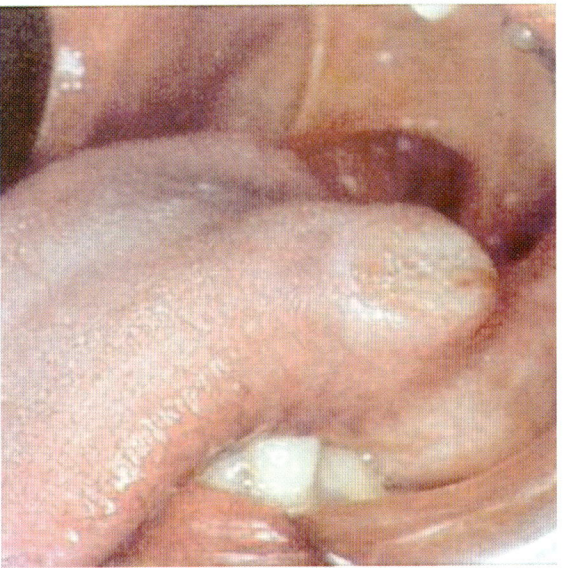

Fig. 6.5: Carcinoma extending into the posterior third of the tongue.

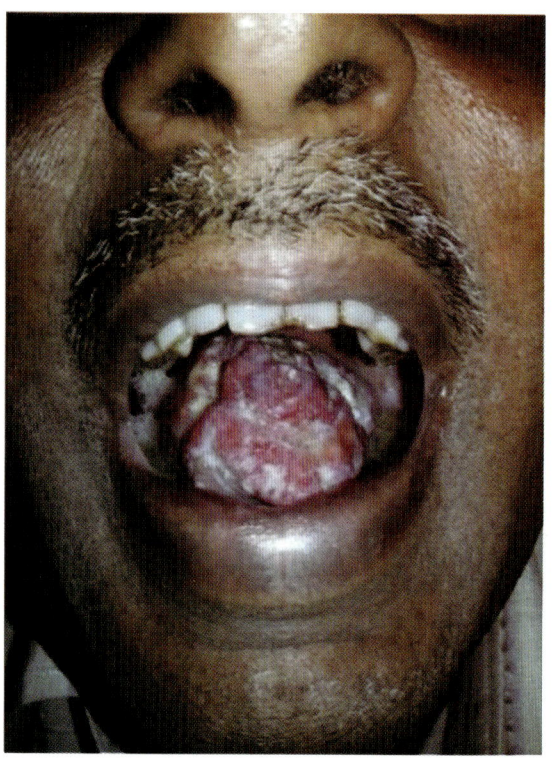

Fig. 6.6: Advanced carcinoma of the tongue with ankyloglossia.

Q. 10. Describe the levels of lymph nodes in the neck.

A **basic knowledge** of the **levels of the nodes in** the **neck** is essential before their **significance** can be discussed. The anatomical boundaries of these levels are described herewith. **Level I.** The level is below the **myelohyoid** muscle and **above** the lower **border** of the **hyoid bone** vertically and limited to the **posterior border of the submandibular triangles** on **either sides** horizontally.

This level is further **subdivided as follows:Level IA: Submental nodes**—Between the **anterior bellies** of the **digastric muscles.**

Level I B: Submandibular nodes—Posterolateral to the **anterior belly** of the **digastric** muscles.

Level II: Internal jugular chain (jugulodigastric)—It extends from the **base of skull** to the **inferior border of the hyoid bone** vertically and **anterior to the posterior border of the sternomastoid** muscles in the horizontal direction.

Level III: Internal jugular chain (jugulo-omohyoid)—It extends from the **lower margin of the hyoid bone** to the **lower border of the cricoid cartilage** vertically, and from the **anterior to the posterior borders of the sternomastoid** muscles, horizontally. **Level II and III** are **deep** to the **muscle.**

Level IV: Supraclavicular nodes—The vertical extension of this space is from the **lower border** of the **cricoid cartilage** to the **clavicle,** and horizontally from an **oblique line** drawn from the **posterior margin of the sternomastoid** to the **posterior edge of the scalenus anterior** muscle.

Level V: Posterior Cervical nodes—These nodes belong to the area of the **posterior triangle** of the neck overlying the **trapezius muscle**.

Level VI: Prelaryngeal and pretracheal nodes (central compartment nodes)—The level extends from the **inferior margin of the cricoid** to the **manubrium** sterni. The nodes are present within the **pretracheal fascia**.

Level VII: Superior mediastinal nodes.

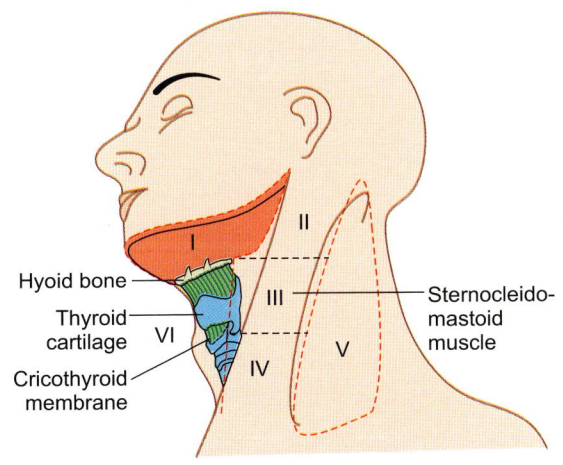

Hyoid bone
Thyroid cartilage
Cricothyroid membrane
Sternocleido-mastoid muscle

Fig. 6.7: Levels of cervical lymph nodes.

Lymph node enlargement in oral cancers can be due to **infection** since the **primary tumour** has an **element of sepsis**. These nodes tend to be **painful, tender, soft and mobile.**

Unfortunately, **most** of **our patients** present with **metastatic nodes**.

Metastatic spread produces **nodes** that are **hard, nontender and mobile**. Once **extracapsular extension** occurs, they are **fixed to each other** as well as to **adjacent structures** like the **sternomastoid** muscle. This is a clear indicator of **poor prognosis**.

Q. 11. Describe the lymph node enlargement in cancers of the lip, cheek and tongue.

Lip cancers primarily drain into **level IA and IB** as well as level II groups. Tumours present in the **central portion** or those **crossing the midline** can produce **contralateral node** enlargement.

Cancer cheek: The nodes frequently enlarged belong to **IB, II and III** groups. **Spread** of the cancer **beyond** these groups occurs only in **delayed** or **recurrent** cases.

Cancers of the tongue: The lymphatic drainage is **more complex** and needs to be studied in detail. The **tip** drains into the **level IA** node. The **lateral margins** of the **anterior two-thirds** of the tongue drain into level **IB, II and III** nodes. If a tumour spreads to **within 1 cm.** of **midline** on the **dorsum** of the tongue, the **nodes on the opposite side** may also be **involved** due to the **free crossing**

of the **lymphatic vessels**. In addition, **level IV nodes** may be enlarged as **skip lesions** even in the **absence of palpable II and III nodes**.

Cancers arising on the **posterior one-third** of the tongue cause **bilateral node** enlargement.

Again a **set of lymphatics** from the **lateral margin** of the tongue **runs deep** to the **periosteum** of the **horizontal ramus** of the **mandible** to reach **IB nodes**. Though its **importance is** being **questioned**, it would **explain** the **spread** of a cancer of the tongue to the **mandible**, when the **tumour does not show** clinical evidence of a **direct spread across the floor of the mouth.**

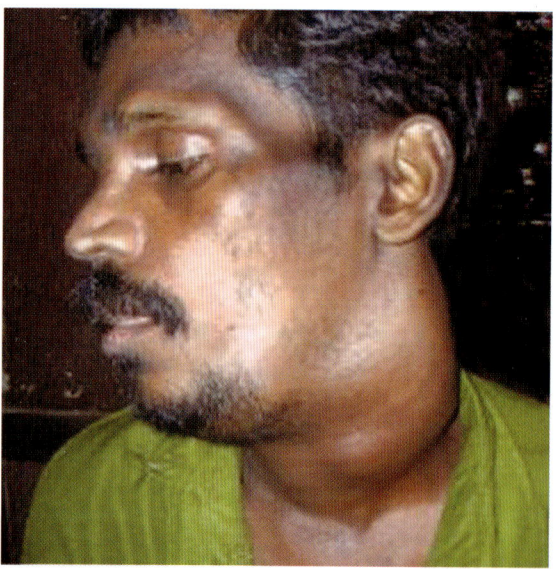

Fig. 6.8: Massive secondary lymph nodes in the neck.

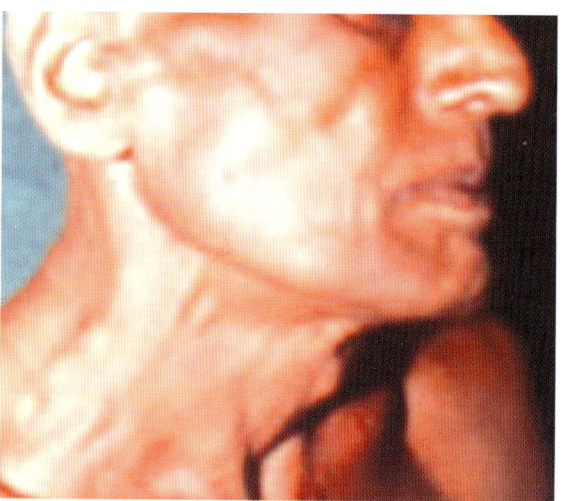

Fig. 6.9: Multiple secondary lymph nodes in the neck.

Q. 12. How common is haematogenous spread in oral cancer?

This **mode of spread** is **extremely uncommon**. Essentially **oral cancers** are **loco-regional** in their **behaviour**, though **lung metastases** have been described in **malignancies of the tongue.**

Q. 13. What is a verrucous carcinoma and what are its special characteristics?

It is a **special form** of a **well-differentiated squamous cell carcinoma** with **specific clinical features**. It appears as a **thick white warty plaque** resembling a **cauliflower.** It is seen in the **cheek, gingivolabial sulcus** and **lip**. It is a **slow growing** tumour that is **locally invasive,** but **spread** to the **lymph nodes** is **rare. Histopathology** shows **well-differentiated hyperplastic** squamous epithelial **cells** with **orderly maturation** and **extensive fibrosis**. All these contribute towards a far **better prognosis** as compared to other oral cancers.

Q. 14. What are the details of the TNM classification?

Primary tumour T.

Tx Tumour **cannot be assessed.**

T0 Clinically **no evidence** of the **tumour**.

T1 Tumour **less than 2 cm in size.**

T2 Size between **2 cm and 4 cm.**

T3 Tumour **more than 4 cm.**

T4 Infiltration of **adjacent structures**. This group is further **classified** into

T4 A) **Moderately advanced local cancer.**

This includes **involvement** of **adjacent structures** like the **overlying skin**, **deeper bone** and muscles. Infiltration of the inferior dental nerve is also included in this group.

T4 B) **Very advanced local disease**, with involvement of the **base of the skull, medial pterygoid muscle and internal carotid artery.**

Nodal status N.

N0 No palpable nodes in the neck.

N1 One node less than 3 cm in size on the same side.

N2 Further classified as follows.

N2 A) One node between 3 cm and 6 cm in size, on the same side.

N2 B) Ipsilateral multiple nodes but less than 6 cm in size.

N2 C) Ipsilateral and contralateral nodes less than 6 cm in size.

N3 Nodes more than 6 cm on any side.

Distant metastases M.

MX Status cannot be assessed.

M0 No evidence of distant metastases.

M1 Distant metastases present.

Q. 15. How is oral cancer staged clinically?

Stage I T1, N0, M0.

Stage II T2, N0, M0.

Stage III T1 to T3, N0, N1, N2, M0.

Stage IV Further divided into 3 groups.

IV A) T4 A, NI to N2C, M0.

IV B) T4 B, any N, M0 and any T, N3, M0.

IV C) Any T, any N, M1.

Q. 16. **What are the investigations done in oral cancer?**

The **basic rule** to remember is that **any ulcer** in the **oral cavity** that does **not heal** within **three weeks** of **adequate treatment**, is to be considered **malignant** until **proved otherwise**. This is the only method to arrive at an **early diagnosis** and thereby ensure a **better outcome** for this group of cancers.

1. **Multiple edge biopsies** are confirmatory. Nearly **90% to 95%** are **squamous cell carcinomas**. **Broder's classification** depends on the **degree of differentiation** seen on **histopathology.** The classification runs as follows.

   Grade I. More than 75% of the cells in a smear are well differentiated.

   Grade II. 50% to 75% of the cells are well differentiated.

   Grade III. 25% to 50% of the cells show differentiation.

   Grade IV. Less than 25% of the cells are differentiated.

   But the **more recent classifications** define the **tumour grade** more **accurately** by including the **degree of mitosis** and evidence of **lymphovascular invasion**.

2. **Orthopantomogram (OPG) X-ray of the jaw bones**. If the **mandible** or less commonly, the **maxilla** is involved, there will be **multiple osteolytic lesions**.

3. **Chest X-ray**. This may show evidence of **infection. Rarely metastases** may be seen.

4. **US** of the neck may show **nodes** that are **not clinically palpable**.

5. **CT scan of the head and neck** is indicated in **locally advanced disease (T4A and T4B)** or in the presence of **recurrent disease**, especially when **radical resections** are **planned. A RO resection** (microscopic **margins free of cancer**) can be **better planned** with the help of **CT**. Further, **CT Dental scans** are useful to plan **curative surgery** with **minimal resections** of the **mandible**.

6. **FNAC of the lymph node** in the neck. This investigation is frequently performed to **detect metastases**. When the **nodes are less than .5 cm** in size, an **ultrasound-guided biopsy** is preferable. But this procedure has **certain limitations**. The node **aspirated** may **not show malignancy**, giving a

sense of **complacency.** Again a node may be the seat of both **sepsis and malignancy,** and the aspirate may not represent the true situation. Hence the **treatment options** in general are **based** on the **clinical findings** rather than the **FNAC reports**.

Q. 17. Name the complications of oral cancers.

(*a*) **Malignant cachexia. Progressive trismus** or a **large proliferative growth,** and uncommonly, an **orocutaneous fistula,** all lead to **grossly reduced food intake** leading to **extreme emaciation and death**. This is more often seen in **recurrent tumours.**

(*b*) **Aspiration bronchopneumonia. Aspiration** is **physiological,** occurring during **deep sleep** when **cough reflex is abolished**. This allows **contents** from **the oral cavity** to slip down the **tracheobronchial tree**. In patients with **oral cancer,** the **contents** are **infective**. Associated with a **poor nutritional status** of these patients, the resulting **pneumonia** can be **fatal.**

(*c*) **Level II, III and IV nodes** are in **close proximity** to the **great vessels** in the **neck.**

Extracapsular spread can cause **erosion** of these vessels leading to **exsanguinating haemorrhage and death**.

(*d*) Recently **death** due to **distant metastases** is also being described, especially in **tongue cancers.**

Q. 18. What are the prognostic factors in oral cancers?

Oral cancers are considered to be **loco-regional cancers** due to their **biological behavior**. This is in contradistinction **to breast cancers,** which are **systemic** in their **nature** from the **very beginning**. Hence **adequate loco-regional treatment** will result in a **good prognosis**. But most of **our patients** report rather **late** to the **hospital.** Even **death** is commonly due to **loco-regional complications** as mentioned above, rather than due to **distant metastases** like in **kidney and testicular cancers.**

The following are the **important prognostic factors.**

(*a*) **Site:** Tumours of the **lip** have the **best outlook** followed by those of the **cheek. Tongue cancers** have a **poorer prognosis** followed by those involving the **floor of the mouth and palate.**

(*b*) **Clinical Stage:** The prognosis depends on the **clinical stage** of the tumour. **TI tumours** obviously have a far **better prognosis** compared to **TIV lesions**. But unlike **many other cancers** a **TIV stage** does not necessarily mean **palliative treatment**, thanks to the tumours being locoregional in their behaviour and **advances** in **radiotherapy** and **radical surgery** with excellent **plastic surgical reconstruction**.

(*c*) **Degree of differentiation** as per **Broder's classification**. **Grade I** cancers behave **much better** than **Grade IV cancers**. In addition evidence of **lymphovascular** and **perineural invasion** indicates a **poor prognosis**.

(*d*) **Type of tumour:** As mentioned earlier, **verrucous cancers** have a good prognosis. **Proliferative type** of tumours have a **better prognosis** as compared with an **excavating type**.

(*e*) **Depth of the tumour: Tumours** having a **depth of more than 5 mm** have a **poor prognosis**.

(*f*) Following **dramatic improvement** in the **various modalities of treatment** during the last **two decades, three additional factors** are to be considered in relation to the **prognosis**.

1. As a result of **early diagnosis** and **adequate treatment**, primarily in the **developed countries**, **patients live long enough** to develop **distant metastases**, especially in the **lungs.**

2. The **effects** of **both tobacco and smoking** are seen in the **entire proximal aerodigestive tract**. Hence **patients** are likely to develop **metachronous cancers** in these areas even **years later.**

3. The **longevity** provided by the **treatment** makes it **possible** for the **patients** to have **secondary malignancies** in **other parts** of the **body** at a **later period**. The higher risk is partly due to the chemoradiation received by the patient for the primary disease.

Q. 19. **What is the rationale behind the treatment protocols of oral cancers?**

The oral **cavity** plays an important part in **chewing, swallowing and talking**. In addition, **externally** it forms an **integral part of the cosmetic appearance** of the **face**. Though the **primary aim** of treating any cancer is to **cure the disease,** the **quality of life** after treatment is **equally important**. One must also remember that those **patients** with **early cancers** have an almost **normal life span**. The aim should be **to minimise the functional disability** and **cosmetic disfigurement** while **treating these cancers**.

The **treatment** involves **multiple disciplines**. They include mainly **surgery** and **radiotherapy** with **chemotherapy** playing a **minor role**. Except in the **group** of patients with **distant metastases** or with **recurrent disease**, the **primary tumour** and the **regional nodes** are treated on their **individual merits.**

Q. 20. Describe the principles of treatment of the primary tumour.

For **TI and TII cancers**, both **surgery and radiotherapy** give **equally good** results. But in carcinoma of the tongue even for **TI and T2 tumours, surgery** is **preferred,** since this is a **mobile structure** and **radiotherapy** is **technically** more **difficult**. In patients with **verrucous carcinoma, surgery** is the preferred line of treatment since **radiation converts** the tumour into an **aggressive one.**

But once we reach **T3 and T4 stages, combined modalities** of **treatment** are needed. The usual pattern is to **operate first** and **offer radiotherapy later**. If **radiotherapy** is administered **first, reconstructive surgery** becomes more **difficult** because of **reduced vascularity** and **fibrosis induced by radiation**. But this may have to be **reversed** in some patients depending on the **location**, **size and depth** of the **tumour.**

Neoadjuvant chemotherapy is advised to **downstage a stage 4 tumour**. Once the **tumour** is **down staged**, **radical surgery** is performed. It is then followed by **radiotherapy.**

The **final decision** however depends on the **following factors**.

(*a*) **Availability of radiotherapy**.

(*b*) **Excisional surgery** is always combined with **reconstruction.** Hence **radical surgery** needs **expert reconstructive surgical facilities**.

(*c*) **Patient preference.** The **cost and the duration** of treatment may **influence** the patient in **deciding the mode** of **treatment.**

Q. 21. Discuss the role of radiotherapy in oral cancer.

The **advantage** of **radiotherapy** over **surgery** is the **minimal disturbance** as far as both cosmesis and functions are concerned. The dose is between **50** and **60 Gy** given in **fractions** over a period of five to six weeks. The **dosage** depends on the **size and the location** of the **tumour. External beam radiotherapy (EBRT)** is the mode most **frequently** preferred at the **present time**. The availability of the modern **IGRT (image-guided radiotherapy)** has **minimised** the **damage** to the **surrounding normal tissues**. Radiotherapy has certain **side effects**. They include **nausea and vomiting** as well as **mucositis and dryness of the mouth**. In the **past**, when **radiotherapy** was used to **treat tumours in close proximity** of a **bone (mandible)**, there was a **risk of producing** a very unfortunate **complication,** namely, **septic osteoradionecrosis. Ionising radiation** produces **endarteritis obliterans** in a **blood vessel**. If the **nutrient artery** to the **mandible** is **thrombosed,** the **bone** undergoes **avascular necrosis**. The **necrotic bone** is **invaded** by **bacteria.** The result is an **extremely painful condition**. The patient has **multiple sinuses** discharging **foul-smelling pus,** a picture of absolute **misery**. Luckily, in **recent times** this complication is **rare.**

Q. 22. Discuss the role of surgery in oral cancer.

Three-dimensional wide excision is the operation of choice. It would mean **excision** of the **mucosa, submucosa, underlying muscle** and **involved bone depending** on the **stage of the cancer**. A **clearance of 1 cm** margin from the **edge of induration,** usually ensures **R 0 resection**. When in doubt, **frozen-section studies** will be of help. If **mandible** is involved, depending upon the **extent of involvement** of the **bone, 3 types** of **resections** are available

(a) **Marginal mandibulectomy:** This is indicated for **cancers** arising from the **mucoperiosteum** of the **horizontal ramus** of the **mandible** with **no evidence** of **bony involvement** on **OPG X-ray** or **CT scan**. In this procedure, a **rim of the horizontal ramus** in relation to the **tumour** is **removed** along with the **primary tumour**. The **advantage** of this operation is that **no reconstructive surgery** is **needed**, and there is **no cosmetic disfigurement**.

(b) **Segmental resections of the mandible:** Once the

imaging studies show **bone involvement**, the **particular segment** is **removed.** This operation causes a **significant cosmetic** and **functional disability.** Hence **reconstructive surgery** is performed **after the resection.**

(*c*) **Hemi-mandibulectomy:** The involved **half of the mandible** including the **vertical ramus** is **removed** in this procedure. The **symphysis menti** is always **preserved.** Tumours of the **cheek** extending **deep into the underlying muscles** and the **vertical ramus of the mandible** need this **major operation.** It is to be noted that **removal of the mandible** produces a very **grave cosmetic deformity** in comparison with a **maxillectomy.** The **latter operation** leaves behind **minimal deformity** with a **flattened malar region.** The **function** of the **oral cavity** is also **severely compromised** following this operation. Hence **reconstruction** is **mandatory.**

Following an **excision, immediate reconstructive surgery** needs to be performed. This would mean **replacement** of the **inner lining (mucosa)**, the bulk of **tissue** including **muscle**, the **skin** and when needed **bone.** Extensive **radical resections** are now **possible** thanks to the **development** of **sophisticated plastic surgical operations.** It is the availability of **myocutaneous** or **osteomyocutaneous flaps** as well as **free vascularised flaps** that has revolutionised **reconstructive surgery** for **oral cancer**, leading to **excellent cosmetic** and **functional results**.

Q. 23. Give a brief description of reconstructive surgery in oral cancers.

Lip: Small lesions can be **excised** and the defect **closed by primary suturing**, provided it does **not** produce a **microstoma.** If the **excision** leaves behind a **defect** of **less** than **one-third of the lip**, **local flaps** raised from the **other lip** like **Abbe** or **Estlander** flaps are **adequate. Larger defects** are treated by **rotating cheek flaps** either on **one side** or **bilaterally** depending on the **size of the defect.** A **forehead flap** based on the **superficial temporal artery** can also be used.

Tongue: A **V-excision** of a cancer of the **tip** of the tongue can be managed by a **primary closure** of the defect. A **partial glossectomy** also does not need any **reconstruction**, though it results in an **alteration of**

the shape. But defects arising from a **hemi, subtotal and total glossectomy** always need to be **corrected**. A **pectoralis major myocutaneous flap** or a **microvascular forearm flap** based on the **radial artery** is commonly used.

Cheek: Small defects can be **closed primarily** or left to **heal spontaneously**. But **larger defects including the skin** are covered by a **pectoralis major myocutaneous** flap. If an **extended resection** is done wherein the **mandible** also is **resected**, a **free vascular fibular graft** is ideal for **replacing the mandible**. The **advantages** of using the **fibula** are

(*a*) It is a **non–weight-bearing bone**.

(*b*)   The **length is adequate** to **replace** the **resected mandible**.

(*c*) The **blood vessel** runs **longitudinally in the fibula**.

Surgical expertise has **advanced** to the extent of even creating a **neotemporomandibular joint, improving** the **functional status** considerably.

Q. 24. **How are the regional lymph nodes treated?**

The **treatment** depends on the **clinical staging**.

Patients presenting with **N0** status pose **certain problems**. If the site of the primary tumour is in the **lip or the cheek** and is of a **low grade, surveillance** is advised. As and when the **lymph nodes become palpable**, they **need treatment**. But in the case of the **tongue**, the risk of **occult metastases in the nodes** is **high**. Hence a **supraomohyoid block dissection** is performed as a **diagnostic procedure**. The nodes removed, are **level I (both A and B), level II and level III**. A **frozen-section report** is always asked for. If the report shows **malignancy**, a **functional neck dissection** is performed. If the **report is negative**, the patients are kept under **observation**.

Enlarged lymph nodes due to **infection** are soft and **tender** and are **rarely** seen in **our patients**. These nodes **resolve completely** with **antimicrobial therapy**. Such patients need only **surveillance** later. **Nodes persisting** after **antimicrobial therapy** are presumed to be **malignant** and **treated accordingly**.

NI and NII nodes (hard and mobile) are treated by a **radical neck dissection**. The **rationale** is to **remove** the **lymph nodes, lymphatic vessels** and the **adjacent structures,** which may contain **malignant cells**. The **following structures** are **removed en bloc** in the **classical (Crile's) operation**.

(*a*) **Subcutaneous fat** on the same side of the neck.

(*b*) **Fascia**. The **investing layer** of the deep **cervical fascia** and the **carotid sheath.**

(*c*) **All the lymph nodes from level I to V.**

(*d*) The **sternomastoid**, the **omohyoid** and the **posterior belly** of the **digastric** muscles.

(*e*) The **internal jugular vein**.

(*f*) The **lower pole of the parotid** and the **submandibular salivary gland**. The indication to **remove the salivary gland** is that **lymphatic tissue** is found **inside the gland.**

MacFee's incision is commonly employed for this operation. It consists of **two transverse incisions** on the **side of the neck**. The **upper incision** is placed 2 **cm parallel** and **below the lower border of the mandible**. The **lower one** is made **2 cm above and parallel to the clavicle**. The **flaps** are raised including the **skin and platysma** for **complete exposure** of the **structures** on **that side of the neck**. The **advantage** of this **incision** is the **absence** of postoperative **skin necrosis**.

But this **formidable operation** has **significant morbidity**. Postoperative **infection** may lead to a **fatal carotid blow out**, since all the **overlying tissues** protecting the **artery have been removed**. Again **division** of the **spinal accessory nerve** leads to **paralysis of the trapezius**. A **drooping** of the **shoulder** causes **traction on the brachial plexus**. The patient will complain of **severe pain radiating down the limb**. A **frozen shoulder** is often **seen** after this procedure.

A set of **modifications** have been introduced to **reduce the morbidity** and **improve the function**. They include **conserving the internal jugular vein**, the **digastric and sternomastoid** muscles and the **spinal accessory nerve**. These operations are also known as functional neck resections. It must be **stressed t**hat these **modifications** should **not undermine** the **oncological principles** of **adequate clearance.**

N3 nodes: A course of **chemoradiation** is given to **downstage the tumour**. **Three weeks** after the **last cycle**, a **radical lymphadenectomy** is performed. **Chemoradiation** is **continued** once the **incisions have healed**. But the **incidence**

of **postoperative morbidity** is **much higher** in this group.

NII C lymph nodes. Once **contralateral nodes** are **enlarged,** the patient needs a **bilateral block dissection**. Operation on the **opposite side** is spaced **after 2 to 3 weeks**. Usually a **modified resection** is performed. If this is not possible, **at least the internal jugular vein** is to be **retained**. Since the **internal jugular vein** is the **main route** for **venous drainage** from the **brain, removal** of **both the veins** is likely to produce **raised intracranial pressure (ICP)**. Measures to **reduce the ICP** include **intravenous mannitol or hypertonic urea.** Over a period of time, **the venous drainage** is taken over by the **vertebral veins**.

Fixed lymph nodes. These are patients with **enlarged nodes fixed to the deeper structures**, especially the **carotid arteries**. The treatment is **essentially palliative** and consists of EBRT As expected, the **prognosis** is very **poor.**

Composite resections (known as a **Commando operation** in the **past). In a small number of patients** the **primary tumour** and the **involved nodes** are removed at the **same time.** An **example** would be **excision** of a **cancer** in the **cheek** with the **involved muscles** and the **mandible** with a **radical lymphadenectomy.**

Q. 25. What is the role of role of chemotherapy in oral cancer?

This modality of treatment has a **very little role** in the management of oral cancer. As mentioned earlier, **neoadjuvant chemotherapy** is used for patients with **stage IV disease** for **down staging** the **cancer**. More often this regime is **used along with radiation**. The drugs used are **Cisplatin** and **5-Fluorouracil**.

■■■

Cystic Swellings in the Neck

7

A CASE OF BRANCHIAL CYST

Setting

- Outpatient department (OPD).

Chief Complaint

- Swelling in the upper part of the neck.
- A **thirty**-year-old **man** presented to the OPD with complaint of a **swelling** in the **upper** part of the **neck** of **four years** duration. He noticed a **pea size** swelling just **below the mandible** on the right side of the neck about four years ago. Since then it has been **gradually increasing in size**. He did not complain of **pain**. There was no history of **fever or cough**. He was not aware of **simila**r **swellings** in other parts of the body.
- His past and personal histories were insignificant.
- General physical examination was normal.

Local Examination

Inspection

There was an **obliquely** placed swelling situated in front of the **sternomastoid** and below the lower border of the **mandible** on the right side of the neck. The swelling was **oval** in shape, measuring 5 cm by 3 cm in size. Except for the **posterior** border, the **other borders** were well **defined**. The **surface** was **smooth**. The **skin** over the swelling was **normal.** The surrounding area did not show any abnormality.

Palpation

The swelling was in the **upper part** of the right side of the neck, extending from the **sternomastoid** to about 5 cm **anteriorly**. The **vertical** extension was about 3 cm from the lower border of the **mandible**. It was neither warm nor tender. The consistency was **soft**. It was **fluctuant but not transilluminant**. The skin could be lifted off the swelling. There was **transverse mobility**. On

contracting the **sternomastoid** against resistance, the mobility became **restricted**. The **posterior** part of the swelling appeared to be **deep** to the **sternomastoid**. Hence most of the swelling was in the subcutaneous plane. Examination of the neck did not reveal any enlarged lymph nodes. Examination of the oral cavity was normal. No similar swellings were noted elsewhere in the body.

Q. 1. What are possible clinical diagnoses?

(a) Branchial cyst.

(b) Tuberculous cold abscess.

(c) Lymph cyst.

(d) Secondary metastatic lymph node.

The correct answer is (a). A history of **four years** rules out **malignancy.** In addition, **secondary nodes** from a squamous cell carcinoma are **hard** in consistency. **Cysts** in relation to the **lymphatic system** are seen in **infancy.** They are also **brilliantly transilluminant**. In **tuberculosis**, usually **multiple** nodes are involved. Once **cold abscess** forms, the **skin** is likely to be **adherent** to the swelling. **Matting** is an important feature of tuberculous lymph nodes. **Branchial cyst** usually presents in an adult as an **asymptomatic swelling** of **several years** duration. The clinical findings are typical of a branchial cyst.

Box 7.1:	Points to be noted in history

- Swelling in the upper part of the neck
- Duration – Rate of growth
- Pain
- Fever and cough
- Similar swellings

Box 7.2:	Points to be noted on clinical examination

- Site and extent – Margins
- Size and shape
- Skin over the swelling – Surface
- Surrounding area
- Warmth and tenderness
- Consistency – Mobility – Anatomical plane
- Regional nodes
- Oral cavity

Q. 2. What were the investigations done in this patient?

Most cases are diagnosed on the basis of **clinical findings**. Ultrasound (**US**) and **fine needle aspiration cytology** (**FNAC**) confirm the diagnosis. **US** showed a sharply **delineated oval mass** that was **anechoic** and lined by a **thin** peripheral wall. During **FNAC, yellow turbid** fluid was aspirated. **Microscopy** showed **cholesterol** crystals (characteristic of a branchial cyst), keratin and lymphocytes.

Q. 3. What is the common complication and what is the treatment?

Infection is the commonest complication of a branchial cyst. This occurs due to the spread of infection from the **oral cavity**

via the **lymphatics,** since these are in **communication** with the **lymphoid tissue** within the **cyst**. The patient develops **pain and fever**. The cyst becomes **warm and tender**. Aspiration yields **purulent** fluid. **Aspiration** under **antimicrobial cover** is successful if the diagnosis is made **early**. Frank **suppuration** needs an **incision** and **drainage**. An **excision** can be performed about **3 months** later. **Rarely** a branchial **fistula** may result following an incision and drainage procedure.

Setting: A week later the patient was posted for surgery.

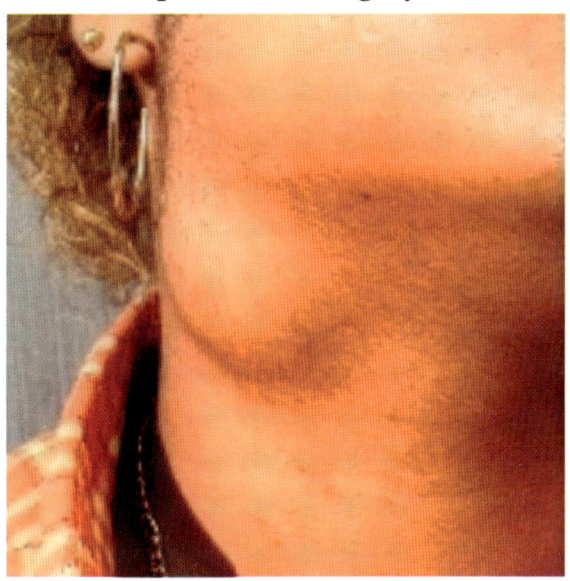

Fig. 7.1: Branchial cyst.

Excision of the cyst was the treatment. An **incision** was made over the cyst, dividing the **skin and platysma**. The cyst was dissected from the surrounding soft tissues taking care not to injure the nerves in close proximity. **Retraction** of the **sternomastoid** helped in removing the **posterior** part of the cyst. If there are dense adhesions, especially following previous **sepsis**, a part of the **sternomastoid** is **divided** for better exposure.

Q. 4. What is the embryological basis for the formation of a branchial cyst?

Both a **branchial cyst and a fistula** result from **congenital** anomalies in relation to the **second branchial arch.** During the **sixth week** of intrauterine life, the **neck** resembles a **tube**, comprising of **six ectoderm**-lined branchial **arches**. The gaps between these arches are termed as **clefts** on the **inner** aspect and pouches on the outside, lined by **endoderm** and ectoderm, respectively. The **fifth arch involutes** by the **seventh week**. The **second arch** grows **caudally** overlapping the third and the fourth arches to join the **sixth arch**. This produces a **blind space** lined by **ectoderm** known as a **cervical sinus**. In most instances, this space is completely **obliterated. Persistence** of this space results in a **branchial cyst.**

A CASE OF BRANCHIAL FISTULA

Setting

- Paediatric surgery OPD.

Chief Complaint

- A **six**-year-old **boy** was brought to the OPD with the complaint of a **discharging sinus** in the **lower** part of the **front** of the **neck that had been present** since **birth**. The **discharge** was **intermittent** and was either **mucoid** or **purulent**. It was not foul smelling. The mother gave a history of **intermittent attacks** of low-grade **fever** lasting for a few days. There were no other complaints.
- **Past and family histories** were insignificant.
- **General physical examination** was normal.

Local Examination

Inspection

A **sinus** was present in the lower part of the **neck** at the level of the **junction** of the **upper-two thirds** and the **lower one-third** of the right **sternomastoid** muscle. It was located at the **anterior border** of the muscle. The sinus was **circular** in shape measuring about 0.75 cm in size. The **upper margin** had a **crescentic** appearance. The sinus was lined by pink **granulation tissue**. There was a small quantity of **purulent**

discharge. It was not foul smelling. The surrounding area appeared normal.

Palpation

The sinus had **sloping edges**. There was no induration. A **fibrous band** like structure could be felt extending **upwards** from the sinus. The amount of discharge increased when **pressure** was applied. No lymph nodes were palpable in the neck.

Q. 1. What are the possibilities in this case?

(a) Branchial sinus.

(b) Tuberculous sinus.

The **right answer is (a). Tuberculosis** usually involves **older** children. The sinus has **undermined edges. Matted lymph nodes** are felt in close proximity to the sinus.

Since the sinus has been present from **birth**, it suggests a branchial sinus. Its anatomical **location** is diagnostic. A **crescentic** upper border is **typical**. It is the result of **repeated** attacks of **infection** leading to **fibrosis**. This pulls the **skin** margin in an **upward** direction.

Box 7.3:	Points to be noted in the history
• Sinus in the neck since birth	
• Discharge – Mucoid or purulent	
• Fever intermittent – Low grade	
• Family history of similar complaints	

Box 7.4:	Points to be noted on clinical examination

- Site – Along the anterior border of the sternomastoid
- Junction of the upper two-thirds and lower one-third of the muscle
- Size and shape – Circular – Less than 1 cm in size
- Margin – Upper – Crescentic
- Fibrous track extending upwards from the sinus
- Regional nodes may be palpable
- The condition may be bilateral

Q. 2. **What is the embryological origin of the branchial fistula?**

The aetiology is the **same** as that of a **branchial cyst**. If the **endothelium** lining the **cervical sinus** gives way, a complete **fistula** is the result. The **internal opening** is in the **supratonsillar fossa**. But **true** fistulae are **rare**. Most are true **sinuses, that is,** blind tracks lined by **ectoderm** terminating at the lateral **pharyngeal** wall. During its course it runs **between** the **carotid bifurcation** and in close **proximity** to the **ninth, eleventh, and twelfth cranial** nerves and the **lingual nerves**.

Q. 3. **What are the investigations?**

Contrast-enhanced computerised tomography (CECT) demonstrates the **entire track** and its **relation** with **important** adjacent **structures**. **Contrast-enhanced MRI** is another option. These investigations have drastically **reduced** the risk of **recurrence**. Intraoperatively, **methylene blue** is used to make **identification** of the **track** easy.

Setting: A week later the case was posted for surgery.

A complete excision of the sinus with the track ensures good results. An **elliptical incision** was made around the sinus. A skin flap containing the skin and platysma was raised. The track was seen to be **extending upwards** on the deep **fascia.** The dissection was carried till the level of the **thyroid cartilage**. A second transverse incision was made at this level (**step ladder** approach). The track was found to be extending **medially and upwards**. The sternomastoid was retracted laterally, and the dissection was continued taking care not to **injure** important **structures** in close **proximity.** Once the **lateral wall** of the pharynx was reached, the **track** was completely **excised**. If it is a **fistula**, the **internal opening** is **closed** with an absorbable suture and the track is excised.

| **B o x 7.5:** | Points regarding treatment |

- Injection of methylene blue
- Elliptical incision around the sinus
- Second incision at the level of thyroid cartilage
- Complete excision of the track
- Avoid injury to important neurovascular structures
- Internal opening if present closed with an absorbable suture

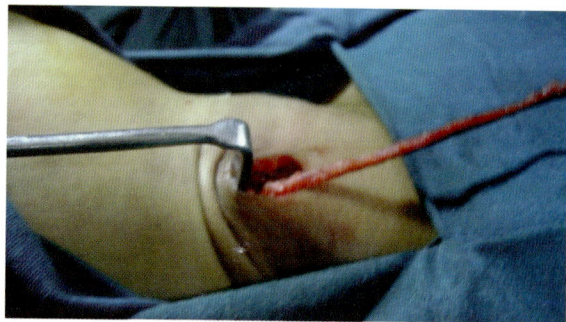

Fig. 7.4: Branchial fistulous track being excised.

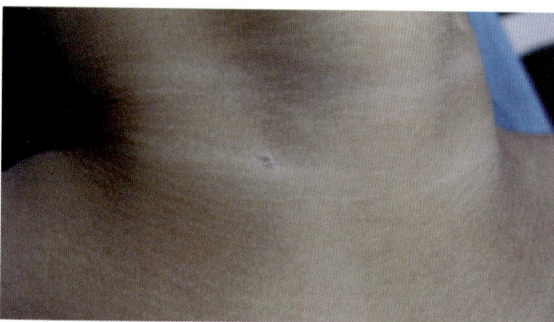

Fig. 7.2: Branchial fistula.

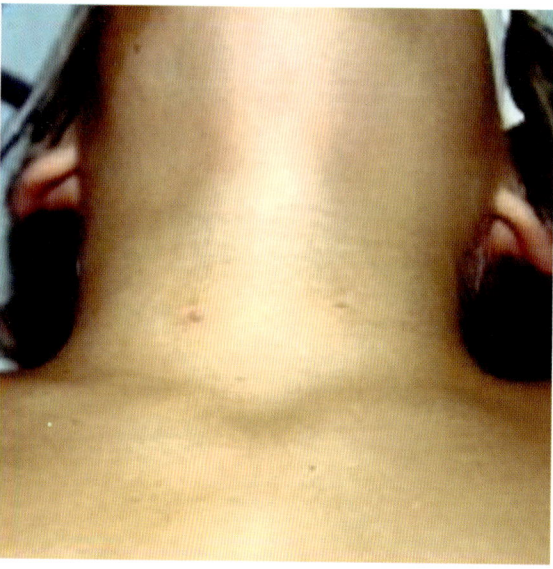

FIg. 7.3: Bilateral branchial fistulae.

A CASE OF THYROGLOSSAL CYST

Setting

- Surgical OPD.

Chief Complaint

- **Swelling** in the **upper part of the neck** of **2 years** duration.

- A 12-year-old girl was brought to the OPD with the complaint of a **swelling** in the **upper** part of the **front** of the **neck**. The mother had noticed a **small swelling** in that region about **two years** ago. The **rate** of growth has been **slow**. Since the swelling has become **large** and noticeable, the mother has brought the patient to the hospital. There was **no** history of **pain**. The patient did not have any **fever** or chronic **cough**.

- **Past, personal and family histories** were insignificant. She had not attained menarche.

Local Examination

Inspection

A swelling was seen in the **anterior** aspect of the neck in the **midline** at the level of the **hyoid** cartilage. The swelling was transversely **oval** measuring 4 cm by 3 cm. All the **margins** could be **clearly** made out. The **skin** over the swelling was **stretched**. The **surface** was **smooth.** The **swelling** was seen to **move upwards** with **deglutition** and forward **protrusion of the tongue**.

Palpation

The swelling did not have warmth and was not tender. It was situated about 0.5 cm **below** the **hyoid** cartilage extending to about **2 cm** on **either side** of the midline. The consistency was **soft.** It was **fluctuant** but **not transilluminant**. There was **restricted** horizontal **mobility**. The anatomical **plane** was **deep** to the **skin** and the cervical **fascia.** **Upward movement** with **deglutition** and forward **protrusion** of the **tongue** was confirmed. The swelling was **free** from the **hyoid** cartilage.

Examination of the **anterior** aspect of the **neck** suggested the presence of the **thyroid** gland in relation to the trachea. **Fullness** was noted in this area and a **few rings** of the trachea were **not easily palpable.**

No enlarged lymph **nodes** were palpable in the neck. Examination of the **oral cavity** did not show any abnormality. Systemic examination was within normal limits.

Q. 1. What was the differential diagnosis in this case?

(*a*) Thyroglossal cyst.

(*b*) Enlarged subhyoid bursa.

These are only **two swellings** that move upwards with **deglutition** and **protrusion** of the **tongue**. The correct diagnosis was a **thyroglossal cyst.** An enlarged **subhyoid bursa** is a **rare** condition at the **present time**. In the past due to **chronic inflammation** caused by **tuberculosis,** the **bursa** became **enlarged**. It was also responsible for **widening** the **thyrohyoid** space.

Hence in practice the only diagnosis to be offered with this clinical presentation will be a **thyroglossal cyst.** It moves **up** with **deglutition** because it is **within** the **pretracheal fascia,** which is attached to the **hyoid** cartilage. The **thyrohyoid apparatus** moves up during **deglutition.** The **cyst** is attached to the **foramen caecum** area of the tongue by the remnants of the **thyroglossal duct.** Hence when the **tongue** is **protruded** forward, the swelling moves **upwards.**

Q. 2. **What is the aetiology of a thyroglossal cyst?**

A **thyroglossal cyst** is considered to be an **embryological** malformation due to **failure** of **obliteration** of the **thyroglossal duct.** The **thyroid gland** is originally located in the **floor** of the **pharynx** between the **tuberculum impar** (first pharyngeal arch) and the **cupola** (second and third arches). This site corresponds to the **foramen caecum** on the dorsum of the **tongue,** at the junction of the anterior two-thirds and the posterior one-third. At this stage it is very **close** to the **pericardial sac.** As the gland develops, it **descends down** into the neck to its final position in **front of the trachea.** During this descent, it leaves behind a narrow **epithelium-lined duct,** namely, the **thyroglossal duct.** In most instances, the duct is **obliterated** by the **tenth week** of **intrauterine life.** The **pyramidal lobe** or the **pyramidalis** muscle is the common **remnant** of the duct. **Persistence** of the **epithelial elements** of the **duct** results in the **formation** of the **cyst.** Due to its **embryological origin,** the **cyst** may be **present** at **any level** between the **hyoid** bone and the **pericardium.** But **most** occur in **relation** with the **hyoid cartilage.**

The **infrahyoid** position is the most **common** site.

Box 7.6: Points to be noted in history
- Age – Childhood – Also seen in adults
- Main complaint – A midline swelling in the front and upper part of the neck
- Duration – Several years
- Rate of growth – Slow
- Pain – Absent
- Fever and cough – Absent

The body of the **hyoid** develops at a **later period** from the **mesoderm.** The **mesoderm** grows from the **lateral to the medial** aspect from the **second and third branchial arches** on both sides and these **join** with **each other** to form the **hyoid cartilage.** This explains the **intimate relation** of the duct with the hyoid cartilage. Occasionally the duct may be **incorporated** into the **substance** of the hyoid. In some instances, the **suprahyoid** portion of the duct may have a **branching** pattern like the tips of a broom.

Box 7.7: Points to be noted on inspection
- Site and extent – Infrahyoid – Midline
- Moves upwards with deglutition and forward protrusion of the tongue
- Margins – Well defined
- Size – Variable
- Shape – Transversely oval
- Skin over the swelling – May be stretched
- Surrounding area – Normal

Box 7.8:	Points to be noted during palpation

- Warmth and tenderness – Absent
- Site, extent and margins confirmed
- Consistency – Soft or tensely cystic
- Fluctuation +ve – Transillumination –ve
- Restricted mobility
- Anatomical plane – Deep to skin and fascia
- Palpation for thyroid gland in front of the trachea
- Lymph nodes – Not palpable
- Oral cavity – Normal

Q. 3. Why are investigations needed in a case of thyroglossal cyst?

(*a*) To **confirm** the diagnosis.

(*b*) To confirm the presence of **normal thyroid** tissue in front of the trachea.

(*c*) **Papillary carcinoma** is a known complication of the cyst.

Q. 4. What are the investigations done in these cases?

US and FNAC are both helpful to arrive at a diagnosis.

US study: The findings are of a **cystic lesion** with a **thin** wall. Occasionally few **semisolid** areas may be seen within the cyst. Presence of **microcalcification** suggests **papillary carcinoma**.

FNAC: The smear shows abundant **colloid** with **ciliated or squamous** epithelium. **Macrophages** and **lymphocytes** are also frequently seen.

Thyroid cells are seen only in a **small percentage** of cases.

Malignancy is more often a **histopathological** diagnosis made **after the operation**.

Q. 5. What is the indication for radio-iodine (RI) studies in these cases?

If after a **clinical examination** and **US** study, the presence of the **thyroid** gland in the **neck** cannot be clearly **established**, this study is required. In a small number of patients the **mass** may be the only **functioning thyroid tissue** in the body.

Box 7.9:	Points to be noted about investigations

- US – Cystic lesion with a thin wall – Semisolid areas
- Microcalcification – Suggestive of malignancy
- FNAC – Colloid with ciliated or squamous epithelium
- Lymphocytes and macrophages
- Thyroid cells – Uncommon
- Malignancy – Needs histopathology
- RI study – To detect normal thyroid tissue in the neck

Q. 6. What are the indications for treatment?

(*a*) Risk of **infection.** But it is less common compared to a branchial cyst.

(*b*) Infection may lead to the development of a **fistula.** It may be the result of a **spontaneous rupture** or a **surgical drainage and is more difficult to treat**.

(*c*) Rarely a **papillary carcinoma** may develop within the cyst.

(*d*) **Cosmetic** disfigurement.

Q. 7. Why does a simple excision lead to a recurrence?

Since the **remnants** of the **thyroglossal duct** are **left behind**, a **recurrence** is common.

Q. 8. What is the rationale behind excision of the central portion of the hyoid cartilage in the management of a thyroglossal cyst?

The **hyoid cartilage** develops from **mesoderm** at a **later period** of foetal life. When the **two** mesodermal elements **join** together in the midline, the **thyroglossal duct** comes into **intimate relation** with these elements. In some cases, the duct is **incorporated** within the cartilage. If the **hyoid** is **spared** during surgery, the chances of **recurrence** are high.

Setting: A week later the patient was posted for Sistrunk's operation.

Q. 9. Describe Sistrunk's operation.

Sistrunk's operation aims at **removal** of the **cyst** along with the **remnants** of the **duct** till the **foramen caecum** of the tongue along with the **body** of the **hyoid** cartilage. A **transverse incision** is made at the level of the cyst. The **skin, platysma and the investing fascia** are incised. The **strap muscles** are **retracted** and the **cyst** is dissected off the **thyrohyoid membrane**. The **ductal component** above the cyst is identified and the **operation proceeds** in an **upward** direction. The **central** piece of the **hyoid** cartilage is **removed** along with the **duct** for reasons explained earlier. The **suprahyoid** part of the duct is very **ill defined** and may have **branches**. Hence a **core of tissue** about **1 cm** in diameter to include the **duct** along with the **surrounding muscles** is excised till the **submucous layer** of the **tongue** is reached. A **finger** placed at the **foramen caecum** area of the **tongue** intraorally **helps the surgeon** at this stage of the operation. An **incomplete removal** will lead to **recurrence** of the **cyst** or formation of a **fistula**. Both these conditions make the **second operation** technically more **difficult.**

Box 7.10:	Points regarding Sistrunk's operation

- Excision of the cyst along with the central portion of hyoid cartilage and the remnants of the duct till the level of the foramen caecum of the tongue
- Incomplete removal leads to either a recurrence or uncommonly a thyroglossal fistula – Second operation – Difficult

Q. 10. Mention one other operation described by Sistrunk.

Sistrunk described an open cystogastros-tomy for a pseudo pancreatic cyst.

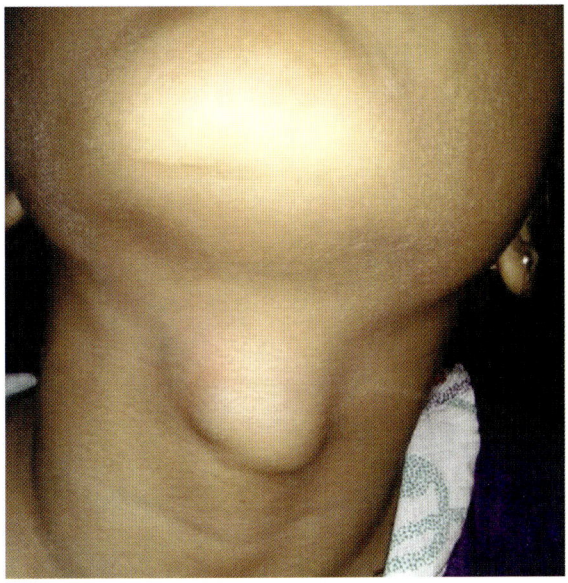

Fig. 7.5: Thyroglossal cyst.

A CASE OF CYSTIC HYGROMA

Setting

- Surgical OPD

Chief Complaint

- A **5-year**-old boy was brought by the father with the complaint of a **large swelling** on the right side of the **neck.** The swelling was noticed at **birth** and was the **size** of a **gooseberry**. Since then there had been a **gradual increase in size**. But the mother noticed that for the previous **six months**, there was a **rapid** increase in size. The sheer **size** of the swelling had made the parents bring the child to the **hospital.** There was no history suggestive of **pain.** The child did not have any **respiratory** symptoms.

- **Past history and family** history were non-contributory.

- **General physical examination** showed a healthy child.

Local Examination

Inspection

- A **swelling** was visible on the **right** side of the **neck**. It was occupying the **lower two-thirds** of the lateral aspect of the neck. It was extending from the **posterior border** of the right **sternomastoid** to about 2 cm from the **midline posteriorly**.

- The **size** measured 10 cm by 8 cm.

- The **shape** was irregular. The **margins** were ill defined.

- The **skin** over the swelling was stretched and thin. There were no dilated veins on the surface.

- The **surrounding area** looked normal.

Palpation

- The swelling was **not warm or tender**.

- The **site** and **size** were confirmed. The **borders** were **indistinct.**

- The **consistency** was **soft**. It was **fluctuant** and **brilliantly transilluminant**.

- The **skin** was **free** from the swelling.

- It had **mobility** both in the transverse and vertical directions.

- The plane was **subcutaneous**.

- **Two small** and **soft** lymph **nodes** were palpable at level III on the right side of the neck.

- **Examination of the oral cavity** did not show any abnormality.

- Rest of the **clinical examination** was **normal.**

Box 7.11:	Points to be noted in the history

- Swelling in the neck
- Age – Infancy and childhood
- Duration – Present since birth
- Rate of growth – Variable
- Pressure symptoms – Depend on location
- Tracheal compression due to large swelling in infants

Box 7.12:	Points to be noted on inspection

- Site – Posterior triangle of the neck – Commonest site
- Size – Variable – Can assume a huge size
- Shape – Irregular
- Margins – Indistinct
- Surface – Smooth or lobular
- Skin over the swelling – Stretched
- Surrounding area – Normal

Box 7.13:	Points to be mentioned on palpation

- Warmth and tenderness
- Site and extent – Larger on palpation
- Borderers – Ill defined
- Consistency – Soft - Fluctuation – Present
- Transillumination – Positive
- Plane subcutaneous – Deep extensions – Restricted mobility
- Extensions into axilla and mediastinum – Restricted mobility
- Lymph nodes – Palpable

Q. 1. What was the clinical diagnosis?

The diagnosis was a **cystic hygroma**. The clinical picture was so **typical** that no other condition needed to be discussed.

Q. 2. What were the indications for investigations in this case?

US examination was done to determine the **entire extent** of the cyst. The tendency of the cyst to spread into the **deeper planes** would make the findings on clinical examination inadequate. US also ruled out extensions into the **axilla** or the **mediastinum**. The appearance was that of a **multilocular** cyst with **clear** contents and a very **thin wall** located in the subcutaneous plane.

Setting: A few days later the child was posted for **surgery.**

A **complete surgical excision** was the treatment performed. The very **thin wall** and extension into various **tissue planes** made the operation slightly **difficult**. **Care** was taken to **make sure** that the **cyst wall did not rupture** during the **operation**. The child had an uneventful recovery.

Q. 3. What is the aetiology of a cystic hygroma?

The cyst is considered to be a **congenital** malformation of the **lymphatic** system. It results from the **lack of communications** between the jugular **lymphatic** and **venous** systems. These are **fluid-filled sacs** lined by an extremely thin wall comprising of a **single** layer of **endothelial cells.** These are multilocular cysts. **Two** types of the cysts have been described. The **superficial** type is in the **subcutaneous** plane. The **deeper** variety lies deep to the **muscles** and can **spread** far and wide in the loose **areolar tissues** and may be intimately related to **vital structures**. Some of the cysts have both of these components.

An association with **chromosomal abnormalities** has been described in some of these cases. **Turner's syndrome** is one such abnormality.

Q. 4. What are the investigations done in cases of cystic hygroma?

US is the investigation that is routinely performed. It will show a **multilocular cyst** with a **very thin wall** containing **clear fluid**.

US detects a **cystic hygroma** in a **foetus at** as early as **six weeks** of **intrauterine** life. This has made a tremendous **difference** in the **management**.

MRI scans. These are needed to rule out **extensions** into the axilla or the **mediastinum**. A **cyst** confined to the **mediastinum** is an **absolute indication** for **MRI**. It is also helpful to **identify** the important **neurovascular structures** in **close proximity to** the cyst, especially in **recurrent cases**.

Q. 5. What is the treatment of a cystic hygroma?

Surgical excision is the **ideal treatment**. But the **very thin wall** along with **multilocularity** makes the operation rather **difficult**. Hence **recurrences** cannot be completely **prevented**. Those lying in the superficial planes can be excised with a degree of **certainty**. But those cysts **extending** into the **deeper planes** and lying close to important structures can pose difficult **problems** during

surgery. A **mediastinal cyst** needs a **median sternotomy** for excision.

Q.6. What is the role of sclerotherapy in cystic hygroma?

Injection of a **sclerosing agent** into the cyst induces an **aseptic inflammation** resulting in **fibrosis.** This helps in obliteration of the cyst. **Bleomycin** and **OK 432** are the agents used for this purpose. The advantages are that a **major surgery** with the **risk of injuring vital structures** is **avoided.** But **recurrences** are more **common** because of **multilocularity. Recurrent cysts** are more **difficult** to treat due to adhesions resulting from the treatment.

Q.7. How are antenatal cystic hygromas treated?

As mentioned above, the diagnosis may be made at as early as **six weeks** of foetal life**. Amniocentesis or chorionic** villous **biopsy** has been advised to rule out **chromosomal** abnormalities. **Repeated US** examinations are necessary to study the **increase** in size during the **gestation period**. Occasionally, the cyst **enlarges** to more than the size of the **foetus** leading to **hydrops and death**. Injections of **sclerosing agents** under expert **US guidance** have

been advised to **reduce the size** of the cyst. A **caesarean** section may be needed for safe delivery. **Expert neonatal** care should also be available.

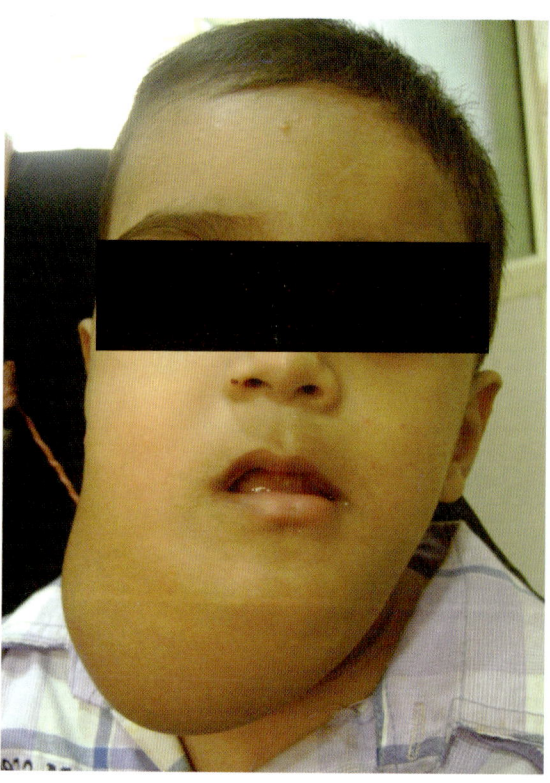

Fig. 7.6: Cystic hygroma in a child.

Multiple Choice Questions

1. During surgery of Branchial fistula which of the following CRANIAL NERVES are at risk of injury?

   (*a*) 9th 10th 11th

   (*b*) 10th 11th 12th

   (*c*) 8th 10th 11th

   (*d*) 9th 11th 12th

   Answer (*d*)

2. In a Sistrunk operation for Thyroglossal cyst a portion of what is removed?

   (*a*) Cricoid Cartilage

   (*b*) Hyoid Bone

   (*c*) Thyroid Cartilage

   (*d*) 1ˢᵗ Ring of Trachea

   Answer (*b*)

3. The MOST COMMON site of a Branchial Fistula in relation to the Sternomastoid Muscle is

   (*a*) Anterior Border of Middle Third

   (*b*) Posterior Border Middle Third

   (*c*) Anterior Border Upper Third

   (*d*) Posterior Border Upper Third

   Answer (*a*)

4. A Branchial Cyst usually arises as a remnant of which BRANCHIAL ARCH?

   (*a*) FIRST

   (*b*) SECOND

   (*c*) THIRD

   (*d*) FIFTH

   Answer (*b*)

5. The most common location for a Thyroglosssal Cyst is

   (*a*) Midline and Suprahyoid

   (*b*) Midline and Subhyoid

   (*c*) Right Lateral and Suprahyoid

   (*d*) Right Lateral and Subhyoid

   Answer (*b*)

6. Complications of a Thyroglossal Cyst will include all of the Following **EXCEPT**

   (*a*) Infection

   (*b*) Thyroglossal Fistula

   (*c*) Compression of Trachea

   (*d*) Malignancy

   Answer (*c*)

7. The usual relation of a Branchial Cyst to the STERNOMASTOID muscle is

   (*a*) Anterior and Deep

   (*b*) Anterior and Superficial

   (*c*) Posterior and Deep

   (*d*) Posterior and Superficial

   Answer (*a*)

8. The INTERNAL OPENING of a Branchial Fistula can be seen at

   (*a*) Foramen Caecum

   (*b*) Tonsillar Fossa

   (*c*) Anterior Tracheal Wall

   (*d*) Lateral Oesophageal Wall

   Answer (*b*)

A CASE OF THORACIC OUTLET SYNDROME

Chief Complaint

Pain radiating along the **left upper limb** of **six months** duration and **blackish discoloration** of the **left index finger** of **one month** duration.

Occupation

- **Home maker**.

History of Present Illness

A **32-year-old woman** presented to the Surgical OPD with the complaints of **pain** along the **left upper limb** of **six months** duration. Initially, the **pain** used to appear on **doing work** at home. It was **cramp** like and was felt in the **fore arm and the hand**. The pain was **relieved** on **taking rest**. The **intensity** of pain gradually **increased** over a **period of time**. She also felt that the **pain** was **radiating** from the **shoulder till her fingers**. The pain was **severe** enough to **disturb her sleep**.

About a **month** ago she developed **pain** even at **rest**. The pain was **very severe** and she was **not able** to do any **work** with the **left hand**. She noticed **darkening** of the **tip** of the **left index finger** at the same time. Over the period of **one month**, the **entire finger** had become **black.**

Further questioning revealed that she used to get **attacks of tingling** and **numbness** in **left upper limb** for the last **one year**. She had also noticed some **weakness** of her **left hand**.

Past, personal and family histories were insignificant.

Treatment History

She was taking **analgesics** regularly. She also had several **injections (combination of Vit.B1, B6 and B12) without** any **relief.** When the **finger** appeared **dark,** her **doctor advised** her to attend a **major hospital**, but she **delayed matters** by one more **month.**

General physical examination was essentially **normal.**

Local Examination of Left Upper Limb

There was **wasting** of the **muscles** of the **forearm and hand**. The **power** was **Grade 3**. There were areas of **paraesthesia** along the **medial aspect** of the **forearm** and **hand.** There was **no sensory deficit**.

Signs of **ischaemia** were present, such as loss of hair, irregular nails and **loss of fat** in the pulp of the fingers. The **limb** below the elbow was **cooler**, compared to the right side. The **subclavian, brachial and radial pulsations** were **weak.** There was no palpable thrill in the supraclavicular region.

The **index finger** showed signs of **dry gangrene** with a **well-defined line of demarcation.**

Examination of the **neck** revealed a **hard, irregular fixed swelling** at the **root** of the neck placed **above the clavicle**. The **supraclavicular region** was slightly **tender.**

There was no palpable thrill in this region.

Examination of the cardiovascular system (**CVS**) was **normal.**

Q. 1. **What was the clinical diagnosis?**

The presence of **neurovascular symptoms and signs** along with a **palpable hard fixed swelling** at the root of the neck, probably a **cervical rib,** made the diagnosis of **thoracic outlet syndrome** easy.

Q. 2. **What were the investigations done in this patient?**

X-ray of the neck showed **bilateral complete cervical ribs**.

Duplex US. The **lumen** of the **subclavian artery** was **narrowed by 90%.** There was a **post-stenotic dilatation** with a **mural thrombus**. There was **minimal flow** in the **brachial and radial** arteries.

CT angiogram was done. It **confirmed** the **US findings**. **Grossly dilated collaterals** were seen in the **scapular** and **shoulder regions.**

Setting: A week later.

Q. 3. **What was the treatment planned for the patient?**

Excision of the **cervical rib** along with **excision** of the **involved segment** of the **subclavian artery** and **replacement** by a **long saphenous vein graft** was planned. A **supraclavicular incision** was made dividing the **skin and platysma**. **Division** of the **scalenus anterior** muscle **exposed** all the **important structures**. Taking **care** not to **injure** the **vital structures,** the **cervical rib** was **excised**. The **diseased segment** of the **subclavian artery** was **excised** and **replaced** with an **autogenous saphenous vein** graft. The patient showed **remarkable improvement** after **surgery**. A **week** later, the **gangrenous index finger** was removed by **disarticulation** at the **metacarpophalangeal joint.**

The **patient** was asked to attend the **physiotherapy department** after all the **incisions had healed.** **She** was to be **trained** to use the **hand without the index finger.** **She** had to learn **exercises** to improve **the power** of the **wasted muscles.**

Q. 4. **What is thoracic outlet syndrome (TOS)?**

It is a **classical misnomer** in surgery. It is a **clinical condition** resulting from **compression** of the **neurovascular structures** at the **thoracic inlet.** It should have been rightly called as a **thoracic inlet syndrome (TIS).**

Q. 5. What is the surgical anatomy of this region?

The **space** basically consists of the **cervicoaxillary canal** for the **passage** of **neurovascular structures** from the **neck** to the **upper limb.** It is broadly divided into **three anatomical spaces.** They are from **medial to lateral,** the **interscalene triangle,** the **costoclavicular triangle** and the **subcoracoid** or the **postpectoralis minor space.** Since the **clinical presentation** of **TOS is** due to **changes** in the **interscalene triangle,** it will be explained in **detail.** The **space** is **bound** by the **scalenus muscle anteriorly.** The muscle **arises** from the **anterior tubercles** of the **transverse processes of C III, IV, V and VI** vertebrae and is **inserted** to the **scalene tubercle** in the **first rib.** The **posterior wall** is formed by the **scalenus medius** muscle. It **originates** from the **posterior tubercles** of the **lower six cervical vertebrae** and is **inserted** to the **first rib behind** the **scalene tubercle.** The **scalenus posterior** is the **smallest** of the three scalene muscles and is **placed**

posteriorly. It arises from the **posterior tubercles** of the **lower two or three cervical vertebrae** and is **inserted** to the **second rib.** It is **occasionally fused** with the **medius muscle.** The **floor** is **formed** by the **first rib.** It is a **narrow triangular dynamic space.** This **narrow space** may be the **price a human being probably pays** for assuming a **biped position** as compared with the **four legged animals.** The **vertical posture** has resulted in **a posterior shift** of the **scapulohumeral region,** causing **narrowing** of the **cervicoaxillary canal.** The **space contains** the **brachial plexus** and the **subclavian artery.** The **trunks** of the plexus arising from **C8 and T1 nerves** are **within this space.** The **subclavian vein** lies in a more **anterior plane** and is **not affected** by **changes in the interscalene triangle. Various anatomical abnormalities** have been **described that** result in **neurovascular compression** within **the triangle. Imaging studies** even in **normal persons** have **shown** that **changes in the position of the shoulder joint** may cause **narrowing** of the **space,** especially during **hyperabduction and extension.**

Box 7.14:	Points regarding the interscalene triangle

- Most medial part of the cervicoaxillary canal
- Narrow triangular space
- Boundaries –
  - Anterior: Scalenus anterior muscle
  - Posterior: Scalenus medius muscle
  - Floor: First rib
- Contents – Trunks of C8 and T1 – Subclavian artery
- Dynamic space – Further narrowing with postural changes

Q. 6. What are the abnormalities associated with TOS?

They may be classified as **congenital** and **acquired. Acquired** causes are uncommon. They include **exostosis** or **fracture** of the **first rib.**

Congenital causes:

(*a*) **Bone:** A **complete cervical rib** extending from the **transverse process of C7** vertebra to the **first rib.**

An **incomplete rib** with an enlarged **bulbous tip.**

An **incomplete rib** with a **fibrous band** connecting it to the **first rib.**

A very **prominent transverse process** of **C7** vertebra.

(*b*) **Muscle: Hypertrophied** or **prominent scalenus anterior** muscle (**scalenus anticus syndrome**).

Abnormal anterior insertion of the **scalenus medius,** close to the **scalene tubercle.**

The **nerves** passing through the **substance** of the **scalene muscles.**

(*c*) **Soft tissues:** Various types of **abnormal fibrous bands** have been described in this region **in isolation** or associated with **scalene abnormalities**.

A **post-fixed brachial plexus** is more prone to develop this condition.

But the **mere presence** of these abnormalities **may not result** in **TOS.** For example, **1% of the population** has a **cervical rib. Neurological symptoms** are seen in **10% of these persons. Vascular symptoms** occur only in **1%.**

Box 7.15:	Points regarding the factors associated with TOS

- Acquired – Uncommon – Exostosis or fracture first rib
- Congenital – Bone – Complete cervical rib – Incomplete – Bulbous tip – Fibrous band
- Muscle – Prominent scalenus anterior – Anterior insertion of scalenus medius – Nerves passing through the substance of the muscles
- Anomalous fibrous bands
- Post-fixed brachial plexus – More likely to have symptoms

Q. 7. What are the symptoms of TOS?

The **symptoms** may be **grouped** under **three heads.**

1. **Nonspecific symptoms:** Patients have **pain radiating down** the **shoulder**. It is often **dragging** in nature. Movements like **hyperabduction** may make the **symptoms worse.** Many patients complain that the **intensity of pain** is more **severe at night. Certain occupations** are commonly **associated** with this **clinical picture. Carrying heavy loads overhead** is one such example. In **thin women, carrying heavy weights by both hands** causes **drooping of the shoulder** and may **precipitate** the **symptoms**. At this stage, most **often signs** are **conspicuous** by their **absence.**

2. **Neurological symptoms:** These are **more frequently** seen **than vascular** symptoms.

   Pain along the **inner aspect** of the **limb** is a **common complaint**. It may be quite **severe**. In addition they have **tingling sensation** along this region. Some patients show areas of **numbness** in the limb. At a **later stage** they have **weakness** of the **muscles**

   especially of the **hand** and the **forearm.** They may find it **difficult** to continue to do their **daily activities**.

3. **Vascular symptoms:** These patients have **cramp** like **pain** involving the **muscles** of the **distal part of the limb**. They may have severe **night cramps. Rest pain** develops at a **later stage. Untreated patients** go on to the stage of **gangrene**. It is usually limited to the **digits** and is the result of **repeated attacks** of **microembolisation** from a **thrombus** in the **subclavian artery**. There may be a palpable thrill or a bruit on auscultation in the supraclavicular region.

Box 7.16: Points regarding history in TOS
• Nonspecific – Dragging pain down the shoulder – Worse at night
• Related to occupation
• Neurogenic – Pain – Medial aspect – Tingling and numbness – Weakness of muscles
• Vascular – Cramps during muscular activity – Rest pain – Gangrene

Q. 8. What are the clinical findings in TOS?

Cervical rib: It is felt as a **bony-hard, fixed and irregular swelling** above the **medial part** of the **clavicle. The upper and lower borders** are **well felt**. There may be **tenderness** around the swelling.

In the **nonspecific group**, there may **not** be any **clinical signs**. **Vague tenderness** may be present in the **supraclavicular region**. There may be **limitation** of **movements** of the **shoulder joint** and **scapula** due to **pain**. Most of the **special tests** described below are **negative** in this group.

Neurological signs: There may be **areas of paraesthesia** along the **medial aspect** of **the limb.** The **power** in the **small muscles** of the **hand** may be **grade 4 or 3.** **Wasting** of the **small muscles** of the **hand** is a **cardinal feature**. **Sensory deficit** is either **absent** or may be **confined** to the **medial aspect** of the **hand** and the **medial two fingers**. This is due to the **overlapping** of **sensory areas** in this region.

Vascular signs: These are the **result of ischaemia** in the limb. This group has the **maximum morbidity** due to **TOS**. It could be due to a **thrombotic** or **embolic phenomenon** in the **subclavian artery. Ischaemic neuritis** of the **brachial plexus** may produce a **mixture** of **neurogenic** and **vascular signs**. The **skin** appears **shiny. Hair loss** is often present. The **nails** are **misshapen. Capillary filling time** is **prolonged.** The **pulp** of the fingers appears **flattened** due to **loss of fat.**

The **distal part** of the **limb** may feel **cooler** as compared with the normal side.

Weak or absent pulses are **important clinical features**. The pulsations of the **radial, brachial** and **subclavian** arteries are to be examined. There may be a palpable thrill or a bruit on auscultation in the supraclavicular region. The **BP** may be less by **20 mm hg** as compared to the **opposite side**.

Patients presenting **late** to the hospital have **dry gangrene**. It is usually confined to the **digits**. The **index finger** is most **often involved**. In **fully evolved cases** a **line** of **demarcation** is seen at the **base of the finger**. It is the **presence** of an **excellent collateral circulation** that **minimises** the **tissue loss** to the **fingers**.

Box 7.17:	Points regarding the clinical findings

- Palpable cervical rib – Supraclavicular tenderness
- Paraesthesia – Reduced muscular power – Wasting – Sensory deficit – Absent or minimal
- Weak or absent peripheral pulses – BP 20 mmHg less
- Thrill and bruit in the supraclavicular region.
- Signs of ischaemia – Dry gangrene – Digits

Q. 9. What are the special tests performed in cases of TOS?

Adson's test: The patient is made to **sit** and **turn his face** to the **affected side**. The **radial pulsations** are felt at the wrist. It may be **normal or weak**. The patient is asked to take a **deep breath**. The **limb** is then **hyperabducted** and **extended**. **Loss** of **radial pulsations** is taken as a **positive result**.

Roo's test: The patient is made to **sit** with the **shoulders abducted to 90%** and the **elbows flexed** to the **same extent**. The patient is asked to **open and close the hand** repeatedly for about 2 to 3 minutes. Appearance of symptoms indicates a positive test.

Wright's test: With the **patient sitting**, the **limb** is **hyperabducted overhead**. The patient is asked to take a deep breath and rotate the neck to the opposite side. At a certain **position**, the **radial pulsations** may become **weak** or **absent**. At this stage, the **symptoms** also become **worse**.

Halstead's test: The **examiner** palpates the **radial pulse** and **applies downward traction** on the **extremity**. The patient is made **to extend the neck** and

rotate it to the **opposite side**. **Absence** of the **radial pulse** is taken as a **positive result**.

Cyriax's release test: All the **tests** mentioned **earlier** are **provocative tests**. This **test** is **performed** to bring about **relief of symptoms**. The **examiner stands behind** a **sitting patient**. The **elbows** are **flexed at 90%**. The **examiner lifts both elbows raising** the **shoulders,** thus **relaxing** the **neck muscles**. **Relief** of **symptoms** is taken as a **positive result**.

Box 7.18:	Points regarding the special tests
• Adson's test	
• Roo's test	
• Wright's test	
• Halstead's test	
• Cyriax's release test	

Q. 10. What are the limitations of the special tests?

None of the **tests** are **reliable totally**. **Both false negatives** and **false positives** are **very common**. A **diagnosis of TOS** is made by **excluding other conditions** with a **similar clinical presentation**. **Specific investigations** are needed to **confirm** that the **clinical picture** is due to **TOS**. Hence with the **availability** of various **imaging modalities**, the **significance** of these **tests** is **markedly reduced**.

Q. 11. What are the changes in the subclavian artery in the presence of a cervical rib?

It is very important to **understand these changes** before proceeding to **investigations** and **management of TOS**. The **second part** of the **artery** lies immediately **behind** the **scalenus anterior muscle**. When a **rib is present**, it **encroaches** on **this space** and causes **compression** of the **vessel**. In addition, due to **constant mechanical irritation** there is **intimal damage**. This may lead to an **inflammatory reaction,** leading to **fibrosis** and **thickening** of the **arterial wall. Compression** along with **thickened wall reduces the lumen** to a **great extent. Intimal damage** may also **result** in **thrombosis** of the vessel. If the **thrombus gets organised**, there is **total obliteration** of the **lumen** distal to the **origins** of the **vertebral** and **internal thoracic (mammary) arteries.**

The **changes** in the **artery distal to the stenotic segment** are more **interesting.** One would expect a **proximal dilatation.** But the **artery** commonly shows a **post-stenotic dilatation. The exact mechanism** for this change is **not known.** The following are the **three explanations** offered for this phenomenon.

1. The **vasoconstrictor sympathetic fibres** are found in the form of a **plexus** around the **adventitial coat** of the vessel. Due to **constant mechanical rub** of the **artery** against the **rib,** these **fibres** may be **destroyed,** resulting in a **reflex dilatation** of the **distal segment.**

2. When **blood exits** the **narrow segment** of the artery, it is at a **higher velocity (Venturi effect).** This **narrow jet-**like stream **hits the arterial wall** at a **particular point.** The **wall becomes weaker** at this point and **undergoes dilatation.**

3. When **blood flows** through the **stenotic segment** it **induces vibrations.** These **vibrations** are known to **weaken the elastin fibres** and may **destroy links** between the **collagen fibres weakening the arterial wall.** The artery becomes **more distensible** resulting in **dilatation.**

The process of continous dilatation ultimately leads to the formation of an **aneurysm. Eddying and pooling** of blood **within** the **aneurysm** leads to the formation of a mural thrombus. **Microemboli** derived from this **thrombus** may **block the digital** arteries, which are **end arteries,** resulting in **gangrene.** In many **patients digital gangrene** may be the **first manifestation of TOS.**

Q. 12. Why are the investigations needed in TOS?

A **diagnosis** of TOS is made by a **process of exclusion.** **Neurological symptoms** may be due to **diseases** of the **cervical vertebrae** such as **intervertebral disc (IVD) prolapse** or **spondylitis with radiculitis.** Carpel tunnel **syndrome** may cause **wasting** of the **small muscles of the hand. Atherosclerosis** is a very **common disease.** If it **involves** the **subclavian artery,** the **vascular symptoms** may be the **same** as of **TOS. Vasculitis** as a part of **connective tissue disorders** may also cause some **confusion.**

Q. 13. What are the investigations?

1. **X-ray of the neck.** It may show a **complete or incomplete rib.**

2. **X-ray AP and Lateral views** of **cervical vertebra** to rule out **IVD prolapse** and **spondylitis** is a **very important investigation.**

3. **Patients** with **neurogenic symptoms** need **nerve conduction studies.** A **conduction deficit** across the **diseased segment** provides **objective proof** of nerve compression in TOS. This is **mandatory** before **cervical explorations** are carried out.

In patients with **vascular symptoms,** the **following investigations** are performed.

4. **Duplex US.** It demonstrates the **state of the subclavian artery. Stenosis** as well as **post-stenotic dilatation** with an **aneurysm** formation is identified. Presence of a **thrombus** in the **aneurysm** is also made out. The **diminished flow** in the **distal arteries** is demonstrated. It can also be used **postoperatively** to study the **patency** of a **graft or stent,** if they have been used during the **operation.**

5. **CT angiogram:** The **arterial system** is **clearly defined** by this **investigation.** It is **needed** if **interventional measures** on the subclavian **artery** are being **planned.** The changes in the subclavian artery described above are more accurately defined. Presence of **dilated collateral vessels** is well **detected** by this investigation.

6. **MRI angiogram** is the **preferred modality** of **imaging** preoperatively. It not only demonstrates the **state of the blood vessels,** but also gives a clear **picture** of the **soft tissue abnormalities** in the region. It is the **template** on which the **treatment strategies** are planned.

Box 7.19:	Points regarding investigations

- X-ray neck – Cervical rib – Complete or incomplete
- AP and lateral X-ray cervical vertebra – IVD prolapse – Spondylitis – Osteophytes
- Nerve conduction studies
- Duplex ultrasound
- CT angiogram
- MRI angiogram

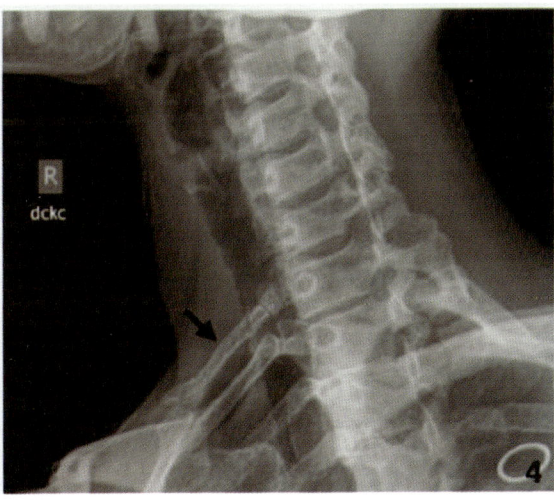

Fig. 7.8: X-ray showing a cervical rib.

Q. 14. Is the presence of a cervical rib an indication for treatment?

The answer is **no. Most persons** with **cervical ribs** pass through a **normal life span without** having any **problem.** Even when a **rib is present**, it is necessary to **prove** that the **symptoms are due to the rib** in the **nonspecific group**. The **rib** is to be **treated** in the **neurogenic** and **vascular groups**, after establishing the diagnosis.

Q. 15. What are the treatment strategies?

In the **nonspecific group**, the treatment is **conservative**. **Physiotherapy** and **exercises** to **improve the shoulder girdle muscles** play an integral part in the treatment. **Measures to relax the neck muscles** are helpful. **NSAIDS** may be needed for **pain relief**. The **sleeping posture** should avoid **abduction** and **extension** at the shoulder. **Change of occupation** becomes necessary for a **few patients.**

Neurogenic group: **Decompression** is obtained by **excision** of the **first rib**. A **transaxillary approach** (Roo's) avoids important structures like the **subclavian artery** and **T1 nerve**. **Postoperative physiotherapy** is advised for these patients. If **abnormalities** in relation to the **scalene muscles** or **fibrous bands** have been demonstrated on **MRI scan**, a **supraclavicular incision** is preferred. A **scalenotomy** and division of the **fibrous bands** relieve the **pressure** on the **nerves.**

Vascular group: The **operation** is carried out via the **supraclavicular route**. An **incision** is **made above and parallel** to the **clavicle.** The **skin and platysma** are incised. The **supraclavicular fat** is dissected. The **external jugular vein** is **ligated** and **divided. Incising** the **investing layer** of the **deep fascia** exposes the **scalenus anterior muscle**. The **phrenic nerve** running downwards on the muscle is **retracted** and the **muscle is divided**. The **cervical rib,** the **subclavian artery** and the **T1** nerve are now **visible.** The **rib is resected**. The **diseased segment** of the subclavian artery (**stenotic and post-stenotic dilated segment**) is **excised** and **replaced** by an **autogenous saphenous vein graft.** A **prosthetic graft** can also be used.

Q. 16. **What are the recent advances in the management of TOS?**

For patients belonging to the **neurogenic group,** **injections of botulinum toxin** into the **scalenus anterior and medius muscles** under

electromyographic guidance have been **tried.** It causes **paralysis of the muscles** for a period of about **six months**. It has shown **good results** in some centres.

Percutaneous endovascular stent placement has shown **good response** in patients having **vascular symptoms** with a **short segment stenosis** of the **subclavian artery**.

Box 7.20: Points regarding treatment
• Nonspecific – Conservative – Physiotherapy – Relaxation exercises – NSAID
• Neurogenic – Cervical rib – Transaxillary resection of first rib
• Scalene abnormality and fibrous bands – Scalenotomy – Release of bands
• Vascular – Scalenotomy – Cervical rib resection – Excision of segment of subclavian artery
• Reconstruction – Replacement graft – Saphenous Vein – prosthetic
• Recent trends – Botulinum toxin injection – Endovascular stent

■ ■ ■

Abdomen

8

EXAMINATION OF AN ABDOMINAL LUMP

The abdomen is the seat of many **important structures;** therefore, the **clinical presentations** of different **diseases** are likely to be very **varied.** In many instances a **lump** is noticed only at a **late stage** of the **disease.** It is likely that in the **times to come, patients** may present only with **symptoms and** hardly any **clinical signs.** Hence **imaging** and other **investigations** will be needed to come to a **diagnosis. A detailed history** therefore becomes **very important. Choosing** the appropriate **investigation** and **planning the management** depends to a large extent on the history obtained from the patient. Abdomen is a vast topic and in this chapter only a **general list** of **symptoms** and **signs** are described.

Pain

This is the **commonest symptom**

Site

Epigastric pain suggests diseases of the **stomach and duodenum. Pancreatic** **pain** is seen in the **epigastrium** and around the **umbilicus**.

Right hypochondrium. Diseases of the **liver, gall bladder** and **head of pancreas** lead to pain in this **quadrant**.

Lumbar pain usually refers to diseases of the **kidney.**

Periumbilical pain occurs in **small bowel disease.** When the **transverse colon** is the seat of disease, the **pain** is felt in the **same region**.

Right iliac fossa (RIF). Pain in this region is the result of diseases of the **right side of** the **colon.**

When the **sigmoid colon** is involved in a **disease process,** the pain is felt in the **left iliac fossa.**

Hypogastric pain is associated with diseases of the **urinary bladder**.

Nature of Pain

Colicky pain is most frequent. It suggests **spasm** of the **circular muscle** fibres of a **hollow viscus. Periumbilical**

colic is felt when the **small bowel** is **affected**.

Biliary colic is felt in the **right hypochondrium** and lasts for **several hours**.

Renal colic, on the other hand, is felt in the **lumbar region** and is transient lasting for a **few minutes**.

Burning pain is a manifestation of **acid peptic disease**. These patients are seen in the surgical wards only when complications like **penetration** of an **ulcer** to the underlying **pancreas** or **gastric** outlet **obstruction** (GOO) occurs. **Dull aching** or **dragging pain** suggests **gradual enlargement** of a **solid** organ like **liver** due to **stretching** of the **capsule.**

(*a*) **Constant unbearable** pain occurs in **late stages** of **intra-abdominal malignancy.**

(*b*) A **ball-rolling sensation** may be mentioned by some patients. This usually **precedes attacks** of **vomiting**.

Intensity

Intensity of pain may be described as **mild, moderate or severe**.

Radiation of Pain

Radiation is described as **extension** of pain from the original site to **another area**, and is due to **reference** along the **nerves. Pancreatic** pain **radiates** to the **back** when the **splanchnic plexus** is involved.

Referred Pain

Biliary pain is referred to the **shoulder** because the **diaphragm,** which is in **close proximity** to a **diseased gall bladder,** and the skin over the **shoulder** have the **same innervation** from **C4 nerve**.

Renal colic radiates from the **loin to the groin. Testicular pain** radiates to the area around the **umbilicus**. The **testis originates** at

T10 level and therefore the pain is **referred** to this **region.**

Aggravating Factors

(*a*) **Food** is the most **common aggravating factor** for diseases involving the **upper abdominal** organs. **Chronic gastric ulcer** and **carcinoma** of the **stomach** produce this **symptom. Fatty food** is said to aggravate the **pain** in **gall bladder disease,** but this is an **unreliable symptom.**

(*b*) **Posture: Pancreatic pain** is worse in the **supine position** due to the **close proximity** of the **pancreas** to the **splanchnic plexus** of nerves.

(*c*) **Jolting movements** make **pain** due to **renal calculi worse**.

Relieving Factors

The commonest is **medication. Antispasmodics** relieve most types of fcolicky pain.

(*a*) **Change of posture:** Patients with **chronic pancreatitis** feel much

better when they are made to **sit bent well forward**, since the **pancreas falls away** from the **splanchnic plexus.**

(*b*) **Vomiting** may **relieve** the pain **partially**, if there is an **obstructive element.**

Vomiting

This symptom is often **associated** with **obstruction** to **a hollow viscus**.

1. **Vomiting** can either be **spontaneous** or **induced.**

   Some **patients** realise that **vomiting relieves** their **symptoms** and hence **induce vomiting** by **tickling** the **fauces,** thereby **stimulating** the **vagus** nerve. But in **most patients** it is **spontaneous.**

2. **Contents:**

   (*a*) The **vomitus** may contain **food** that is **undigested** or **partially digested** as seen in patients with GOO**.**

   (*b*) If the **contents** are **retained in the stomach** for a long time, **bacterial action** leads to **foul-smelling contents**.

   (*c*) **Quantity:** The quantity is **large** in the presence of **obstruction**.

   (*d*) **Presence of bile: Nonbilious** vomiting suggests an **obstruction** in the **stomach** or proximal **duodenum. Bilious** vomiting is a manifestation of an **obstruction** distal to the **ampulla of Vater**.

   (*e*) **Faeculent** vomiting seen more often in **acute situations** and is the result of **ileal obstruction**.

   (*f*) **Presence of blood: Coffee ground** vomitus is a classical finding in **diseases** of the **stomach.** The **colour** resembles that of coffee due to the **action of acid on haemoglobin**. But **bright red blood** is seen in massive bleeds.

   (*g*) **Relief of symptoms:** As mentioned earlier, the symptoms may be **relieved partially** or **completely** following **episodes** of **vomiting**.

Abdominal Distension

This could be the result of **either gas or fluid** retained in a part of the gastrointestinal (**GI) tract** or **ascites**. **Upper abdominal distension** is described in GOO. **Distension around the umbilicus** is the complaint seen in **small bowel obstruction**. In **chronic large bowel obstruction**, the distension is usually **generalised,** but more **pronounced along the flanks. Ascitis** leads to **distension of the whole abdomen** unless there is a **localised collection** of fluid as seen in **tuberculous abdomen**.

Bowel Habits

Constipation

Constipation associated with a **malignancy** reflects an **obstructive element**. **Alternating constipation with diarrhoea** is the classical symptom of a **colonic malignancy**. **Constipation** is easily explained by the **retention** of **faecal matter proximal to a growth**. But **bacterial action** leads to **liquefaction** of the **accumulated contents** resulting in **diarrhoea**. **Increasing constipation** leading to a **consumption** of **higher dose of laxatives** is described in **cancers** of the **left side of the colon**. But this is not commonly seen in our patients. **Patients** with **rectal cancer** complain of tenesmus.

Diarrhoea

It is a **nonspecific symptom**. **Carcinoma of the right colon** may manifest with this **symptom**. More often **small bowel disease** produces diarrhoea. "**Spurious**" **diarrhoea** is seen in patients with **rectal cancers.**

Malaena

Black-coloured, tarry semisolid stools with a **typical foul smell** define **malaena. Bleeding from lesions** of the **proximal part of the GI tract** gives sufficient time for **bacteria** to act on this **blood** to produce **malaena**. It is **difficult** to **localise the site of bleed**

from this **symptom** alone. **Carcinoma of** the **right side** of the **colon** is a possibility, especially in the presence of a **lump.**

Lump

A small group of **patients** present with a **lump** as the only complaint. These **lumps** are associated with **either minimal** or **no symptoms. Hepatocellular** and renal carcinomas top the list. Gastrointestinal stromal tumours (**GIST**) and **Neuroendocrine tumours** of the **small intestine** are **rare conditions** that also present with a lump. **Secondary deposits** or nonHodgkins lymphoma (**NHL**) involving the **para-aortic and pre-aortic** group of **lymph nodes** can manifest as a **lump.** In some of these cases, the **secondaries** may be from a **small tumour** of the **testis.**

Jaundice

Jaundice is an important symptom. It suggests **hepatobiliary** or **pancreatic** disease. **Progressive painless jaundice** is a classical manifestation of **malignancy. Intermittent jaundice** suggests **choledocholithiasis.** But there are **exceptions** to this rule.

Fever

High fever with chills indicates **ascending cholangitis** often associated with **biliary stone disease**. Since **tuberculosis of the abdomen is**

still seen in **our country, evening rise of temperature** with **night sweats** may be complained of by these patients. Patients with **renal carcinoma** may present with **fever** as the **main complaint**.

Chronic Cough

Associated **pulmonary tuberculosis** will result in the patient having **chronic cough** and other symptoms **referable** to the **chest**.

Back Pain

Pain in the **lumbar region** could be the result of **two conditions** presenting with an **abdominal lump. Tuberculosis** of the **lumbar vertebrae** could present with a **lump in the iliac fossa** due to a **cold abscess** along the **psoas major** muscle. Again certain **abdominal malignancies** like **renal carcinomas** can **spread** to the **lumbar vertebrae,** leading to **back pain**.

The **list of symptoms** described so far is **not complete**. Additional **information** will be needed **depending on the system** involved in the **disease process** and the **findings** obtained during the **clinical examination**.

EXAMINATION OF THE ABDOMEN

This part of the examination is a **perfect example** for the famous statement made by **Sir William Osler** that medicine is "**ART BASED ON SCIENCE**". A certain degree of **rapport** with the **patient** is an **absolute requisite** for an **accurate examination**.

Inspection

Patient is examined in the supine position.

Proper Exposure

The **entire abdomen** and the **external genitalia** in the **male** should be available for **inspection** in **good light**.

Shape of the Abdomen

This tends to vary with **age and sex.** A **multiparous female** may have a **slightly distended lower abdomen**. **Scaphoid abdomen** is **not** considered to be the **normal shape**.

Umbilicus

The position may be **shifted** and may show **eversion** in the presence of **distension**.

Swelling

A **swelling** may be **visible**. The abdomen is divided into **nine quadrants** for ease of description. The **site and extent** of the swelling is **described** in **relation** to these **quadrants**. The **margins** can be made out in **lesions** that are **superficially placed**. Then the **size and shape** can also be detected. The other inspection findings include the nature of the **surface** of the **lump** and the state of the **overlying skin**.

Fullness in the Abdomen

This term is used when the **margins** of a suspected swelling are **not made out** clearly. The **surface**, **size** and **extent also** cannot be made out clearly.

Dilated Veins in the Abdominal Wall

Periumbilical veins are a manifestation of **portal hypertension**. Grossly **dilated veins** along the **flanks** suggest **inferior venacaval** obstruction. In this case the flow of blood is from below upwards , the veins being connected to the intercostal veins draining to the superior venacava via the azygos system.

Presence of Scars

If present, the nature of the scar is described in detail. **Healing** by **primary intention** results in a **thin linear scar**. If the **scar** is **broad**, **puckered**, **irregular** and **thickened** it indicates healing by **secondary intention**, usually the result of **postoperative sepsis.** Uncommonly, a keloid may be seen. Rarely, in cases of **total wound dehiscence**, the **area** might have been **covered** by a **split-skin graft** (known as healing by **tertiary intention**).

Hernial Orifices

The patient must be made to **stand up** and **cough vigorously**. The appearance of a **swelling** indicates the **presence** of a **hernia**. The **inguinal, umbilical, epigastric** and **paraumbilical regions** are the **common** sites. **Divarication** of the **recti** produces a **diffuse bulge** below the **umbilicus**. If there is a **swelling** in relation to a **scar**, it indicates an **incisional hernia**.

External Genitalia

The presence of both the **testes** must be **noted**. An **absent testis** with a **poorly developed hemiscrotum** suggests an **undescended testis.**

Palpation

This part of the **examination determines** the **expertise** of the **clinician**. **Voluntary guarding** of the **abdominal muscle** makes **palpation difficult.** A patient with an "**interesting**" **lump** becomes a **victim** of a **large number of students**. Such patients tend to become **uncooperative** within a **short period of time**. Few **basic rules** need to be remembered at all times.

(**a**) As mentioned earlier, a **good rapport** with the patient is the **foundation** on which the **entire examination** is based. It is better to **distract** the patient's **attention** with some **interesting conversation**. It may take **some time** to achieve **this goal.**

(**b**) It is always better to **start from an area** that is **farthest** from the likely **site of the disease**.

(**c**) Palpation should be **gentle**.

(**d**) The palpation can be either **superficial** or **deep**. It depends upon the amount of **pressure** applied by the **fingers. Retroperitoneal structures** are deeply placed, and hence need **more pressure** during **palpation** to identify **lumps** located in this **region**.

(*e*) **Lumps deep** to **recti** are **more difficult** to **feel, especially in men** with **muscles** that are very **well developed**.

(*f*) The appearance of a **lump** in many instances indicates a **late stage** of the disease, especially in cases of **malignancy.**

Palpation of the abdomen must be made in a **systematic manner.**

Tenderness

Tenderness is felt more often in **acute situations**. But a **tender lump** demands **extra gentleness** on the part of the **examiner**.

Site, Size and Extent

These three parameters of the lump are **accurately defined** by palpation.

Borders

The borders are **better identified** by palpation. The **upper border** is **not felt** in many swellings arising from organs like liver and spleen because they extend **beyond the costal margin**. **Borders** are **difficult** to feel in **retroperitoneal lumps**.

Surface

It could be **smooth, lobular or nodular** depending on the pathology.

Consistency

A lump could be soft, firm or hard. Deeply placed **soft lumps** are likely to be **missed by a novice**.

Mobility and Anatomical Plane

(*a*) **Intrinsic mobility:** Lumps arising from organs in **direct contact** with or in **close proximity** of the **diaphragm** move **downwards** during **inspiration**. The **liver, spleen, and stomach and the two kidneys** are **directly related to the diaphragm,** and hence demonstrate this **sign clearly**. Both the **greater omentum** attached to the **greater curvature of the stomach** and the **gall bladder** on the **inferior surface of the liver move with respiration** as they are **indirectly related** to the **diaphragm**. This is referred to as **indirect mobility. Lumps in the retroperitoneal** plane are usually **fixed Bulky tumours** arising from the **body or tail of pancreas** may **displace the stomach** and come in contact with the **left dome of the diaphragm** and hence move **downwards** during **inspiration.** But this **movement disappears** usually when the **position of the** patient is **changed**. This has been called as **tree-top mobility.**

(*b*) **Extrinsic mobility:** If the **clinician** is able to **move the swelling** during **palpation,** it is known as **extrinsic mobility. Retroperitoneal lumps** usually have **no mobility.** Mobility is tested both in the **vertical and transverse** directions. It could be either **free or restricted**.

(*c*) **Anatomical plane:** A **swelling** could be **arising** from the **anterior abdominal wall, intra-abdominal or intraperitoneal contents** or the **retroperitoneum.** The **head raising test** or the **straight lower limb raising test** is the first step. If the **swelling becomes more prominent** with **restricted mobility,** it indicates that the plane is the **abdominal wall.** But **swellings deep to the recti** may **cause confusion** and this is **best exemplified** by a **desmoid tumour.** If a **lump falls forward** when the patient is put in the **knee–elbow position,** the plane is **intra-abdominal.** If it retains its **original position,** it is likely to be **retroperitoneal.** But it is now believed that the **test disregards human dignity** and has been **practically given up.** To a large extent, the **same result** can be achieved by **changing the position** of the patient from **supine** to the **right and left lateral positions.** If the lump **shifts** during this manoeuvre, it is likely to be **intra-abdominal.** But these **tests** have **certain limitations**. If an **intra-abdominal lump extends** into the **retroperitoneum,** it may be interpreted as **retroperitoneal** and vice versa.

(*d*) **Palpation of additional lumps** in the rest of the abdomen. **Hepatosplenomegaly** is a **common combination.**

(*e*) **Free fluid in the abdomen:** This is demonstrated by a **fluid thrill.** It is important to keep a **hand** at the **midline** around the **umbilicus** to prevent the **transmission** of the thrill across the **subcutaneous fat** of the **abdominal wall.**

Percussion

Percussion as an aid in the diagnosis of surgical diseases is **under-utilised. Solid organs** like **liver and spleen** are **dul**l on percussion. **Stomach and intestine** are **resonant.** A **dilated stomach** has a **tympanitic** note. An **enlarged kidney** being **covered** by the **colon anteriorly** may have a **band of resonance** across the **lump.**

Shifting dullness is a sign employed to **demonstrate free fluid** in the abdomen. It is based on the fact that **gas-containing bowel** will be **lighter** and will occupy the **central part of the abdomen** and be **resonant** on percussion. The **flanks are dull** due to the **presence of fluid**. When the patient is **turned** to a **lateral position,** the intestines will **move** towards the **flank.** Hence the **flank becomes resonant** and the **dullness shifts** towards the **centre of the abdomen**.

Auscultation

This sign is more **pertinent** in an **acute situation. Normal bowel** sounds are heard in **most of the patients** under discussion. **Auscultopercussion test** is useful in demonstrating a **dilated stomach**. A word of **caution** must be mentioned regarding a "**silent abdomen**". It **occurs** in the presence of **paralytic ileus**. Hence **bowel sounds** are **not heard** on auscultation. But it is not a **silent abdomen** in the **true sense** of the word. The **breath sounds** are **clearly heard** during **auscultation** of the **abdomen**.

Scrotum, Supraclavicular Region and Lumbar Spine (3S)

No examination of the abdomen is **complet**e, if these **three areas** are **not palpated**. The importance of the examination of the **scrotal contents** has already been **stressed**. A **malignant tumour** of the testis can give rise to a **retroperitoneal lump** due to **enlargement** of **pre-** and **para-aortic lymph nodes**.

The **supraclavicular region** is examined for **enlarged nodes**. **Carcinoma of the stomach** is one of the **common malignancies** spreading to the **left supraclavicular node**. The **pathway** of the malignant cells **to**

reach this site runs as follows. All the **lymph** from the **stomach** drains into the **coeliac group** of lymph nodes. This **lymph** in turn is drained into the **cisterna chyli**. The **thoracic duct originating** from this cyst runs across the **left side of the chest** to **drain** into the **circulatory system** at the **junction** of the **left internal jugular vein** and the **left subclavian vein** on **the left side of the neck**. The presence of a **valve** to **prevent reflux** of **blood** into the **duct** acts as a **barrier** for **further spread** of the **malignant cells. Proliferation** of **these cells** leads to the development of a **supraclavicular node**. Since the **cisterna chyli** drains **lymph** from **all the abdominal contents**, the **primary tumour** may also be **arising from other organs**.

In some patients, the **lymphatic drainage** from the **cisterna chyli** occurs along the **right lymphatic duct**. This duct passes via the **right** side of the **chest** to join the **circulatory system** in the **neck** at the **same junction** as described on the left side. Thus the **right supraclavicular region** may show an **enlarged node**. Hence **all patients** with an **abdominal lump** need a **careful examination** of **both sides** of the **neck**.

If the **primary tumour** is in the **testis,** the **route** taken by the **malignant cells** to give rise to a **supraclavicular node** is **different**. The **spread occurs** via the **retroperitoneal and mediastinal nodes**.

Examination of the **spine,** especially the **lumbar** portion, is needed for **two reasons.** A **lump** in the **iliac fossa** could be due to a **cold abscess** secondary to **tuberculosis** of the **spine.** Again certain **abdominal malignancies** like that of the **kidney** can **spread** via the **blood stream** to the **lumbar spine.** The basic examination of the **spine** includes looking for **tenderness, deformity, limitation of movement and spasm of the sacrospinalis** muscle.

Rectal Examination

The **importance** of this test cannot be **overemphasised. Cancers** of the **stomach** and other **intra-abdominal malignancies** spread **transcoelomically** to give rise to **secondary deposits** in the **rectovesical pouch** in the male and the **pouch of Douglas** in a female. They appear as **hard nodular masses** with an **intact mucosal covering.**

Pelvic Examination

It has a **limited role** in general. It is indicated in **multiparous women** with **lower abdominal lumps.**

A **brief description** of the **clinical findings** in relation to the **common viscera** in the **abdomen** is described herewith.

Liver

A **swelling** is seen in the **right hypochondrium** extending to the **epigastrium, umbilicus, left hypochondrium** and the **right lumbar quadrants.** More often only a **fullness is noted**

On **palpation,** the swelling is **located superficially** just **underneath** the **abdominal wall.** It **moves** well with **respiration.**

Since the **liver enlarges vertically** in a **downward direction,** the **palpation** starts in the RIF and then to the **hypochondrium.** It is a **paradox** that **massive enlargements** are **missed** if this **method is not followed.**

The **lower border** is **clearly felt.** It could be **rounded or sharp.**

The **upper border** is **not felt** since the **swelling extends** beyond the **costal margin.** Hence it is **not possible** to insinuate the **fingers between** the costal margin and the **swelling.**

The **consistency varies** with the underlying **pathology.** It is usually **firm or hard.**

The **surface is** either **smooth or nodular.**

It is **dull** on percussion and this **dullness is continuous** with that of the **liver** under the **right costal margin.**

A **bruit** may be heard on auscultation in some **vascular hepatocellular carcinomas.**

Gall Bladder

In **emaciated patients,** it may be **visible** as a **globular** swelling in the **right hypochondrium.**

It is palpable as a **spherical swelling** in relation to the **lower border** of the **liver,** beyond the **lateral margin** of the right rectus muscle.

It feels **firm** but the **consistency** is **different** from that of the **solid liver**. **Independent transverse mobility** is an **important clinical sign.**

It is **dull** on percussion.

Stomach

A **visible gastric peristaltic wave** is seen in the presence of GOO.

On palpation the **lump** is felt in the epigastrium. It may **extend** into the **left hypochondrium and the umbilical regions.**

The **swelling** moves with **respiration.**

The **lower border** is **easily palpable**. The **upper border** may be felt in the **epigastrium**. It is **not felt** if the swelling extends to the **left hypochondrium**.

The **consistency** may vary from **firm to hard** and the **surface** is usually **irregular**.

The **dilated stomach proximal** to a **cancer** of the **pyloric region** may be felt as a **soft boggy** mass.

On **turning the patient** to the **left lateral position**, the **swelling** usually **shifts** towards the **left side** indicating its **intra-abdominal plane**.

On percussion the **lump** is **resonant** or shows **impaired resonance**. In the **epigastrium** this **sign** is **important** to identify a **swelling** arising from the **left lobe of the liver,** which is **dull to percussion**. A **grossly dilated stomach** shows a **tympanitic note** on **percussion**.

Auscultopercussion test is useful to identify a **dilated stomach**.

Spleen

On inspection a **swelling or fullness** is seen in the **left hypochondrium**.

On **palpation,** the swelling is felt in the **left hypochondrium** and appears to be **superficial**. To be **palpable**, the spleen must be **enlarged** at least **three times** its **normal size**. As it **enlarges further**, the **direction is oblique**, towards the **umbilicus** and the RIF. Hence **palpation** for **splenomegaly** also **starts** from the RIF. To identify a **minimal enlargement**, the patient is **turned** on to the **right lateral position**. The **fingers** are placed at the **left costal margin** and the **patient** is asked to take a **deep breath**. The **lower pole** of the spleen may **touch the fingers** at the **height of inspiration.**

The **swelling** moves with **respiration.**

The **anterior border** is **felt clearly**. A **notch** when **felt** along this **border** confirms the **anatomical origin**.

The **swelling** is **dull on percussion** and this **dullness extends** to the **Traube's area** lined by the **left sixth rib** superiorly, the **left anterior axillary line laterally** and the **left costal margin inferiorly**.

Kidney

Inspection

Bulge of the loin. In this examination, the **patient** is made to **sit** and **attention is focused** on the **area** between the **12th rib** and **iliac crest posteriorly**. Normally it is **either concave** or **straight**. A **bulge** at this site **indicates** a **kidney swelling**. In the **supine position**, **fullness** may be seen in the **lumbar region anteriorly**.

Palpation

The **lump** is felt in the **lumbar quadrant**. It may **extend** to the **neighbouring quadrants**. A **large Wilm's tumour** or a **huge hydronephrosis** may occupy **all the quadrants** of the **abdomen**.

The **swelling** moves with **respiration**.

The **lower** and the **anterior borders** are well **made out**. But in **large swellings** especially on the **right side**, the **upper border** may be **under the costal margin** and thus **not palpable**.

The **surface** may be **smooth (hydronephrosis)**, **nodular (malignancy)** or **bosselated (polycystic kidney)**.

The **consistency** is either **firm (hydronephrosis) or hard (malignancy)**.

Kidney swellings in general are **better felt posteriorly** in the **renal angle**, bounded by the **12th rib** and the **lateral border of sacrospinalis**. Since it is also **palpable** in the **lumbar**

region anteriorly, it is **bimanually palpable**. **Ballotability** is a **specific sign** for a **kidney swelling**. The **left hand** is kept in the **renal angle** and is used to **push** the **swelling**. The **lump moves forwards** and is **felt** by the **right hand** placed in the **lumbar region**. The **reasons** for **ballotability** are as follows. The **kidney** has a **narrow pedicle** of **attachment** at the **hilum** consisting of the **renal vessels** and the **renal pelvis.** It is **surrounded by perirenal fat**, which at **body temperature** is **liquid.**

On **percussion** the **renal angle** is **dull. Normally**, this is **resonant** due to the **presence** of the **colon**. As the **kidney enlarges**, it displaces the **colon** and the **area becomes dull**. A **band of resonance** due to the **presence of colon in front** of the kidney is described, but more often the **note** is one of **impaired resonance** thanks to the **small bowel loops** occupying this **region.**

Enlargement of the **opposite kidney** must be **specifically looked for. Polycystic disease** is essentially **bilateral. Obstructions below** the **ureterovesical junction** tend to produce **bilateral hydronephrosis** and **uncommonly,** patients have **bilateral malignant kidney tumours**.

Rectal examination in a male is mandatory. A **benign hypertrophy** of the prostate in an **elderly male** is the **commonest finding.**

Pancreas

Lumps resulting from **pancreatic disease** are either due to a **tumour** or **pseudocysts.**

Tumours

Adenocarcinomas are usually of the **scirrhous type** and a **palpable lump** is seen only in the **late stage** of the disease. These are **deeply placed** with an **irregular surface**. They are **immobile** and show **impaired resonance** on **percussion**. Lesions in the **head of** pancreas appear as **lumps** in the **right hypochondrium** or **umbilical region** and are mostly associated with **obstructive jaundice**, due to **blockage of the common bile duct (CBD).** **Courvoisier's law** is of great help in the diagnosis. Occasionally the **lesions** in the **head** may be **away** from the **CBD** and hence **may not be** associated with **jaundice.** On **percussion,** there is **impaired resonance. Tumours** of the **body** present as **lumps** in the **umbilical** or **left hypochondriac** regions. **Compression** of the **distal stomach** or the **duodenum** may produce the **picture** of GOO. **Transmitted pulsations** of the **abdominal aorta** may be a **helpful sign. Palpable tumours** of the **body and tail** of the pancreas have a **poor prognosis**, since they indicate **advanced malignancy.**

Bulky tumours of the **pancreas** are either **cystadenoma** (**serous,** mostly **benign**) or **cystadenocarcinoma** (**usually mucinous**). They may assume a **large size** to **occupy the entire upper abdomen**. They are **usually fixed,** but may occasionally show **tree-top mobility**. They tend to **remain asymptomatic** until they assume a **large size.**

Computerized tomography (CT) and **endoscopic ultrasonography (US),** when available, are **useful tools** in the **diagnosis**. Accurate **preoperative biopsies** are **feasible** with these **investigations**. In addition, **operability** can also be decided on **CT findings**.

Cancers of the **head of pancreas** need a **Whipple's radical pancreatoduodenectomy**. The **palliative operation** is a **cholecysto-jejunostomy. Tumours** of the **body and tail** of the pancreas are treated by a **distal pancreactetomy** and **splenectomy** along with dissection of the **regional lymph nodes**. The **extent** of pancreatic **resection depends** upon the **location** of the **tumour**. But most of **our patients** reach the **hospital** at an **inoperable stage. Palliative pain relief** can be obtained by **injection of absolute alcohol** into the **splanchnic plexus. Radical total pancreatectomy** is indicated in a **small number** of patients with **multifocal tumours**.

Pseudocysts

These lumps are **commonly** seen in **diseases** of the **pancreas**. Most patients give a **history** suggestive of **acute pancreatitis.** The **time interval** between the **acute stage** and the appearance of the **cyst** is usually a **few weeks. Disruption** of the pancreatic **duct system** due to **autodigestion** by the **proteolytic** pancreatic **enzymes** leads to the **collection** of a **large amount of fluid rich** in these **enzyme**s. The **common site** for such a **collection** is the **lesser sac** of the **peritoneal cavity**. The **communication** between this **sac** and the **main cavity** is via the **foramen of Winslow** (**epiploic foramen**) bounded by the **free border of the lesser omentum** anteriorly, the **inferior vena cava** posteriorly and the **caudate lobe** of the **liver** on the superior aspect, with the **duodenum** forming the lower border. This **opening** is **obliterated** during the **inflammatory process**. Thus a **pseudocyst** is formed. The **absence** of an **epithelial lining** along the **cyst wall differentiates it from a true cyst**. The **anatomical structures surrounding** the **space** form the **boundaries,** and a **thin wall** of **granulation tissue** forms the **lining** of the **cyst** at a **later stage**. This **process** is known as **maturation** of the **cyst**. A typical **pseudocyst lies behind** the **posterior wall** of the **stomach** and the **gastrohepatic omentum.**

The patient **presents** with a **gradually enlarging swelling** in the **upper abdomen,** as the **symptoms** of **acute pancreatitis settle down.** The **epigastrium** and the **left hypochondrium** are the **common sites**. But **bigger cysts** may extend to the **umbilical** and **lumbar** regions.

A **cyst** in relation to the **head of the pancreas** may be felt in the **right hypochondrium**. The swelling has **ill-defined margins**. It is **firm** in **consistency**. It is **immobile**. **Fluid thrill** can be elicited in **most** of these **swellings**. **US** and **CT** are diagnostic. **CT** is more **accurate** in **identifying** the **changes** in the **pancreas** caused by the **previous inflammation**.

A large **majority** of these **cysts undergo spontaneous resolution**. Once the **inflammation resolves**, the **disrupted duct** tends to **heal preventing further secretion,** and the **contents are absorbed**. But **several complications** are described in relation to a **persisting pseudocyst. Secondary infection** is a **dangerous complication. Erosion** of the **splenic vessels** following **sepsis** can be **fatal. Rupture** can lead to **general peritonitis** and a **gradual leak** to the development of **pancreatic ascites**. A **cyst** that **persists** for more than **6 weeks** and is more than **6 cm** in size **needs treatment. Internal drainage** is the **preferred** mode of **treatment. External drainage** has the **risk** of producing a **pancreatic fistula. Endoscopic cystogastrostomy** is the **common method. Laparoscopic** or **open cystogastrostomy** are done **infrequently. Pseudocysts** in relation to the **head of the pancreas** are treated by a **cystoduodenostomy.** If the **cyst is not related** to the **stomach** or the **duodenum,** a **Roux-en-Y cystojejunostomy** is performed. **US-**

guided **catheter drainage externally** is an option in **very sick patients**.

LUMP IN THE RIGHT ILIAC FOSSA

In the **past** these **lumps** posed several **problems** as far as **diagnosis** and **treatment** were **concerned.** The availability of **endoscopy** and **imaging** has made their **management** much **simpler**. Acute conditions like an **appendicular mass or an abscess** are **not discussed** in this section.

Carcinoma of Caecum

There is an **alarming increase** in the **incidence** of **colonic cancer** in **this country** over the **last few decades.** The **rectosigmoid** is the **most common** site followed by the **transverse colon** and **caecum. Malaena** and alteration in the bowel habits with **diarrhoea** are **common symptoms.** A **lump** may be the **presenting feature** in **some** of these **patients. Colonic symptoms** may be **conspicuous** by their **absence** in a **small number of patients. Anorexia, anaemia and asthenia,** described as the classical triad of symptoms of a **carcinoma of the stomach**, may also be **manifestations** of a **right-sided colonic cancer. Pain** occurs at a **late stage** of the disease. **Obstructive symptoms** are **uncommon** because the **lumen is large, the contents are liquid** in **consistency** and the **tumour** is often of the **ulcerative type.**

Clinical Examination

There may be **fullness** in the RIF.

A **lump** is palpable in the **RIF.** It is **not tender.** It is **hard** in consistency. The **surface** is **irregular**. There may be **transverse mobility.** But in **advanced cancers**, the mass is **fixed.**

Free fluid and **liver metastases** may be present in **late stages**

Investigations include a **barium enema** study, which shows an **irregular filling defect** in the **caecum. Colonoscopy and CT scan** have **replaced barium enema** as **investigations of choice. CT scan** is needed to **decide** about **operability. Operable cases** are treated by a **radical right hemicolectomy**. The **structures removed** include about **20 cm** of the terminal ileum, the **caecum, the ascending colon, the hepatic flexure** and the **right one-third** of the **transverse colon.** The **ileocolic and the right colic arteries** are **ligated and divided** close to their **origin** from the **superior mesenteric artery.** The **right branch** of the **middle colic artery** is **divided** close to its **origin**. These measures are **needed** for **complete nodal clearance. The ileal mesentery** and the **mesocolon** of the **involved segment** is **removed,** thus clearing the **epicolic, paracolic, intermediate** and **central group** of **lymph nodes** in **relation** to the **arteries mentioned above.** Since the **ileocolic artery** is **divided**, the segment of the **terminal ileum needs** to be **removed.** The intestinal continuity is established by an anastomosis between the remaining ileum and the transverse colon. In patients with histologically proved positive lymph nodes, postoperative chemotherapy is advised. Gemcitabine and 5-Fluorouracil are the drugs commonly used.

Patients presenting with obstruction are treated by a radical right hemicolectomy if the patient is considered fit for such a procedure. Otherwise, a bypass surgery (ileotransverse-colostomy) is done to relieve the obstruction, followed by a radical resection a few weeks later.

Inoperable cases are treated by an anastomosis between the ileum and the transverse colon to prevent a possible obstruction at a later date, followed by palliative chemotherapy.

Hypertrophic Ileocaecal Tuberculosis

A condition seen frequently in the past, its incidence has come down considerably at the present time. Ingestion of bovine type of M. tuberculosis is said to be the causative factor. Hence it is often not associated with pulmonary tuberculosis. Systemic symptoms may or may not be present. The clinical picture is very similar to that of a carcinoma. Abdominal pain and attacks of diarrhoea are common. Loss of appetite and weight are frequently noted. Fever may not be present in all cases. Before colonoscopy became available it was very difficult to distinguish these two conditions. Barium studies were not always conclusive. An alteration of the ileocaecal angle from that of acute to obtuse was considered diagnostic. This occurs because the caecum is pulled up by the fibrosis induced by chronic inflammation. In addition there is irregular narrowing of the lumen of the terminal ileum and caecum. CT and colonoscopy are performed to rule out malignancy. The treatment is to perform a local resection of the involved ileum and the caecum under antitubercular treatment (ATT) cover. The common combination consists of Rifampicin, INAH and Ethambutol. Anastamosing the ileum with the ascending colon establishes the continuity of the bowel. ATT is continued for about 6 months after the operation.

The pathological picture differs to a large extent from tuberculous lesions in other parts of the body. Caseation is conspicuous by its absence. Intense fibrosis causes marked thickening of the wall of the caecum and narrowing of the lumen. It also results in a palpable mass in the RIF. Ulceration is minimal and superficial. Associated enlarged nodes also do not show caseation. The fibrosis is said to indicate either a less virulent strain of the bacterium or increased resistance on the part of the body.

Amoeboma of Caecum

This also has now become a **rare** condition following **efficient treatment of amoebiasis**. It is a **granuloma** of the **caecum** caused by an **amoebic infestation associated** with **secondary bacterial infection**. The main complaint is **pain in the RIF** associated with **diarrhoea**. Passage of **mucus with blood** is also seen. **On examination,** a tender firm longitudinal **lump** is seen in the **RIF.** The **surface** of the lump is **smooth**. **Demonstration** of *E histolytica* is **not conclusive** of the **diagnosis,** since amoebiasis is **endemic in our country.** If the **mass does not resolve** with **antiamoebic treatment** combined with **antimicrobials**, a **colonoscopy** is **needed. Resections** with a **mistaken diagnosis** are a **thing** of the **past.**

Lymph Node Mass

Enlarged common iliac and **external iliac group** of **lymph nodes** can be felt as a **mass in the RIF. Secondary deposits** are **more common** than NHL. The **primary tumour** may be in the **lower limb (melanoma)** or **external genitalia (carcinoma of the penis).** **Diagnosis** in this group is **easy** because the **primary either** has **obvious symptoms and signs when present or has been treated earlier.** The **mass is present** in the **RIF,** extending down to the **inguinal ligament.** The surface is nodular. The **consistency is variable**. The mass is **fixed. Associated inguinal node enlargement** is very **common**. Evidence of **lymphatic or venous obstruction** in the **lower limb** is seen in the presence of **massive enlargement** of **nodes. External compression** of the **iliac arteries** may produce **weak pulsations** in the **femoral artery.** If needed, a **CT scan** and a **guided core-needle biopsy** may be performed to **confirm the diagnosis**.

Psoas Abscess

Active tuberculosis involving the **lumbar vertebrae** can result in a **cold abscess** tracking along the **psoas major muscle**. This produces a **lump obliquely placed** in the **RIF**. It has a **longitudinal shape** and is **immobile.** The **consistency is soft**. There may be an **extension** into the **inguinal region behind** the **inguinal ligament** due to the **insertion** of the muscle to the **lesser trochanter** of the femur. **Cross fluctuation** can be **elicited** across the **abdominal** and **inguinal components** of the **abscess** under these circumstances. **Examination of the lumbar spine** will demonstrate enough **signs** to clinch the **diagnosis.** Treatment of the **spinal disease** is the **first priority.** The **cold abscess** needs **aspiration. Surgical treatment** of the **primary disease** may also **include** the **complete evacuation** of all the **contents** of the **psoas abscess.**

In **females** a tubo-ovarian (TU) mass is to be **considered** in the **differential diagnosis**. They are associated with **gynaecological symptoms** such as **vaginal discharge** and **menstrual irregularities**. Fever and **chronic right iliac pain** may be **additional symptoms**. US is **beneficial** in the **diagnosis**. Occasionally a **CT** is performed to **rule out malignancy**.

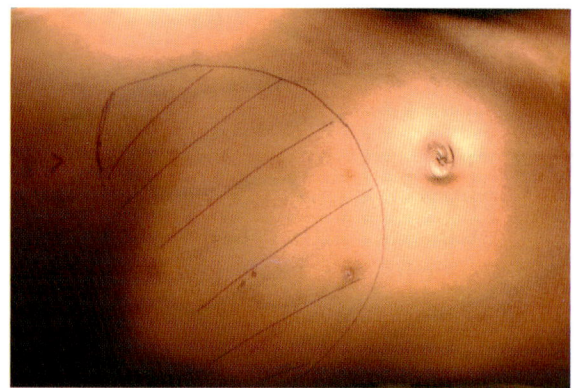

Fig. 8.1: Large retroperitoneal tumour.

Retroperitoneal Sarcoma

An **uncommon condition**, they often present as **large tumours** extending to the **adjacent quadrants**. They remain **asymptomatic** till a **late stage**. **External compression** of the **bowel** or the **ureter** may produce **relevant symptoms**. On **examination,** there is a **lump** of **variable size and consistency**. It is **fixed** to the **deeper structures**. US **followed by CT** is useful in the **diagnosis. CT-guided core-needle biopsy** confirms the **pathological nature** of the tumour. **Liposarcoma** is a **common** variety in this **location. CT chest** may show **secondary deposits. Operable cases** are treated by **wide excision.** But **most patients** have **inoperable tumours** at **presentation.**

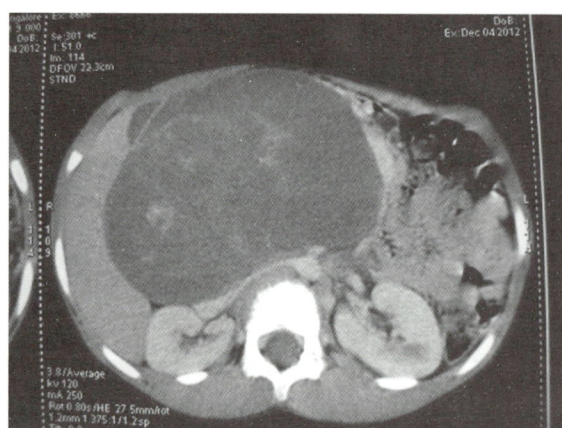

Fig. 8.2: CT scan showing a large retroperitoneal sarcoma.

Aneurysm of the **external iliac artery** and **GIST** are mentioned only to **complete the list.**

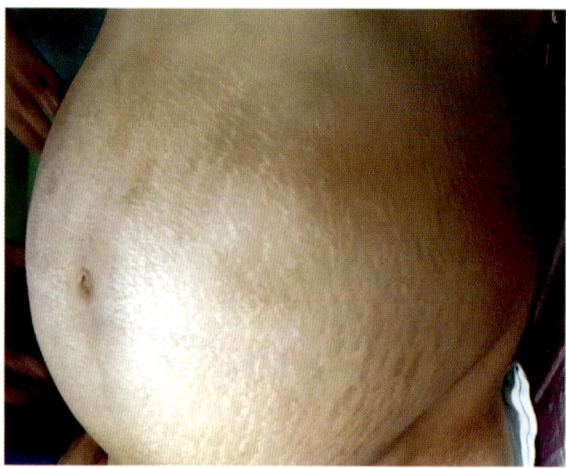

Fig. 8.3: Giant hydronephrosis.

A CASE OF CARCINOMA OF THE STOMACH

Setting

- Surgical outpatient department (OPD).
- A **58-year-old man** presented himself to the OPD with the **following complaints**.
- **Loss of appetite**- 6 months.
- **Upper abdominal distension**- 3 months.
- **Vomiting** – 2 months
- **Loss of weight** – 2 months.

History of Present Illness

This 58-year-old man was having **loss of appetite** for the last **six months**. It was **gradually** becoming **worse**. He had no **special distaste** for any **particular** type of **food.**

He noticed that he was getting **distension of the upper abdomen** after intake of **small quantity** of food. He experienced **early satiety**.

He had been **vomiting** for the last **two months**. Initially the **episodes** used to occur **once in 2 or 3 days**. Recently he has been **vomiting** almost **daily**, about **60 to 90 minutes** after **intake of food**. The **vomiting** was preceded by a **ball-rolling sensation** in the upper abdomen. The **vomitus** contained **partially digested food** and was occasionally **foul smelling. Vomiting** relieved the **upper abdominal distension** to a large extent. There was **no** history of **haematemesis.**

He had **lost weight** in the last **two months**, but was unable to quantify it.

Patient had **mild pain in the upper abdomen** aggravated **after intake of food**. There was no history of **radiation of pain to the back**.

There was no history of **malaena.**

He was **constipated** for the previous two months.

Patient did not give a history of **jaundice**, **fever** or **chronic cough**.

There was no history of **back pain**.

Past History

There was no history of **jaundice** or **acid peptic disease** in the past.

Personal History

He was a **smoker** and used to consume **alcohol** on a daily basis.

Family History

No significant family history.

Treatment History

He had received multiple courses of **H2 blockers, proton pump inhibitors (PPIs)** and **antiemetics without any relief**.

General Physical Examination

Patient was **anaemic** and appeared **poorly nourished**. There were **signs of** dehydration. There was no evidence of **jaundice**, **clubbing of fingers** or **pedal oedema.**

Local Examination

Inspection

The **upper abdomen** appeared **distended. Fullness** was noted in the epigastrium. There were **no dilated veins**. The **umbilicus** was centrally placed and did not show any abnormality.

Succussion splash was heard above the umbilicus.

Following intake of **water**, a **visible gastric wave** was demonstrated moving from the **left to the right** across the upper abdomen, **above the umbilicus.**

The **hernia orifices** and **external genitalia** were normal.

Palpation

A **mass** was palpable in the **epigastrium** extending from 1 cm below the **xiphisternum** to the level of the **umbilicus**. It extended from the **midline** to 2 cm below the **left costal margin** horizontally.

The **upper and lower borders** could be easily **felt,** but the **right** and **left** borders were **ill defined.**

- The **size** was 5 cm by 4 cm.
- The **shape** was **irregular**.
- The **surface** was **irregular** and the **consistency was hard.**

- The mass was seen to **move** with **respiration**.
- There was minimal **transverse mobility**.
- The **plane** was **intra-abdominal**.
- **Liver and spleen** were not palpable.
- A **soft boggy mass** could be palpated to the left of the epigastric mass **below** the **left costal** margin.
- **Fluid thrill** was absent.

Percussion

- The **lump** was **resonant** on percussion. **Shifting dullness** was **absent**.
- **Auscultopercussion** test revealed that the **greater curvature** was about 2 cm **below the umbilicus**.
- Palpation of both **testes** did not reveal any abnormality.
- **Both** the **supraclavicular fossae** did not have any **palpable nodes**
- The **lumbar spine** was normal.
- **Per rectal (PR)** examination was normal.

Box 8.1:	Points to be noted in history

- Loss of appetite - Distaste for a particular type of food.
- Epigastric distension - Early satiety.
- Vomiting – Contents – Relief from symptoms.
- Haematemesis – Malaena.
- Pain – Aggravating and relieving factors – Radiation.
- Loss of weight.
- Jaundice, fever and cough.
- Back pain.

> **Box 8.2:** Points to be noted on inspection
> - Shape and contour of the abdomen.
> - Visible lump or fullness – Site, margins, shape and size.
> - Visible gastric peristaltic wave – Site – Direction – Ingestion of water.
> - Umbilicus – Dilated veins.
> - Hernial orifices and external genitalia.

> **Box 8.3:** Points to be noted regarding rest of the clinical examination
> - Supraclavicular fossae on either side for palpable lymph nodes.
> - PR – Secondaries in rectovesical pouch.
> - Other systems.

Q. 1. What was the clinical diagnosis?

(a) Duodenal stenosis with GOO.

(b) Carcinoma of the pyloric region of the stomach with GOO.

(c) Carcinoma of the head of pancreas with GOO.

(d) GIST in the stomach with GOO.

The correct answer is (**b**).

A chronic duodenal ulcer leading on to **stenosis** was **common in the past.** But most **ulcers** are now **controlled** by drugs like **H2 blockers** and **PPIs. Control of H. pylori** infection has also contributed towards **healing** of duodenal ulcers. The **duration** of the illness is measured in **years.** Hence **duodenal stenosis** causing **GOO** is very **uncommon** at the **present time.**

The **cardinal symptoms** of a **carcinoma of the head of pancreas** are **progressive jaundice** and **itching.** The **lump** when present is **deeply placed** to the **right of the midline** and does **not move with respiration. Liver** is usually enlarged and **palpable** due to **hydrohepatosis.** Symptoms of **GOO** occur at a **late stage. Pain** when present, often **radiates** to **the back.**

GIST is a **rare** condition. But the **stomach** is one of the **commonest organs** involved in this disease. A **large lump** with **minimal symptoms** is a regular feature. A **submucous** GIST can produce **GOO.** But either **haematemesis or malaena** are prominent features at this location.

Carcinoma is the most likely clinical diagnosis. A **short history** of **loss of appetite** along with **epigastric distension** and **vomiting** support the same. The clinical findings of a **lump and visible gastric peristalsis (VGP)** clinch the diagnosis.

Q. 2. What were the investigations done on this patient?

An **upper GI scopy** was performed. It showed a **proliferative growth obstructing the pyloric lumen.** The scope could not be passed beyond this point. The **stomach** was dilated and showed evidence of **gastritis. Residual food** was seen in the lumen. **Multiple biopsies** were taken from the growth.

US abdomen showed **thickening** of the **distal part of the stomach**. No enlarged nodes could be visualised. **Liver** was normal. There was **no free fluid.**

Chest X-ray was normal.

CECT abdomen showed a lesion in the **pyloric region** of the stomach with **enlarged perigastric nodes**. The **fat planes** posterior to the stomach were **intact.**

Blood tests. Hb was 7 gm%. **Serum albumen** was 2.7 gm%

Serum sodium–123 meq. **Chlorides**–72 meq. **Creatinine**–1.4 mg%.

Setting: 3 days later the **biopsy report** was received. It was an **adenocarcinoma.**

Q. 3. **What was the treatment planned for this patient?**

A **lower radical gastrectomy** was the operation of **choice.**

The **patient** as well as the **stomach** was **prepared** for the next **10 days.**

Q. 4. **How was the patient prepared for the operation?**

Dehydration was corrected by **glucose saline** infusions daily. **Urinary output** and **creatinine**

levels were used as guidelines. **Multivitamins** and trace elements were added to these infusions.

Packed red cells were given to bring Hb to **11 gm%**

Albumen was given IV till serum levels were **3.2 gm%.**

Orally, only **fluids** were permitted.

Q. 5. **How was the stomach prepared for surgery?**

Stomach washes were given **twice daily** with a **wide-bore tube. Normal saline** was used for these washes. They were continued till **returns** were **clear.**

Setting: Ten days later.

Both the **patient** and the **stomach** were **fit for surgery**.

Q. 6. **What surgery was conducted on this patient?**

The patient underwent a **lower radical gastrectomy**. The structures removed included the following: the **proximal duodenum**, the **pylorus** and a part of the **body**, **five fingers breadth** beyond the **palpable edge of induration, greater and lesser omenta** and **level I and II lymph nodes. A Billroth II** type of **reconstruction** completed the operation. The patient had a **smooth postoperative** period.

Q. 7. What is the frequency of cancers of the stomach? Cancers of the **stomach** are the **fifth most common** cancers. But they are the **second** most **common** cause of **cancer-related deaths**. Compared to the **West**, gastric cancer is **less frequent** in **India.** But with the **huge population** that we have, the **tumour burden** is quite **large.** Paradoxically, at the **global** level, the **frequency** of this tumour is showing a **downward trend**. Again **unlike** in the West, **distal gastric cancers** are more **common** in our country than the **proximal type**.

Q. 8. What is the frequency of this cancer within the country?

Within the **country**, there is a **marked variation** in its occurrence. The **Northeastern** and **Southern** parts have a much **higher incidence**. This is probably **related** to the **dietary habits** of these people.

Q. 9. What are the important aetiological factors?

1. The disease is more common in **males.**

2. The common age group is between **35 and 55 years**, a **decade younger** compared to the **Western figures**.

3. There is a higher susceptibility in persons of **blood group A.**

4. A **spicy diet** with greater consumption of **chillies** and the intake of **hot food** are factors blamed for the high incidence in our country. The intake of **salted and pickled** food as well as **smoked meat** is an additional factor implicated in the **aetiology**.

5. There is an **increased incidence** in persons who use **tobacco** or consume **alcohol.**

6. Exposure to **H. pylori infection** in the stomach is considered to be an **important factor** in the **causation** of this cancer. But most **Indians** are infected **asymptomatically** in **childhood.** Hence **serological tests** for *H pylori* are **positive** in a **high percentage** of our **population.** Therefore to prove a **cause** and **effect** with reference to H. pylori in gastric cancer is **difficult**. However this **bacterium** has been **proved** to be **significant** in the aetiology of mucosa-associated lymphoid tissue (**MALT**) **lymphoma** of the stomach.

7. **Chronic atrophic gastritis**, which is often associated with **pernicious anaemia,** is a known **premalignant condition**.

8. The risk of a **benign gastric ulcer** undergoing a **malignant change** is now considered to be **very low (0.2%)** probably because of the effective **treatment** of the ulcer by **medication**. **Previous gastric surgery** for **benign disease increases** the **risk.** If a **gastrojejunostomy** or a **Billroth II** type of gastrectomy has been done earlier, the **entry of bile** into the **stomach** has **two deleterious effects**. It **neutralises the acid,** and leads to an increase in the **bacterial flora.** These **bacteria** convert the **dietary nitrates** (from meat etc.) into **nitrosamines**, which are known to be **carcinogenic**. In addition, the **bile** has a **damaging effect** on the **gastric mucosa**, making it more **prone** for a **malignant change**

9. **Menetrier's disease** also increases the risk of malignancy.

Box 8.4:	Points regarding aetiology

- Male preponderance.
- Common in the fourth and fifth decade.
- Blood group A.
- H pylori infection.
- Smoking and consumption of alcohol.
- Spicy diet
- Benign gastric ulcer.
- Menetrier's disease.
- Chronic atrophic gastritis.

Q. 10. Why is family history important in these cases?

An **increase** incidence in other **members of the family** has been described. A **genetic abnormality** is probably the reason for this phenomenon.

Q. 11. How are gastric cancers classified as per their anatomical location? What is the significance?

The study of the **location** of gastric cancers will help to understand the **clinical features** as well as the **rationale of the operative treatment**. Depending on the **site,** they are classified as **proximal (cardia, fundus and proximal body)** and **distal (distal body, antrum and the pylorus)** gastric cancers. A **line** drawn across the stomach at the **level of the incisura angularis** demarcates these **two divisions**. Their **clinical features**, **treatment protocols** to some extent and the **outlook** are **different**

Q. 12. Describe the macroscopic features of gastric cancers.

Macroscopic appearances. The pattern in early gastric cancer (EGC) will be described in detail later. **Borrmann's classification** is used to describe the remaining gastric cancers.

Type I Polypoid growth.

Type II Fungating growth.

Type III Ulcerative growth.

Type IV Diffuse infiltrating type. The tumour **spreads** mostly along the **submucous and subserous** planes of the stomach. It is known as linitis **plastica** and can involve the **entire organ** (**leather bottle stomach**) or can be localised to the **pyloric region** producing a GOO.

Q. 13. What are the histological types of this cancer?

Histologically most are **adenocarcinomas,** and they are divided into three types as per **Lauren's classification**.

(*a*) **Diffuse type (50%):** This is often seen in **females** and **young patients**. These tumours are **aggressive** and have a **poor prognosis**.

(*b*) **Intestinal type (30%):** The epithelium undergoes an **intestinal metaplasia** before a **malignant change** occurs in this group. An association with **H. pylori** infection or a pre-existing **benign gastric ulcer** has been described with this type. In general, the **outcome** is **slightly better.**

(*c*) **Indeterminate type** is uncommon.

Q. 14. What are the modes of spread of gastric cancer?

1. **Direct spread:** The tumour in the initial stages is **confined** to the **mucosa and the submucosa (EGC).** It then spreads across the various **layers of the wall** of the stomach. The **submucous and subserous layers** offer **less resistance** for the **spread** of the cancer. The tumour therefore can spread far and wide along these tissue planes. Once the tumour **erupts** on the **serosal surface**, the chances of **peritoneal dissemination** increase **exponentially**. The cancer tends to involve the **adjacent structures** at a **late stage**. The **omenta**, the **pancreas**, and the **transverse mesocolon** with the **middle colic artery** are the common sites of extension. Rarely the tumour may get adherent to the **transverse colon** and **the left lobe of the liver**.

2. **Lymphatic spread:** This mode of spread has a **direct influence** on the type of **radical resections** performed and the **outcome** in gastric cancer. The **Japanese classification** is accepted universally. The **lymph node stations** are numbered **from 1 to 16**. The **rationale** of **radical lymphadenectomy** is based on this **classification**.

Level N 1 Perigastric nodes belong to this group. They are numbered from **1 to 8.** They include the **right and left cardia nodes**, those along the **lesser and greater curvatures**, and the **supra and subpyloric nodes**.

Level N 2 Nodes from number **9 to 11.** These are nodes present along the **named arteries**. Nodes along the left gastric, right gastric, hepatic, and **splenic arteries** and the celiac trunk as well as the nodes at **the splenic hilum** belong to this group.

Level N 3 (Nodes from number **12 to 15**). This group comprises of nodes along the **hepatoduodenal ligament**, on the **posterior surface** of the **pancreas** and at the **root of the mesentery**.

Level N 4 (number 16). Comprised of nodes belonging to the **para-aortic and the paracolic groups**.

Involvement of the **last two** groups indicates a very **late stage** of the disease.

3. **Blood spread:** Venous blood from the stomach drains into the **portal vein**. Hence the **liver** is the common seat of **secondary deposits.** Spread **beyond** the liver **is rare**.

4. **Transcoelomic or transperitoneal spread:** Once the **serosal surface** is involved, the entire **peritoneal cavity** is exposed for **metastases. Peritoneal deposits** can manifest with **ascites** or **small bowel obstruction. Secondary deposits** are frequently felt in the **rectovesical pouch.** In women of the **reproductive age group**, the **ovaries** are involved, resulting in **Krukenberg tumours.** It must be stressed that this route is **more lethal** when compared with **secondaries in lymph nodes.**

Box 8.5:	Points regarding the modes of spread
• Direct spread – Posterior pancreas, transverse mesocolon, middle colic artery, transverse colon and left lobe liver.	
• Lymphatic spread – No. 1 to 16 .Levels I, II, III and IV.	
• Blood spread – Secondaries – Liver.	
• Transcoelomic – Peritoneal secondaries – Recto vesical pouch.	

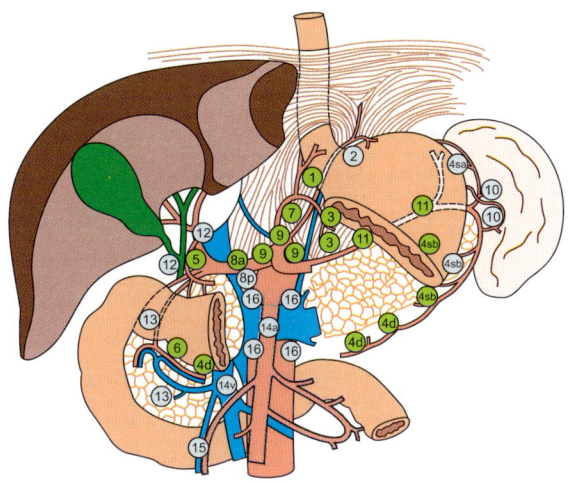

Fig. 8.4: Lymphatic drainage—nodes depicted without the stomach.

Q. 15. What are the changes in the stomach due to gastric outlet obstruction (GOO)?

In patients with GOO resulting from a **pyloric growth**, changes in the **stomach** are **significant**, since all these have to be **corrected before surgical treatment**. The abnormalities seen are as follows.

(*a*) The **ingested food** is **retained in the stomach**. This causes **dilatation of the stomach** resulting in **reduced** muscular **tone**. It sets in a vicious cycle with the stomach becoming **atonic** and **grossly dilated**.

(*b*) In the presence of **achlorhydria,** frequently present in these patients, the **bacteria** tend to **multiply**. These bacteria act on the partially **digested food**

contents, leading to the formation of lactic and butyric acids.

(*c*) The **acids** in turn produce **gastritis.**

(*d*) Due to the **inflammation**, the **mucous and the submucous** layers will become **oedematous,** and the **stomach wall** becomes very **friable**.

If **surgery** is performed at **this stage,** an **anastamotic leak** is very likely, resulting in **fatal peritonitis**.

Box 8.6:	Points regarding changes in the stomach due to GOO

- Retention of food with gastric dilatation.
- Atonic stomach.
- Bacterial action with production of lactic and butyric acids.
- Severe gastritis with oedema and friability of the wall.

Q. 16. What are the clinical features of carcinoma of the stomach?

The symptoms of carcinoma of the stomach are very nonspecific and hence there is invariably a **delay** in the diagnosis. This is especially true in the case of poorly educated **patients who lack health consciousness** and access to **adequate medical resources**.

1. **Dyspepsia de novo in men** after the age of **40 years** should always raise a

suspicion of malignancy. But **dyspepsia i**s such a universal complaint that to **investigate each and every patient** with this complaint is **not practical**.

2. The cardinal symptoms of this malignancy that form the classical triad are **anorexia, asthenia and anaemia.** But the same **objections** mentioned above hold **true** for this group as well.

3. **Feeling of indigestion** with **epigastric discomfort.**

4. Recent **loss of appetite**. A particular **distaste** for **meaty food is** described as an important symptom.

5. **Bloating sensation** in the **epigastrium** after intake of **small quantities** of food (**early satiety**) is frequently seen.

   Most of the **patients** with these set of **vague symptoms** tend to **self-medicate**. Even if they reach the **health professional** at the primary level, **specific investigations** are **rarely performed**, causing further **delay in the diagnosis**.

6. **Unexplained loss of weight** over a **short period** of time.

7. **Pain** is a **late symptom**. It may be the result of a GOO or due to **infiltration of structures in the stomach bed,** leading to **radiation** of the pain to the **back.**

8. **Vomiting**. This is a manifestation of a **distal gastric cancer** producing **obstruction**. The vomiting is **spontaneous** and the contents are **nonbilious**. It may contain **partially digested** food particles and may be **foul smelling**. Vomiting usually **relieves** the pain **partially**. The process is often **preceded** by a **ball-rolling sensation** in the **upper abdomen**.

9. **Haematemesis and malaena** manifest rather **late** in the course of the disease. The **vomitus** is described as **coffee ground** in colour because of the **breakdown of haemoglobin** inside the **stomach**. But **brisk bleeding** results in **bright red blood** in the contents. **Massive haematemesis** is an **uncommon** feature.

10. **Progressive dysphagia** is the primary symptom of a growth in the **cardia.**

11. Some of **our patients** present with a **lump** in the **upper abdomen**.

12. **Symptoms due to metastases** include **jaundice,**

supraclavicular lymph node enlargement and abdominal distension due to ascites.

Q. 17. What are the clinical findings in the abdomen?

(*a*) In the **early stages**, clinical examination does **not** reveal **any abnormality**. **Minimal tenderness** may be felt in the epigastrium. At this stage, the **diagnosis** can only be made with the help of **investigations.** As in the case of many other malignancies, the **number of patients** identified at this level is **extremely low** in **our country**.

(*b*) **Lump in the epigastrium**. Presence of a **lump** is a sign of **advanced disease**. It is described as a **complex mass** because it comprises of a **bulky primary tumour**, **enlarged perigastric nodes** and **secondary deposits in the omentum** in close **proximity** of **the tumour**.

The **clinical features** of the lump are as follows.

(*a*) **Site** The lump is present in the **epigastrium.** If it is **large**, it may extend towards the **left hypochondrium** and the **umbilicus**.

(*b*) The **lower border** is **well defined**. In the epigastrium, the **upper border is palpable**, but if the tumour **extends** to the **left hypochondrium** under the **costal margin**, this is **not possible**.

(*c*) The **consistency** is **hard** and the **surface is irregular**. In patients with a GOO, the dilated proximal stomach may be felt as a **soft boggy mass** to the **left of the primary tumour** in the upper abdomen.

(*d*) The lump usually has **restricted extrinsic mobility**.

(*e*) It is **resonant on percussion**. In the case of a **large epigastric swelling**, this finding is useful to **distinguish** it from an **enlarged left lobe** of the **liver**.

(*f*) On **turning the patient** to the **left lateral position**, the **lump shifts towards the left side,** proving that the plane is **intra-abdominal**.

If the **malignancy arises primarily from the posterior wall of the stomach** and spreads to the posterior abdominal structures, the findings may be **different**. The **lump** may be **fixed, transmitted pulsations** of the **aorta** may be felt and it **may not shift** on turning the patient to the left lateral position.

Box 8.7:	Points regarding the clinical features

Clinical features. Early stages, vague and nonspecific.

- Dyspepsia denovo.
- Loss of appetite.
- Loss of weight.
- Anaemia.
- Early satiety.
- Pain in the epigastrium.
- Vomiting with ball-rolling sensation.
- Haemetemesis and malaena.
- Dysphagia.
- Mass in the epigastrium.
- Symptoms due to metastases.

Q. 18. Describe the clinical features of GOO.

1. **Visible gastric peristalsis:** This is seen as a **wave-**like movement **extending from the left costal margin** towards **the epigastrium or umbilicus**. It is the result of the **contractions of the hypertrophied circular muscle** fibres in the **proximal stomach**, in an effort to **push the contents** across the **obstructed segment**. Since the stomach is basically **hypotonic,** about **300 mL. of water** is given to **act as a stimulus** to **induce the wave.** One has to be **patient** and watch the **upper abdomen** carefully for the **peristaltic movement to develop.** A **vigorous rub** of the **abdominal wall** may initiate the **peristalsis. Pouring of ether on the abdominal wall** to cause a **sudden decrease** in the **temperature** with the same idea is **described** but is **rarely practiced.** A **grossly dilated stomach,** which is **totally atonic,** may **not demonstrate a wave**.

2. **Succussion splash:** The sign is **significant,** only if the **patient's stomach** has been kept **empty for at least two hours**. If a **splashing sound** is heard on **auscultation** while **shaking the abdomen,** the sign is **positive,** indicating the presence of obstruction. **During examination** of the patient, this sign should be **looked** for **before giving water to elicit VGP**.

3. On **percussion,** a **tympanic note** is observed over the **dilated stomach**.

4. **Auscultopercussion:** The chest piece of the **stethoscope** is placed over the **epigastrium**. A **finger** is used to **produce a scratching sound,** by moving it **downwards** from the epigastrium. Once the **finger moves beyond the greater curvature,** the **intensity of the sound** is markedly **reduced.** This point is **marked on the abdominal**

wall. Similar points are marked as the **test is repeated** from the **left hypochondrium** towards the **right side**. The **line** resulting from **joining all these points** indicates the **level of the greater curvature** of the stomach. If it is **below the umbilicus**, it suggests a **dilated stomach**.

The availability of an **endoscope** has made these **tests less important**.

Q. 19. What are the signs of metastatic disease?

1. **Free fluid** in the abdomen. It indicates that the tumour has involved the **serosal surface** of the **stomach.** It is an **ominous sign** since the entire **peritoneal surface** is available for **spread of the tumour.**

2. **Hepatomegaly: Malignant cells** reach the **liver** via the **portal vein.** The enlarged liver is **hard and nodular.** In many instances, **hepatic metastases** appear **after surgery** has been performed for the **primary tumour.**

3. **Enlarged supraclavicular lymph nodes:** Enlarged hard lymph nodes may be palpable in the supraclavicular region either on the left or less commonly on the right side

4. **Tumour cells** spreading along the **lymphatics in the ligamentum teres** produce a hard **indurated nodule** in the **umbilicus (Sr. Joseph's nodule).**

5. **Rectal examination. Transcoe-lomic spread** gives rise to **palpable secondary deposits** in the **rectovesical pouch.**

Q. 20. What are the investigations needed in a case of gastric cancer?

1. **Upper GI scopy:** A **proliferative** or an **ulcerative** lesion is easily identified on **endoscopy.** A minimum of **eight biopsies** should be taken for **histologic diagnosis.** But **detecting** an **early malignancy** needs **experience. Small superficial** lesions can easily be **missed.** Again a **linitis plastica** type of tumour spreads primarily in the **submucosal** layer and the **mucosa** may have a **normal appearance. Lack** of **distensibility** of the stomach during the examination indicates **infiltration** of the wall by **malignancy.**

Repeated **stomach washes** are necessary in patients with GOO, **before endoscopy** is performed. The **large amount of food** remaining in the **stomach** is likely to **mask** the findings. If the **biopsy** reports are **negative** the patient may need a **repeat endoscopy**.

Q. 21. What are the recent advances in the field of endoscopy?

Recent **advances** in **technology** have been applied in this field to **reduce** the chances of **missing early cancers**. They include the following.

(*a*) **Chromoendoscopy:** Spray-ing the stomach wall with **indigocarmine** will help to identify **abnormal mucosa** and sites for **biopsy.**

(*b*) **Narrow band imaging:** The technique uses **filters** to **narrow** the projected light to the **blue and green** part of the spectrum, to **generate** a **coloured image**. The **superficial mucosal capillaries** are **visualised** by this method. The **changes caused by the malignancy** in the **shape and density** of the **capillaries** are likely to **reduce** the **risk of missing a lesion**.

(*c*) **High-definition gastroscopy** aims at increasing the **magnification** to pick up **small tumours** not detected on routine endoscopy.

(*d*) **Conofocal laser endoscopy:** This provides a **histologic** view of the **targeted areas** within the **mucosa.**

Despite all the newer techniques described above, the standard upper **GI scopy** is the one **most frequently** used in clinical practice.

Q. 22. Describe the role of US in gastric cancer.

1. This investigation has a **low sensitivity** in identifying a **primary** tumour. **Thickening of the stomach wall** may be an **indirect evidence** of a **malignant** tumour. But the findings mentioned below are very helpful. The role of **endoscopic US** is described in relation to EGC.

   Enlarged lymph nodes in relation to the stomach are picked up by the ultrasonologist.

2. **Secondary deposits** in the **liver.** They are usually **multiple.** They may appear as **solid areas** or of **mixed echogenicity.** Presence of a **"halo" around the mass** is said to be **diagnostic** of a metastasis.

   Minimal free fluid, not detected during the clinical examination, is picked up on US.

3. **Chest X-ray** is routinely ordered, even though the

incidence of **secondaries** is **very low**.

Additional investigations are needed if at the end of the **clinical examination** and the **investigations** mentioned above, the disease is probably "**curable**".

Presence of the following clearly indicates an **incurable disease**.

Jaundice.

Ascites.

Secondaries in the **liver,** detected either clinically or on US.

Palpable supraclavicular node.

Secondary deposits in the **rectovesical pouch**.

4. **CECT** has come to be the **most important investigation** to decide on the feasibility of **radical surgery**.

   (*a*) The **area of the stomach** involved by **cancer** is defined **accurately**. This helps in planning the **type of surgery** needed for cure. The local **extension** of the tumour by **direct spread** to the **adjacent structures** can be detected by **CT**. This has **brought down** the number of **trial dissections** carried out

during surgery, with the hope of performing a **curative resection**.

   (*b*) **Metastatic** nodes are identified more accurately by CT.

   (*c*) **Secondaries in the liver are detected by CT**.

5. **Diagnostic laparoscopy:** This is usually performed **before** open **surgery** is undertaken. The presence of **surface metastatic** lesions in the **liver** and **peritoneum** are detected **only** by this **investigation**.

6. **Blood investigations:** These patients are **malnourished and hypoproteinaemic,** and if **vomiting** is present, they are also **dehydrated**. Hence the following investigations are required to assess the various abnormalities that may occur and correct them before treatment.

   (*a*) **Haemoglobin** and **haematocrit** values. It should be done **after dehydration** has been **corrected** to **avoid the false values** resulting from **haemoconcentration.** Values above **10 gm%** are satisfactory.

   (*b*) **Serum albumen:** The levels are usually low. Serum

albumen levels **below 3 gm%** need to be corrected before treatment. **Low levels** interfere with **wound healing,** leading to **life-threatening complications** such as **anastomotic leak** and **wound dehiscence**.

(c) **Serum electrolytes:** There is **chloride loss when excessive vomiting is present,** resulting in **hypochloremic metabolic alkalosis**. So estimations of **serum sodium, potassium and chloride** are mandatory.

(d) **Blood urea and creatinine** levels may be **raised** due to **dehydration.**

7. **Paradoxical aciduria:** An interesting **biochemical paradox** is the association of **acidic urine** in the presence of **metabolic alkalosis**. Initially to **compensate** for the metabolic alkalosis, the **kidney secretes more sodium bicarbonate** making the **urine alkaline**. Thus **hyponatraemia** occurs due to **extra loss of sodium**. In turn there is **excessive**

secretion of **aldosterone,** leading to **sodium and water retention**, at the expense of **hydrogen** and **chloride** ions. So the patient develops **hypokalaemia** and the **urine** becomes **acidic** due to the presence of **more hydrogen** ions resulting in **aciduria**.

Box 8.8:	Points regarding investigations

- Upper GI endoscopy and biopsy.
- Abdominal US.
- Chest X-ray.
- CECT abdomen.
- Endoscopic US.
- Laparoscopy.
- Biochemical parameters:
  - Hb.
  - Urea and creatinine.
  - Serum albumen.
  - Serum electrolytes.

Q. 23. What are the factors taken into consideration while planning the treatment?

The success of treatment is based on the following factors.

I. **Adequate pre-** and **postoperative** management.

II. The **extent of gastric resection**.

III. The **extent of lymphadenectomy**.

IV. **Chemotherapy.**

Q. 24. What are the preoperative measures?

Preoperative measures can be divided into the **care of the patient** and **preparation of the stomach**.

Preparation of the patient

(*a*) **Correction of dehydration** is by **intravenous saline** infusion. Measurement of **urinary output** is an easy method of correction of dehydration. But **haematocrit values** are more accurate. **Urea and creatinine levels** also will return to **normal.**

(*b*) **Electrolyte imbalance** is also corrected by IV **saline** infusion.

(*c*) **Packed cell transfusions** are arranged to bring the Hb levels to about **10 gm%.**

(*d*) **Albumen deficiency** is ideally treated by **IV albumen** transfusion. Since the solution is very **expensive, amino acid infusions** are used, but are **poor substitutes.**

(*e*) **Vitamin C and zinc** are needed for proper **wound healing**. So **multivitamins** and **trace elements** are added to the saline **infusion.**

The preoperative preparation usually lasts for about a **week** or **ten days**.

Box 8.9:	Points regarding the preoperative preparation of the patient

- IV fluid infusion.
- Electrolyte infusion.
- Packed cell transfusion.
- Albumen or amino acid infusion.
- Multiple vitamins and trace elements infusion.

Preparation of the stomach. This is specifically needed for patients with GOO**.**

Saline stomach wash. Plain water is not used as further **chloride loss** results in the worsening of the **electrolyte imbalance.** A **wide bore tube** is used for this purpose and the washing is continued till the **returns are clear**. This kind of wash is performed **twice daily**. Several **litres of saline** may be needed since the stomach is **grossly dilated**. In between, the patient is **allowed** to consume only **fluids.**

As a result of these washes, the **stomach** is **emptied** completely. Hence the size becomes **smaller** and the **tone improves. Lactic and butyric acids** are **not** being **produced,** thereby improving the inflammation of the mucosa.

Mucosal oedema and friability of the stomach wall are adequately controlled.

At this stage the stomach is ready for surgical intervention. This period of time usually corresponds to that of preparation of the patient.

Q. 25. What are the surgical procedures employed for gastric cancer?

The aim of surgery is to obtain R0 resection. This would mean that microscopically both the proximal and distal margins are free of the tumour. A 5 cm. clearance from the palpable edge of the induration caused by the tumour usually ensures R0 resection. Proximally, it is often possible to obtain such a clearance. Since only the first few centimetres of the duodenum are free from the pancreas, a tumour-free margin may not be available distally in many instances. The term RI resection is used if the margins show evidence of tumour on histopathological examination. Hence what was planned as R0 resection may turn out be RI resection following the pathology report.

If macroscopic malignant tissue is left behind at the end of the operation, it is known as RII resection (basically a palliative resection).

Distal gastric cancer. The operation usually performed is a subtotal radical gastrectomy. There is a tendency to perform a total radical gastrectomy for this group of patients at the present time in order to improve the prognosis. In a subtotal radical gastrectomy, the proximal part of the duodenum, the pyloric antrum and a portion of the body 5 cm beyond the palpable edge of the cancer, along with the omenta are resected. The extent of lymph node dissection is described in the next section. A Billroth II type of reconstruction is usually performed. This entails closure of the duodenal stump and anastamosing the proximal jejunum to the remaining portion of the stomach. Since a loop of jejunum is brought in front of the transverse colon, it is called as an antecolic type of reconstruction. Alternately, a Roux–en-Y loop of bowel is used occasionally, to reduce the complication of bile gastritis.

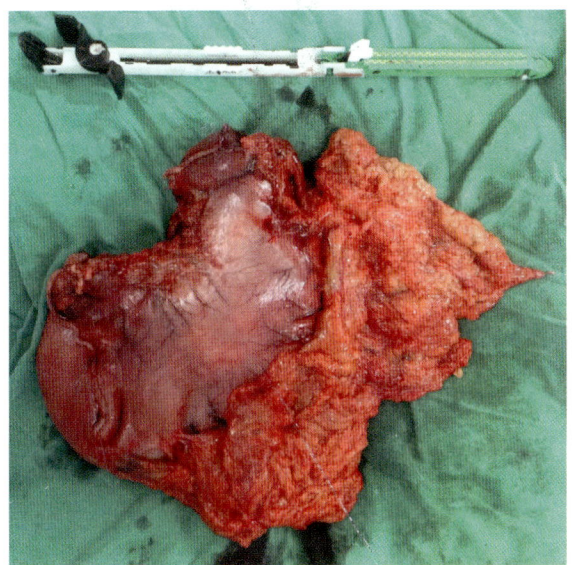

Fig. 8.5: Specimen of a total radical gastrectomy.

Q. 26. **How are proximal gastric cancers treated?**

These cancers are best treated by a **total radical gastrectomy**. The **entire stomach** and the **omenta,** the **distal oesophagus**, the **body and tail** of **pancreas** and the **spleen** are **removed. Resection** of the **pancreas and spleen** are performed to **obtain adequate lymph node clearance**. Certain **modifications** have been introduced in this procedure and they **will be discussed** along with **lymphadenectomy.** A **Roux-en-Y jejuno-oesophagostomy** completes the operation. A **feeding jejunostomy** is added on to ensure adequate **enteral nutrition** early in the **postoperative period**.

In many centres these **operations** are now being performed **laparoscopically**.

Q. 27. **What are the indications for extended radical resections?**

If the **adjoining structures** like the **transverse mesocolon or the colon** itself are **involved,** they are also **removed** along with the **stomach.** But it must be stressed that once the tumour has **breached the serosal surface, aggressive locoregional resections do not** always **result in long-term disease-free intervals**. Sadly, **many of our patients** belong to this group.

Q. 28. **Discuss the role of lymphadenectomy in gastric cancer.**

The **Japanese terminology** has been used to describe this **operation. D1 resections** would mean removal of **perigastric nodes (level 1) en bloc** with the stomach. **D2 radical lymphadenectomy** involves removal of **perigastric nodes** and **those along the main blood vessels (level 2)**, with the primary tumour. This is the **standard operation** for **gastric cancer.** Unfortunately **resections of the pancreas and spleen increase** the **postoperative morbidity** significantly. Hence at present, **modified D2 resections** are being performed **more often** wherein the **lymph nodes** are **removed** but these **two organs are preserved**. This has **not affected** the **long-term survival** to any extent. **D3 (removal of level 3 nodes)** and **D4 type of resections** (level 3 **and level 4 nodes** included in the resection) are **rarely performed**. These **operations** are associated with **significant mortality and morbidity**, but do not **improve** the **outcome** to any extent.

Box 8.10:	Points to be noted in the surgical treatment
	• Total radical gastrectomy.
	• Subtotal radical gastrectomy.
	• D2 lymphadenectomy – Standard operation. D3 and D4 resections rarely performed.

Q. 29. What is the role of chemo-therapy?

Since **adenocarcinomas** are **radio-resistant**, **radiotherapy** is **not used** in the treatment. **Chemotherapy** has a **very limited role.** The **drugs** used are **5 fluorouracil** or **gemcitabine** and **cisplatin**. In the **neoadjuvant setting**, these drugs have been **tried to downstage** the **tumour,** making them **suitable for radical surgery**. But the **results** have **not been encouraging**. They have also been given as **adjuvant therapy** following **radical surgery**, to **reduce the incidence**

of recurrent and **metastatic disease**, with **indifferent results**.

Box 8.11:	Points to be noted regarding chemotherapy
	• 5 fluorouracil, gemcitabine and cisplatin
	• Neoadjuvant setting.
	• Postoperative adjuvant.
	• Palliative – Limited use.

Q. 30. What are the palliative measures available for advanced disease?

Most of **our patients** have either **locally advanced** or **metastatic disease** at **presentation.** In this group, **only palliative treatment** is possible. **Palliative surgery** is the ideal option. **Distal gastric cancers** are more amenable for **palliative surgery**. **Palliative partial gastrectomy** aims at **removal of the portion of the stomach** containing the **tumour.** Since it prevents the **complications** of **obstruction, bleed** and **perforation**, it is considered to be the **best palliative operation.** If **resection** is **not possible** due to **local infiltration** of **important structures** like the **pancreas,** a **bypass surgery** is done only in the **presence of GOO**. A **gastro-jejunostomy** is the operation **commonly performed.** The **anterior wall of the stomach** is used for this operation, since the **posterior wall is infiltrated** by the tumour in this group of patients. Both these operations will only improve the quality of life, but do not keep the patient alive for a longer period of time. Palliative chemotherapy is the only treatment available for patients with recurrent and metastatic disease. But the response is rather poor.

Box 8.12:	Points to be noted regarding palliative surgery

- Palliative partial gastrectomy.
- Palliative anterior gastrojejunostomy in the presence of GOO.

Q. 31. What are the prognostic factors?

The prognosis primarily depends on the site and the stage of the disease. Proximal gastric cancers have a worse prognosis as compared to the distal type. If the cancer has spread to the serosal surface or if the lymph nodes are involved, the outlook is poor. These cancers in general are very aggressive in their behaviour. The five-year disease-free interval quoted often for all patients grouped together is about 30%. But the figures for patients seen in our OPD are much lower, since they present very late in the course of the disease. Most patients develop metastases within two years despite radical surgery. Only about 5% are alive and disease free at the end of five years. The average life span for patients following palliative surgery is between 6 and 9 months. The prognosis of EGC is discussed in the next section.

Q. 32. Discuss the clinical and pathological aspects of Early Gastric Cancers (EGC).

EGCs are defined as cancers involving the mucosa or the submucous layer, with or without extension into the lymph nodes. These were initially identified in Japan following a mass screening programme. It is being repeated to some extent in the developed countries by investigating all patients presenting with minor and vague symptoms referable to the upper abdomen. But it is impractical in our country because of the huge population and the very limited health resources at our disposal. The incidence of lymph node infiltration in mucosal tumours is as low as 3%. If the submucosa is also involved, the risk increases to 15%–20%. These two types of early cancers can only be diagnosed and staged with the help of investigations since the clinical signs are conspicuous by their absence.

(*a*) Upper GI scopy is the most important investigation.

Expertise in performing **endoscopy** is an **absolute requisite**. **Early cancers** are more **difficult** to **identify**, and the **various improvements mentioned earlier** are very **useful** in **diagnosing this condition**. In addition, **endoscopy** has revealed that many of these **cancers** are **multifocal**.

Macroscopically four different types have been described.

1. **Elevated type**
2. **Protruding type**
3. **Flat type**
4. **Excavating type**

Depending on **the size**, they are known as **minute** (less than **5 mm**.) and **small (a few centimetres)**

(b) **Endoscopic US** is an **integral part** in the **diagnosis**. The **depth of invasion** can only be **detected** by this **investigation**. The **distinction** between **cancers** involving the **mucosa** and those extending to the **submucous layer** is **accurately defined**. Once the tumour penetrates the **muscular layer** it is **no longer** considered to be an EGC.

(c) **CECT** is advised if spread into the **regional lymph nodes** is **suspected**.

(d) **Laparoscopy** has also been used to assess the **status of the lymph nodes**.

Box 8.13:	Points to be noted in the diagnosis
• Endoscopic classification:
• Protruding type
• Elevated type
• Flat type
• Excavating type

Q. 33. What are the guidelines for treatment of EGC?

If all the **factors** mentioned above are **taken into consideration**, these **cancers** are **cured by endoscopic procedures**. **Endoscopic mucosal resections (EMR)** are performed for **tumours confined to the mucosa**. If **frozen sections** show evidence of the **tumour at the margin, resection of the surrounding mucosa** is needed.

Cancers involving the **submucosa** are treated **endoscopically** by a **submucosal dissection (SMD)**.

A **frozen section** examination is mandatory. Since **EMR** has shown a **significant rate of recurrence**, even **mucosal tumours** are **now** being **treated by SMD** more **frequently.**

The main **complications** are **bleeding** and **perforation**. If **detected** during the procedure, they can be treated **endoscopically**. The risk of **postoperative bleed** is reduced by **administration** of PPIs for **one week.** If there is evidence of **lymph node involvement**, a **laparoscopic lymphadenectomy** is performed. The **five-year cure** following **EMR is 99%** and **SMD 95%.** But this group needs **regular endoscopic surveillance** to identify **recurrences** and **metachronous tumours**. As far as **our patients** are concerned, it still remains a **distant possibility.**

Box 8.14:	Points to be noted in the treatment of EGC

- Endoscopic mucosal resection.
- Submucosal dissection.
- Laparoscopic lymphadenectomy.
- 5-year DFS 90% to 95%.

Multiple Choice Questions

1. In a patient with Gastric Outlet Obstruction all of the following are true **EXCEPT**—
   - (*a*) Metabolic Acidosis maybe present
   - (*b*) Succussion splash can be elicited
   - (*c*) Vomiting occurs about 2-3 hours. after food intake
   - (*d*) Paradoxical aciduria may be present

   Answer (*a*)

2. All of the following are true about Gastric Outlet Obstruction **EXCEPT**—
   - (*a*) Vomiting is usually preceded by ball-rolling sensation
   - (*b*) Operation without preparation of stomach leads to increased complications
   - (*c*) Stomach washes with distilled water are mandatory for preparation of stomach
   - (*d*) Proton Pump Inhibitors may produce symptomatic relief

   Answer (*c*)

3. All of the following are true about Carcinoma Stomach **EXCEPT—**

(*a*) Presence of an umbilical nodule indicates advanced malignancy

(*b*) Pernicious anaemia is a premalignant condition

(*c*) Right Supraclavicular Lymph Node can be involved indicating metastasis

(*d*) Muscular layer is involved in Early Gastric Cancer

Answer (*d*)

4. Which of the following is **NOT TRUE** about Early Gastric Cancer?

(*a*) Lymph node involvement maybe present

(*b*) Mucosa and submucosa are involved

(*c*) Ascites can be seen in these patients

(*d*) Endoscopic Mucosal resection is a treatment option

Answer (*c*)

5. An R1 resection in Oncological Surgery means—

(*a*) Microscopically margins are Negative

(*b*) Microscopically margins are Positive

(*c*) Macroscopically margins are Negative

(*d*) Macroscopically margins are Positive

Answer (*b*)

6. Which of the following statements is **NOT TRUE** about Duodenal ulcers?

(*a*) The first part is the most common site

(*b*) H pylori is an aetiological agent

(*c*) Proton Pump inhibitors are primarily used in treatment

(*d*) It is a premalignant condition

Answer (*d*)

7. The most common Histological type of Carcinoma Stomach is—

(*a*) Adenocarcinoma

(*b*) Squamous cell carcinoma

(*c*) Adenosquamous carcinoma

(*d*) Melanoma

Answer (*a*)

8. Which of the following is **NOT TRUE** about Carcinoma Stomach?

(*a*) It is usually associated with hyperchlorhydria.

(*b*) Endoscopy maybe normal in linitis plastica.

(*c*) Previous gastrojejunostomy increases the risk.

(*d*) People of blood group A have a slightly increased risk.

Answer (*a*)

■■■

Obstructive Jaundice

9

A CASE OF CARCINOMA OF THE HEAD OF PANCREAS

Setting

- Surgical OPD.

Chief Complaint

- **Yellowish discoloration** of the **eyes** and **itching** of **4 months** duration.

History of Present Illness

A **45-year-old man** was brought to the surgical OPD with complaints of **yellowish discolouration** of the eyes and **itching.** A **close relative** noted that the patient's **eyes** looked **yellow** about **4 months ago**. Since then the **discolouration has been** getting **worse.** He noticed that he was passing **high-coloured urine.** About 3 weeks later he started passing **pale stools.** Patient did not give any history of **malaena.**

- **Itching** also started about **4 months ago.** It was becoming **severe** and was disturbing his **sleep.**

- He had **no pain.**
- There was no history of **vomiting.**
- The patient had **lost appetite** as well as **weight.**
- There was no history of **fever.**

Past History

The patient did not give a history of **previous** episodes of **jaundice.** He did not have any **major illness** in the past.

Personal History

He was a **chronic smoker** and used to **consume alcohol.**

Family History

No member of the family gave a **history of jaundice.**

Treatment History

He had tried some **home remedies** before consulting an **Ayurvedic doctor** for jaundice without any relief.

General Physical Examination

The patient was **deeply jaundiced**. The **sclera**, the **palate** and the **skin** were **tinged deep yellow**. The **skin** showed scratch marks. There was **no pallor or pedal oedema**. Clubbing of the fingers was not present. The **pulse** rate was **66 per minute** and the BP was 136 by 82 mm of Hg.

Examination of Abdomen

Inspection

- A **fullness** was noted in the **right hypochondrium**. The **margins** were **ill defined**.
- The **surface** appeared **smooth**.
- The abdominal **skin** showed **scratch marks**. There were **no dilated veins** in the abdominal wall.
- The **umbilicus** was normal.
- The **hernial orifices** and the **external genitalia** were normal.

Palpation

Liver was palpable **4 finger-breadths** below the **costal margin**. It was **not tender**. The **lower border** was **rounded**. It was not possible to **feel the upper border**. The **surface** was **smooth**. It was **firm** in **consistency**. It was moving **with respiration**

- The **gall bladder** was palpable **below** the **lower border of the liver** to the **right** of the **of the rectus muscle**. It was **not tender**. It was **grossly distended** and **globular** in shape.
- There was **no other palpable mass** in the abdomen.
- **Fluid thrill** was absent.
- The external **genitalia** on **palpation** were found to be **normal**.

Percussion

- The **liver was dull on percussion and the span** measured 18 cm.
- The **gall bladder** was **dull** on percussion.
- **Shifting dullness** was absent.
- Examination of the **supraclavicular region** did not reveal any **lymph node** enlargement.
- Examination of the **lumbar spine** was normal.
- **Rectal examination** was normal.

Box 9.1:	Points to be noted in history

- Jaundice – Duration – Progression – Intensity.
- Itching – Intensity.
- Pain abdomen – Nature – Radiation.
- Vomiting.
- Colour of urine and stools.
- Loss of appetite and weight.
- Treatment history.

Box 9.2:	Points to be noted on inspection of the abdomen

- Fullness or a visible lump.
- Lump – Site – Extent – Margins.
- Size and shape.
- Surface.
- Skin over the abdomen
- Umbilicus – dilated veins around the umbilicus.
- Hernial orifices and external genitalia.

Box 9.3:	Points to be noted in palpation

- Warmth and tenderness.
- Liver – Enlargement – Extent-lower border.
- Movement with respiration.
- Surface – Consistency.
- Gall bladder – Position – Shape – Mobility.
- Other lump – Spleen – Pancreas.
- Fluid thrill.
- External genitalia.

Box 9.4:	Points to be noted regarding rest of examination

- Supraclavicular nodes.
- Lumbar spine.
- Rectal examination.
- Other systems.

Q. 1. What was the clinical diagnosis?

(a) Malignant obstructive jaundice.

(b) Stone in CBD causing obstructive jaundice.

(c) Klatskin's tumour.

(d) Carcinoma of the gall bladder.

The correct diagnosis is (*a*).

Carcinoma of the gallbladder is seen frequently as a **complication** of **gall stone** disease. It is also a **common disease** in parts of **North and Northeast India**. Such patients give a history of **previous** attacks of **biliary colic** with or **without jaundice**. The **lump** arising from a **malignant gall bladder** will be **hard, irregular and fixed**. **Jaundice** is the result of **infiltration** of the **biliary system** by the **tumour**.

Klatskin's tumour is a **malignant tumour** present at the **confluence** of the **two hepatic ducts** to form the common hepatic duct. All **symptoms** of **obstructive jaundice** are present in these patients. Since the obstruction is proximal to the **cystic duct,** bile has **no access** to the **gall bladder,** and hence the gall bladder will **not be palpable**.

As per **Courvoisier's law,** if the **gall bladder is palpable**, the cause is **not gall stone disease**. There are **exceptions** to this rule, but they are **uncommon**. Patients with stones as mentioned above give a history of **biliary colic**. The **jaundice** will be **intermittent** with **fever** and **pain** (**Charcot's triad**).

The **short history** of **painless progressive jaundice** along with **loss** of **weight** and a **palpable gall bladder**, suggest a diagnosis of a **malignancy** causing jaundice.

Q. 2. What were the investigations done on this patient?

1. **Ultrasonogram (US) abdomen**. The **gall bladder** was **grossly distended** with a **thin wall** and contained **clear fluid**. There were **no stones** in the biliary tree. The **intrahepatic biliary ducts** were **dilated**. The common bile duct (**CBD**) was **dilated** till its **termination**. The liver was **enlarged**.

   A **mass** lesion was seen in the **head** of the **pancreas** of **3 cm by 4** cm **size** with **mixed echogenicity**. **No** enlarged lymph **nodes** could be detected.

   There was **no free fluid**.

2. **Liver function tests**.

   Serum bilirubin was 9.8 mg%

   Serum alkaline phosphatase levels were 980 units.

   ALT and AST levels were within normal limits.

   Prothrombin levels were INR 2.2 IU.

3. **Blood tests. Hb%** was 11 gm%.

   Urea and creatinine levels were within normal limits.

   Serum albumen was 3.2 gm%.

   Tests for **hepatitis B and C** were negative.

4. **Urine examination** showed that **bile pigments were present and urobilinogen was absent**.

5. **Magnetic resonance cholangio-pancreatography (MRCP) scan**. The **biliary system** was grossly **dilated**. A **mass** lesion was seen in the **head** of the **pancreas**. The **main pancreatic duct** was measuring 1.5 cm in size. The **body** and **tail** of the **pancreas** appeared **bulky** with a **dilated ductal system**.

6. **Contrast-enhanced computed tomography (CECT) of abdomen confirmed** the findings of **MRI**. The portal vein was found to be **free** of tumour. Few enlarged **lymph nodes** were detected in relation to the tumour. A **CT-guided biopsy** was also performed (following injections of Vitamin K and the INR levels being brought to normal).

Box 9.5: Points regarding investigations

- US – Site, nature of obstruction – Liver and gall bladder.
- MRI – Ideal – Biliary and pancreatic systems well defined.
- CECT – Local extension – Encasement of vessels – Guided biopsy.
- ERCP – Periampullary carcinoma.
- LFT and renal function tests.
- Hb and albumen.
- Tumour marker – CA19/9.

Setting: A week passes.

Biopsy report was an **adenocarcinoma.**

The patient was given **Vitamin K** as mentioned above daily, during this period.

He was also given **IV i**nfusions of **glucose saline** daily.

The **nature** of the **disease** as well as the **gravity** of the **operation** was **explained** in **detail** to the **patient** and the **relatives**. The **possible complications** in the **postoperative period** were explained in detail. The **long-term outcome** was also **discussed** with the group.

The patient was started on **preoperative antimicrobial therapy**.

Q. 3. **What was the treatment strategy adopted for this patient?**

The patient underwent a **Whipple's operation** (**radical pancreatoduo-denectomy {PD}**). The following **structures** were **removed** during the procedure. The **distal part of the stomach**, the **entire duodenum**, the proximal **20 cm of the jejunum**, the **head** of the **pancreas** containing the **tumour,** the **gall bladder and the common bile duct**, and the **lymph nodes** in relation to the tumour were all **resected enbloc**.

Reconstruction consisted of a **hepaticojejunostomy** (anastomosis between the common hepatic duct and the proximal jejunum), a **pancreatojejunos-tomy** (an anastomosis between the pancreatic duct and the jejunum) and a **gastrojejunostomy**. The patient had a smooth postoperative period.

He was given a course of **chemotherapy** consisting of **gemcitabine** and **5 fluorouracil (5 FU)**.

Q. 4. **What is the likely outcome for this patient?**

Pancreatic cancers are very **aggressive cancers** and the **outlook** is **very poor**. Even after **radical surgery**, the prognosis is **gloomy.** It is very likely that he would develop **metastatic disease** within **two years** and **succumb** to the disease.

Q. 5. **What is the incidence of pancreatic cancer?**

It is the **fifth** most common cause of **death** due to **cancers**. The incidence is **increasing** in **our country**. People in our country are usually affected by pancreatic cancer in the fourth and fifth decades of their lives. **Both the sexes** are involved to the same extent.

Q. 6. What are the premalignant conditions?

Chronic pancreatitis is a proved **premalignant** condition. It is very prevalent in **Kerala** and the adjoining parts of **South India**. This could be one of the reasons for the **frequency** seen especially in **young patients** in **India.**

Intraductal papillary mucinous neoplasm (**IPMN**) is a type of **ductal neoplasm** that has a **high propensity** to turn malignant.

Mucinous cystadenoma also increases the **risk of cancer**.

Box 9.6:	Points regarding premalignant conditions

- Tropical pancreatitis.
- IPMN.
- Mucinous cystadenoma.

Q. 7. What are the special problems faced by our patients with jaundice?

Hepatitis A is very **prevalent disease** in our **country**. It is almost **self-limiting** in nature. Hence most patients **do not consider jaundice** as a **serious illness**. A large number of **home remedies** are also available. In addition patients try various **alternative types of treatment**. The concept that **jaundice** can be a **surgical disease** is not known even to the **educated class** of people in our country. Hence most of **our** patients with

malignancy reach the hospital with an **inoperable cancer**.

Q. 8. Explain the cause for itching in these patients.

Itching is an important symptom of **obstructive jaundice** and is caused by **accumulation** of **bile salts** in the **skin**. It is the **symptom** that causes **maximum distress** to the patient. **Removal** of **obstruction** brings **immediate relief** to the patient.

Q. 9. Define Courvoisier's law and explain its rationale.

Courvoisier's law states that in a jaundiced patient if the gall bladder is palpable, the cause is not gallstones. The common type of **gallstones** is the **mixed type** and they occur in an **infected gall bladder. Chronic inflammation** leads to **fibrosis,** and hence the gall bladder is **incapable** of **distension** in the presence of obstruction. But in **malignant obstructions**, the gall bladder is **healthy** and becomes **distended** with **bile**. Hence it is clinically **palpable.**

Q. 10. What are the exceptions to Courvoisier's law?

The law is **valid** in a **majority** of clinical situations. **Exceptions** are **uncommon**. The following are the exceptions.

If there is double impaction of both the **cystic duct** as well as the **common bile duct** with **stones,** the gall bladder will be distended by a **mucocele** and be **palpable.** Again if the **insertion** of the **cystic duct** to the **CBD** is very **low,** a **pancreatic tumour** may block the **cystic duct** **preventing** the entry of **bile.** If **malignancy** of the pancreas develops in a patient with **pre-existing chronic cholecystitis**, the gall bladder **will not** be **palpable.**

Q. 11. What are the common malignancies causing obstructive jaundice?

Carcinoma of the **head of pancreas** and **periampullary carcinoma** are the **common** malignancies. In addition, **cholangiocarcinoma, Klatskin's tumour** and **carcinoma of the gall bladder** also manifest with **jaundice.** But they are **uncommon** and will not be discussed in detail. The term **periampullary carcinoma** includes cancers arising at the following sites.

(*a*) The **ampulla of Vater**.

(*b*) The **terminal part of the CBD**.

(*c*) **Terminal part** of the pancreatic duct.

(*d*) The **duodenal mucosa** in close proximity of the **ampulla.**

It is important to **distinguish** between a carcinoma **head of pancreas** and **periampullary carcinoma,** since the **long-term results** are **better** with the **latter.**

Box 9.7:	Points regarding the anatomical sites

- Head of pancreas.
- Periampullary carcinoma
- Ampulla of Vater.
- Terminal part of CBD.
- Terminal part of the pancreatic duct.
- Duodenal mucosa in proximity.

Q. 12. What are the clinical differences between these two cancers?

Certain differences are mentioned, but **none** of them are **totally accurate,** and **imaging** and endoscopy are required to **localize** the **tumour.**

Carcinoma head of pancreas is said to have **painless progressive jaundice.** But when the **tumour infiltrates the nerves, pain** can be an important complaint.

Intermittent jaundice is said to be a feature of **periampullary** carcinoma. If parts of the **tumour slough off,** the **CBD lumen** is **opened up** leading to **passage of bile. Growth of the tumour** results in **blockage** of the duct again and **deepening of the jaundice.** If **central necrosis** of the tumour in the **head of the pancreas** does occur, the extrinsic pressure on the CBD is reduced allowing passage of bile to the intestine, thereby reducing the intensity of the jaundice. As the tumour grows again, jaundice will become more severe. Thus the jaundice will be intermittent in nature.

Weight loss is said to be an important feature of carcinoma head of pancreas. But if malignancy develops as a complication of chronic pancreatitis, the patient has already lost significant weight due to the previous disease.

Passage of "silvery stools" is a finding described in patients with periampullary carcinoma. Ulceration leads to bleeding. A combination of altered blood (malaena) along with clay-coloured stools is said to produce this silver colour. This is a rare finding though.

Q. 13. What are the details regarding history in a patient with obstructive jaundice?

1. The presenting complaint is jaundice, often severe in nature. The duration varies from several weeks to months. In a majority of cases it is progressive, but an occasional patient may give a history of episodes of remission as mentioned earlier. Unfortunately this causes a false sense of complacency in the patient, thereby delaying medical advice further. Stone in the CBD usually produces intermittent jaundice. But a stone impacted at the opening in the ampulla can give rise to progressive jaundice.

2. Pruritus or itching is an important symptom. It is often serious enough to disturb the sleep at night. But the severity of jaundice and that of itching do not always correspond with each other. Again the relief of obstruction causes an improvement immediately.

3. Classically, cancers are supposed to produce painless progressive jaundice. But infiltration of the splanchnic nerves by a cancer of the head of pancreas will result in intense back pain. Stretching of the capsule of the liver due to hepatomegaly causes a dull dragging pain in the right hypochondrium. Stone disease is exemplified by colicky pain in the right side of the abdomen. The pain may radiate to the interscapular region and tends to last for several hours.

4. Intermittent fever with **chills** and rigors occurs in **stone disease**. Fever is the result of **ascending cholangitis**, since **static bile** acts as a **focus** of infection.

5. These patients complain of passing **high-coloured urine** due to the presence of **bile pigments**. **Absence** of these **pigments** produces **clay-coloured stools**.

6. **Loss of appetite** is seen in most patients.

7. **Loss of weight** is very prominent in **malignant jaundice**.

8. In **late stages**, **symptoms** arise due to the presence of **metastatic disease**. **Ascites** produces **abdominal distension**. An **occasional patient** may present with a **swelling** in the **neck** due to **supraclavicular node** enlargement.

Q. 14. What is the importance of past history?

Patients with **gallstone** disease may give a history of **previous episodes** of **jaundice.** It is more commonly seen in **women.** A **co-morbid** condition such as **diabetes** is common in patients with a previous history of **chronic pancreatitis.**

Q. 15. What are the special features to be looked for in general physical examination?

Presence of **jaundice** should always be checked only in **natural light**. It is difficult to detect **mild jaundice** in **artificial light**. But by the time the patient reaches the **surgical department**, the jaundice is often **severe.** The **sclera** and the **palatal mucosa** are the **common sites** to be looked at. Later, the **palms** as well as the **skin** will show the **yellowish hue**. **Pallor** is also seen in many patients. **Scratch marks** on the skin are an indication of the **severity of pruritus**. Examination of the **skinfold** over the **triceps** on the posterior aspect of the arm confirms the **nutritional status.**

Q. 16. What are the special inspection findings in the abdomen?

1. A **fullness** may be seen in the **right hypochondrium** due to the **hepatomegaly**. Uncommonly in **emaciated patients**, the **gall bladder** is seen as a **globular swelling** in the **right side** of the **upper abdomen**. This swelling **moves with respiration**.

2. In **advanced** cases, **distension** of the abdomen is seen due to **ascites.**

Q. 17. What are the important findings on palpation?

1. **Liver** is palpable in the **right hypochondrium**. It may also extend to the **neighbouring quadrants**. This enlargement is the result of **intrahepatic dilatation** of the **biliary ducts (hydrohepatosis)**. The **consistency** is **soft**-to-**firm** and the **surface is smooth**. The **lower border** is **rounded**. It is **nontender.**

2. But the **liver** may also be the seat of **metastatic disease**. It results in a liver that is **nodular,** and these nodules are **hard** in consistency.

3. A **careful search** for a distended **gall bladder** is essential. The commonest **position** is at the **junction** of the **lateral border** of the **right rectus** abdominis and the **lower border** of the **liver**. But often it is **palpable** more **laterally**. The following **clinical signs** confirm that the palpable **swelling** is the **gall bladder.**

   (*a*) Shape is **globular**.

   (*b*) The **consistency** is **different** from that of the **solid liver**.

   (*c*) It has independent **transverse mobility**.

(*d*) It also **moves with respiration**.

Unfortunately, **all distended gall bladders** are **not palpable** since the **overhanging edge** of the **enlarged liver** can easily **conceal** the **same.**

Box 9.8:	Points regarding a distended gall bladder

- Site – Lower border of the liver – Lateral to right rectus.
- Globular shape.
- Firm but different from the liver.
- Moves with respiration.
- Independent transverse mobility.
- All not palpable clinically – Covered by the enlarged liver.

4. In more **advanced cases**, the following signs may be elicited.

   (*a*) A **palpable mass** in the **right side** of the **upper abdomen** arising from the **head of pancreas**. It is **deeply placed**, **hard** and **nodular**. It is **not mobile** and placed **retroperitoneally.** On **percussion** it shows **impaired resonance**. But a **grossly enlarged liver** may make this **mass difficult** to **palpate.**

   (*b*) **Free fluid** due to **intraperitoneal** spread.

   (*c*) **Splenomegaly.** If the **tumour** in the pancreas **invades the splenic vein**, a **left-sided**

portal hypertension results, giving rise to **splenomegaly.**

(*d*) Palpable **lymph node** in the **left supraclavicular region.**

(*e*) **Rectal examination** may reveal a **secondary deposit** in the **rectovesical pouch.**

Spread beyond the liver is **rare** and hence the other systems are essentially normal.

Q. 18. **What are the investigations done in patients with obstructive jaundice?**

1. **Ultrasonography:** The availability of this investigation has resulted in a **paradigm shift** in the **understanding** and **management** of a **jaundiced** patient.

(*a*) **Presence** of a **dilated biliary system** indicates an **obstructive lesion.**

(*b*) The **level of obstruction** can also be demonstrated. A **distended gall bladder** suggests that the obstruction is **distal** to the **junction** of the **cystic duct** with the **CBD.** But the **terminal part** of the CBD **may not be visualized** due to the **gas-filled duodenum** located **anteriorly.**

(*c*) The **status** of the liver. **Intrahepatic dilatation** of the **biliary ducts** is demonstrated. In **advanced cases, metastatic deposits** are detected in the **liver.**

(*d*) The **nature of obstruction. Calculi** present in the **gall bladder (Mirizzi syndrome)** and the **biliary ducts** are identified easily **except** in the **terminal portion of the duct.**

(*e*) A **mass lesion** in the **head of the pancreas** is detected by US**.** The **pancreatic duct** and its **tributaries** are seen to be **dilate**d due to the **obstruction** caused by the **tumour.**

(*f*) The presence of chronic **calcific** or **calculous pancreatitis,** which is quite **prevalent** in this **part of the country,** is also detected. This is **significant** because it is a premalignant condition. Again when **malignancy** supervenes in a patient with **chronic pancreatitis,** it can be **multicentric.**

(*g*) Presence of **enlarged lymph nodes** along the **pancreas** and the **hepatoduodenal ligament.**

(*h*) **Minimal ascites** not detected clinically.

But this investigation has certain **limitations** .The extent of **local spread** and involvement of the **adjacent structures** like the **portal vein cannot be demonstrated**.

2. **MRCP:** Magnetic resonance imaging has emerged as the most **reliable investigation** in patients with **obstructive jaundice**. It demonstrates both the **biliary and pancreatic duct systems accurately.** Both **calculi** and **malignant tumours** are **detected** easily.

3. **CECT** (performed after ensuring that the renal function is not impaired)**:** CT will help to **distinguish** a **periampullary carcinoma** from a **mass** in the **head of the pancreas**. In addition **metastatic lymph nodes** are detected more **accurately**. Most significantly, the **extent** of **involvement** of the adjacent structures such as the **portal vein** and the **superior mesenteric artery** is identified by **CT. Encasement of these vessels** is considered to be an indication of an **inoperable cancer**.

4. **Tissue diagnosis**: The **distinction** between **calculous** and **malignant** obstruction has now become **simple** thanks to the availability of the **imaging modalities**. In the case of **malignanc**y, it is considered essential to have a **tissue diagnosis** before undertaking a **major surgical procedure. In periampullary carcinoma,** an **endoscopic biopsy** may prove the presence of a **malignant tumour** at the **papilla** or in the **adjacent duodenal mucosa. Brush cytology** can also be performed. But a **negative report** does **not rule out malignancy** in many instances. To prove a **mass** in the head of the **pancreas** to be **malignant** is even **more difficult. Core needle biopsy** (CNB) under **CT guidance** may reveal the **diagnosis.** But **chronic pancreatitis** and **malignancy** can **coexist** in a patient. Again a zone of **inflammation** often **surrounds** the **tumour** and a **biopsy** may show only **inflammation.** Availability of **endoscopic ultrasound** (**EUS**) has **increased** the **success** rate of CNB. But it remains as one of those few situations where the **clinical acumen** of the **surgeon** is considered as the **most**

important factor in deciding the **treatmen**t.

5. **Tumour Marker:** Elevated levels of **CA19/9** are useful more in the **follow-up** of a **treated patient. Normal levels** do **not rule out** pancreatic **malignancy.** If the levels were **raised initially,** they tend to **come down** with **treatment. Increased levels of CA19/9,** occur **before clinical evidence** of either **recurrent** or **metastatic disease** become **manifest.**

6. **Liver Function Tests:** The state of the **liver** also influences the **prognosis** in this group of patients, since **deep jaundice** irrespective of the aetiology, signifies **severe damage** to the **liver.**

   (*a*) **Serum bilirubin** levels of more than **10 mg** are indicative of a **severely damaged** liver and **biliary decompression** may be needed **before major ablative surgery** is planned.

   (*b*) **Raised ALT and AST** again are suggestive of significant **liver damage**.

   (*c*) Raised **prothrombin time** is due to inability to absorb the **fat-soluble Vitamin K** in the **absence of bile** in the **gut.**

Blood tests. **Haemoglobin levels** may be low.

Serum albumen. Albumen is **synthesized** in the liver. It may be **low** in patients with **damaged livers**.

7. **Renal Function Tests:** Patients with deep jaundice are prone to develop acute renal failure in the immediate postoperative period. This complication is known as hepatorenal syndrome.The causative factors are rather complex but dehydration and hypotension are considered important.

Q. 19. **What are the treatment strategies for these patients?**

Whipple's operation offers the best outcome. But the **cancers** of the **head of pancreas** are **very aggressive** tumours. Hence **despite radical surgery** the **outlook** remains **poor**. It is also recognised that the **survival rates** are **better** when surgery is performed in **high-volume centres** by **experienced surgeons.** The **operative mortality** has been brought down to **2%–4%.** The **postoperative complications** are also **less** in this group.

Periampullary carcinoma carries a **better prognosis**. **Jaundice** appears much **earlier** due to the **close proximity** of the

tumour to the **ductal system**. These tumours are also **less aggressive** in their **behaviour.**

Q. 20. **What are the preoperative measures?**

Before **surgical** or **endoscopic inter-ventions** are planned, these patients need **specific** measures to **reduce** the postoperative **morbidity** and **mortality**.

(*a*) IV **10% glucose** to replenish the depleted **glycogen** stored in the **liver.**

(*b*) **Adequate hydration** is needed to prevent dehydration.

(*c*) **Injection Vitamin K** is given IM to bring the **prothrombin time** to **normal** levels. If the liver is **severely damaged**, this treatment may not succeed, and such patients need **fresh frozen plasma (FFP)**

(*d*) **Antimicrobial cover.** The **dilated biliary system** with **static bile** offers an excellent opportunity for **bacterial infections**. A **third-generation cephalosporin** along with **metronidazole** is the combination most often used.

Box 9.9:	Points about preoperative preparation

- 10% glucose to replace depleted glycogen reserves in liver.
- Hydration to reduce the risk of hepatorenal syndrome - IV mannitol.
- Injection Vitamin K to correct prothrombin time.
- Broad spectrum antimicrobials.

Q. 21. **What is the role of preoperative biliary decompression?**

Patients with **impaired liver function** do not **tolerate** major surgery well. Both the postoperative **morbidity and mortality** are much **higher** in this group. The most **popular** method is stenting of the **CBD** across the **obstruction endoscopically.** But this **increases** the risk of **ascending cholangitis,** which can lead to **life-threatening septicaemia.** A **percutaneous US**-guided **catheter** drainage of the **gall bladder** is another option. Hence there is a **personal** preference among **surgeons** in **performing** these **procedures.**

Q. 22. **Describe the operative treatment of these two malignancies.**

The standard operation is a **radical pancreaticoduodenectomy** also known as **Whipple's operation.** The **structures removed** in this operation are the **distal part of the stomach**, the CBD and the **gall bladder**, the **entire duodenum**, the **proximal 20 cm. of the jejunum**, the **head of the pancreas** along with the **lymph nodes**. The **pancreas** is **divided** at the **neck in front** of the **portal vein**. The **proximal jejunum** is removed since its **blood supply** is derived from the **pancreatoduodenal arteries**. The **reconstruction** includes a **hepaticojejunostomy**, a **pancreaticojejunostomy** and a gastrojejunostomy.

The most **important complication** that can be **life threatening** is a **pancreatic fistula** due to a leak at the site of the **pancreatojejunal anastamosis**. This can lead to **secondary peritonitis**, **severe wound disruption** and **multiorgan failure**. **Pancreatic fistula** also causes considerable morbidity because of **autodigestion** of the abdominal wall due to the action of the **proteolytic enzymes**.

Prolonged **gastroparesis** can also be a problem in the immediate **postoperative period**. In properly selected patients, a **pylorus preserving modification** (**PPPD,** also known as **Longmire and Traverso** procedure) is employed to **reduce** the incidence of **gastroparesis**. It is useful for **small** tumours in the **periampullary** region without **suprapancreatic nodal involvement**.

Box 9.10:	Points regarding surgical treatment

- Whipple's radical pancreatoduodenectomy.
- Structures removed – Distal stomach, duodenum, proximal 20 cm jejunum, head of pancreas, gall bladder and CBD along with lymph nodes.
- Reconstruction – Hepatic jejunostomy, pancreatojejunostomy and gastrojejunostomy.
- Modification – Pylorus preserving resection – Periampullary carcinoma with proper selection.
- Extended resections – Portal vein – Replacement with saphenous vein graft.

Chemoradiation. Gemcitabine and 5 FU along with image-guided radiation therapy (**IGRT**) are being used **postoperatively** to improve the **outlook,** but the **cancer** remains one with a **dismal prognosis**.

Again **encasement** of the portal vein is **not** considered to be indicative of **inoperability** in many **advanced oncological centres**. **Extended resections** are being performed with the involved **segment** of the **portal** vein resected along with the specimen and replaced by an autogenous saphenous vein graft.

Q. 23. What are the palliative measure available for these patients?

A vast **majority** of our patients have **advanced disease** where **only palliation** is possible. **Relief** of **jaundice** and the associated **itching** is the primary **objective**. ERCP and **stent** placement in the **CBD** across the **obstruction** results in dramatic **improvement** of the symptoms. If the **patient** were to develop **duodenal obstruction** at a **later period** due to the **encroachment** of the **lumen** of the **second part of the duodenum** by the tumour, an **expandable self-retaining** stent can be placed across the **obstruction endoscopically**.

If **endoscopic expertise** is **not available**, an **open** cholecystojejunostomy to relieve the **biliary obstruction** and a **gastrojejunostomy** to **relieve** a possible **duodenal obstruction** later are performed. A **jejunojejunostomy** between the **afferent** and the **efferent** loops of jejunum involved in

the **cholecystojejunostomy** is added to reduce the **risk** of **ascending cholangitis**. If the **pancreatic duct** is also **dilated**, some surgeons add on a **pancreatojejunostomy.** The procedure is then called as a **triple anastomosis**. All these **operations** can be performed **laparoscopically.**

Box 9.11:	Points regarding palliative treatment

- ERCP – Papillotomy and stent across the obstructed segment of CBD.
- Endoscopic placement of a self-retaining stent across duodenum.
- Palliative cholecystojejunostomy and gastrojejunostomy.
- Addition of pancreatojejunostomy – Triple bypass surgery.

Q. 24. What are methods used for control of pain in advanced malignancies?

Pain control is needed in **advanced cases** as this becomes the most **distressing symptom**. Interventional **radiologists** are able to **inject absolute alcohol** into the **splanchnic plexus** of nerves to reduce the pain. This can also be performed **intraoperatively** during **palliative procedures**.

Q. 25. What is the prognosis?

In general carcinomas of the **head of the pancreas** have a **gloomy** prognosis. The disease is **rarely curable** and the overall **survival** rate at the end of **five years** is about **5%.** In patients with a **tumour** less than **2 cm** in size, confined to **within the capsule** of the **pancreas** and no **lymph node** involvement, the **five year survival** is about **18% to 20%.** Although adjuvant **chemoradiation** is given, the tumour is usually **resistan**t to these modalities. But the **five year cure rate** for **periampullary carcinomas** are much higher being in the range of **50%.** Following **palliative treatment**, the **survival i**s between **6 to 9 months** but there is significant **improvement** in the **quality of life**.

Q. 26. How are obstructions due to stones in the CBD treated?

By comparison the treatment is **simpler** when the obstruction is caused by **calculi.** The **preoperative workup** is the **same**. **Endoscopic stone extraction** is the **treatment** of choice. With the help of a **side viewing gastroduodenoscope,** a **sphincterotomy** of the **ampulla** (also known as **papillotomy**) is performed. **Balloon** or **basket extractions** of the **stones** are two **common** methods employed. **Endoscopic ultrasound** as well as the availability of **choledochoscope** has brought down the **incidence** of **missed stones**. Once **all the stones** have been **removed,** a **cholangiogram i**s done to confirm the same. A temporary **nasobiliary drainage** completes the procedure. Following **improvement** in the **status** of the **liver**, these patients undergo a **laparoscopic cholecystectomy** since most have **stones** in the **gall bladder** as well.

In **properly selected patients**, a **laparoscopic** route is used for **extraction** of the **stone in the CBD** as well as the **removal of the gall bladder** in the same sitting.

Q. 27. What are the open surgical procedures available for these cases?

These procedures are not commonly performed currently. They are indicated only when the **procedures mentioned above** are either **not available** or **not successful**. The **CBD** is exposed at the **free border** of the **lesser**

omentum. A **choledochotomy** is then performed and the **stones** are removed. The **CBD** is **flushed** with **normal saline** to **ensure removal** of **all the stones**. An **operative cholangiogram** is performed to confirm the same. The **incision** in the **CBD is** then **close**d around a **T-tube**. The **long end** of the **T-tube** is **brought out** and connected to a **closed drainage system**. The presence of the **T-tube** minimises the **bile leak around** the **CBD. Bile unfortunately** induces an **inflammatory reaction** and this can lead to a **biliary stricture** at a **later date**. A **cholecystectomy** is carried out **simultaneously.** About a **week later**, a

postoperative cholangiogram is done and if all the **findings are normal**, the **T-tube is removed**. **Open surgery** had the **highest incidence** of **retained stones**, and this has **come down** to a large extent in the **endoscopic era**. But **recurrent stones** can **develop** irrespective of the **modality** of treatment. An **anastomosis** between the **CBD** and the **duodenum** has been suggested to **prevent blockage** of the duct by **recurrent stones**.

■■■

Surgical Diseases of the Liver

10

HEPATO CELLULAR CARCINOMA

Setting

- Surgical OPD.

Chief Complaint

- An **upper abdominal mass** of **8 months** duration.

History of Present Illness

A **48-year-old male** presented to the OPD with the complaint of an **upper abdominal right-sided mass** of **8 months** duration. He had **noticed** a slight **fullness** in the **upper abdomen 8 months** ago. Since then it had been **gradually increasing** in size. The **swelling** had reached a **large size prompting** the patient to take **medical advice**.

- He had **dragging type of pain** in the **upper abdomen** for the last **one month**. There was **no** history of **radiation** of pain.
- He had **lost weight** during this period.

- The **appetite** was **normal,** but he had **early satiety**.
- There was **no** history of **vomiting.**
- There was **no history** of **jaundice**.
- He did **not** have **fever**.
- His **bowel habits** were **normal.** There was **no** history of **malaena.**
- He did **not** have any **respiratory symptoms**.

Past History

There was **no history** of attacks of **jaundice** in the **past.** He did **not suffer** from any **major illness** earlier.

Family History

There was **no history of jaundice** in members of the **family.**

Personal History

He was a **smoker** and used to **consume alcohol** daily.

Treatment History

He was **told** that he had a **liver disease** and hence had consulted an **Ayurvedic doctor**. He had **taken treatment** for **two months**. Since his **condition** had **worsened,** he had **come** to the **Surgical OPD.**

General Physical Examination

The patient appeared **well built** and well **nourished**. There was **no jaundice** or **pallor**. **Pedal oedema** was absent.

Examination of Abdomen

Inspection

- A **swelling** was **visible** occupying the **right hypochondrium** and extending to the **epigastrium**. The **lower border** was **indistinct.**
- The **surface** appeared **smooth.**
- The **swelling** was seen to move with **respiration.**
- The **skin** over the **swelling** was **normal. No dilated veins** were seen in the **abdominal wall.**
- The **hernial orifices** and **external genitalia** were normal.

Palpation

- A **swelling** was palpable in the **right hypochondrium** extending to the **epigastric, right lumbar and umbilical** regions.
- The **lower margin** was **felt,** and was **sharp** in nature and felt about **five finger breadths below** the **costal margin**.
- It was **not possible** to **insinuate** the **fingers** between the **costal margin** and the **swelling.**
- The **surface** was **nodular**. The **largest** nodule was felt to occupy the **epigastrium** and the **umbilical regions,** measuring **5 cm by 4 cm** in size. **Smaller nodules** were felt over the rest of the **swelling.**
- The **consistency** of these nodules was **hard.**
- The swelling was seen to move with **respiration.**
- **The spleen** was **not palpable**.
- **No other mass** was palpable in the abdomen.
- There was **no fluid thrill**.

Percussion

- It was **dull** to percuss and the **dullness** was **continuous** with that of the **liver.**
- The **liver span** measured **20 cm.**
- **Shifting dullness** was **absent.**

Auscultation

- **No bruit** was heard over the swelling.

Examination of Other Systems

- **External genitalia** were normal.
- **Supraclavicular region** did not have any **palpable lymph nodes**.

- Examination of the **spine** did **not** reveal any **abnormality**.
- **Rectal examination** was **normal**.

Q. 1. What was the clinical diagnosis?

(*a*) Hepatocellular carcinoma (HCC).

(*b*) Secondary deposits in the liver.

(*c*) Hydatid cyst of the liver.

The likely diagnosis was a HCC.

The following **clinical findings** proved that the **swelling** was from the **liver.**

Site: The swelling was in the right hypochondrium extending to the **neighbouring quadrants.**

The **lower border** was well **felt.** But it was **not possible** to feel the **upper border** since it was **extending above** the **costal margin.**

It was **seen to move** with **respiration.**

It was **dull to percuss** and the **dullness** was **continuous** with the **liver dullness.**

The **liver span** was **more** than **normal.**

Hydatid cyst of the **liver** was **ruled out because** the **relevant history** usually would be of **several years** duration. The **liver surface** would be **smooth** and **consistency firm.**

A **diagnosis** of a **malignant liver** was easily **made.** The **surface** was **nodular** and the **consistency hard. One nodule** was much **larger compared** with the **others.** The **common sites** for a **primary malignancy** to give rise to **secondaries** in the **liver** are the **stomach and colon.** This **patient** did not have any **symptoms or signs** referable to these **organs. Free fluid** in the **abdomen** is **frequently present** in this **condition.** Usually these **deposits** are **metachronous** in their **appearance.** They become **manifest** after the **primary tumour** has been **treated.** The **time interval** may vary from **months** to **a few years.** At that stage, the **general condition** of the patient is often quite **poor.** But there are **situations** where **distinction** between a **primary malignancy** and **secondary deposits** may be **difficult clinically. Cancers** of the **right colon** may remain **asymptomatic** and the **first manifestation** may be **metastases** in the **liver.**

In this case the **diagnosis of HCC** was made on the following **findings.**

The **general condition** of the patient was **good.**

The **liver** had **multiple hard nodules** with **one** being **much larger** in size.

Q. 2. What were the investigations done in this patient?

Ultrasonogram (US) study. The study showed **multiple masses** with **mixed echogenicity** occupying **both** the **lobes of the liver**. A **central area of necrosis** was noted in the **large mass** situated in the **left lobe**. **Doppler study** did **not** show any **thrombus** in the **portal vein**.

Spleen was **normal** in size.

There was **no free fluid** in the abdomen.

Contrast-enhanced computerised tomography (CECT) abdomen. There was **enhancement** in these lesions during the **arterial phase**. The **late venous phase** showed **wash out** of the **contrast** from the **nodules**.

Liver function tests (LFT). **Serum bilirubin** and **enzyme levels** were within **normal** limits.

Serum albumen was **2.5 gm%**.

Tests for **hepatitis B & C** were **negative.**

Prothrombin time was within **normal** limits.

Serum alpha fetoprotein (AFP) level was **1020** units.

Chest X-ray was normal.

FNAC of the **large nodule** in the **left lobe** was done under **US guidance**.

Setting: A week later.

FNAC report was a HCC.

The **diagnosis as well as** the **state of the disease** was **explained** to the **relatives**. The **futility** of any type of **interventional treatment** was made **very clear** to these **relatives**.

The **patient** was **discharged** with **drugs** to **relieve** the **symptoms**.

Q. 3. What could be the possible outcome for this patient?

The **prognosis** was likely to be **very poor**. He would develop **jaundice** within a **short period**.

Death could be the result of **liver cell failure**. A **second** but an **uncommon cause** of **death** would be a **spontaneous rupture** of one of the **nodules** leading to **exsanguinating intra-abdominal bleed**.

Q. 4. What is the incidence of HCC?

In the past, HCC was considered a rare disease, but it is now being recognised quite frequently in patients. There is a **growing incidence** of **HCC** all over the **world.** It is the **sixth most common cancer** and the **third cause** of **cancer-related deaths**. It accounts for **7%** of all **malignancies**. The **geographical** incidence varies and **East Asia** and the **Subsaharan Africa** have the **highest number**. The **incidence** in the **developed countries** is **low,** but most of the **increasing incidence** has been **reported** from **this part of the world**. Although considered a **disease** of the **elderly** in the **West**, in the **developing countries**, it occurs at a **younger age**. This **cance**r is more common in **males.** In the **West, primary malignancy** is responsible for about **80%** of all cancers and the remaining **20%** are **metastatic** in nature. **In the past,** malignancies seen in the liver were mainly secondaries, but now there is a **change** in favour of **HCC**. This **change** has taken place probably due to **two reasons**. There is a **true increase** in the **incidence** of **HCC**. The **availability** of various **imaging modalities** and **immunohistochemistry** has made the **diagnosis easier**. In addition, **better management** of the various **cancers** especially of the **GI tract** has **brought down** the **number** of **patients** with **hepatic metastases.**

Q. 5. What are the aetiological factors?

More than **50%** of these **cancers** develop in a **cirrhotic liver**.

The **common causes** for **cirrhosis** are as listed below:

(*a*) **Hepatitis B and C viral hepatitis**.

(*b*) **Alcohol abuse.**

(*c*) **Cryptogenic.**

(*d*) **Nonalcoholic steatohepatitis** (**NASH**).

(*e*) **Biliary tract disease** leading to repeated attacks of **cholangitis** can in turn lead to **biliary cirrhosis.**

(*f*) **Haemochromatosis.**

Dietary exposure to **Aflatoxin B1** derived from the fungus *Aspergillus flavus* is an important factor in **our patients**. This is due to ingestion of **food adulterated** with this **toxin.**

Cigarette smokers have a higher risk of developing this cancer.

Chewing **of tobacco and betel leaves** has also been implicated in the aetiology.

The presence of obesity, diabetes and fatty liver has been mentioned as cofactors.

A **few genetic factors** have also been identified recently.

Box 10.1: Points regarding aetiology
• 50% occur in patients with cirrhosis.
• Cirrhosis – Causes – Hepatitis B or C – Alcohol – Nutritional – Cryptogenic – Aflatoxin.
• NASH
• Haemochromatosis.
• ? genetic factors.

Q. 6. **What are the symptoms in a case of HCC?**

The picture is **nonspecific** and only a **high degree of suspicion** will help in arriving at an early diagnosis.

Pain in the right hypochondrium is the **main symptom**. But it tends to occur rather **late** in the **course of the disease**.

There may be **loss of weight** and **appetite. Compression** of the **stomach** may produce early **satiety.**

Some of these **patients** present with a **mass** in the **right upper quadrant** of the abdomen.

Jaundice is a **late symptom**. It could be due to the following factors.

(*a*) **Extensive infiltration** of the **liver** by the tumour with **loss of function**.

(*b*) The **mass** obstructing a **major biliary duct.**

(*c*) **Secondary nodes** at the **porta hepatis** may **block** the **CHD.**

Screening programmes instituted for **cirrhotic patients identify** a large number of **patients** at an **asymptomatic stage** in the **advanced countries.**

Box 10.2:	Points regarding symptoms of HCC

- Picture – Nonspecific – High degree of suspicion needed.
- Pain – Upper abdomen – Late.
- Loss of weight and appetite.
- Mass in upper abdomen.
- Jaundice – Late
- Screening of cirrhotic patients periodically.

General physical examination. Pallor is often present. **Jaundice** as mentioned above is seen at an **advanced stage**. It is surprising to note that in the **noncirrhotic group**, the **patient** appears **fairly healthy** till a **late stage. Signs of liver cell failure** may be present in **patients** with **cirrhosis.**

Q. 7. **What are the clinical findings?**

Hepatomegaly is the prominent sign. **Single** or **multiple nodules** are felt in the **liver.** They are **firm-to-hard** in **consistency** with **clear-cut borders**. They are **nontender.** Their **size** varies from **1–2 cm** to **several centimetres**. A few of them may be much **larger** having a **bosselated appearance**.

The **spleen** may be palpable in patients with **associated cirrhosis** or **secondary** to a **tumour thrombus** blocking the **portal vein.**

Ascites is present in many of these **patients.** It could either be due to **portal hypertension** or **peritoneal secondaries**.

Features of **portal hypertension** may be present in **cirrhotic patients.**

Spread beyond the **abdomen** is uncommon in HCC.

Box 10.3:	Points regarding clinical findings in HCC

- Hepatomegaly – Single or multiple nodules – Hard.
- Ascites – Peritoneal secondaries or portal hypertension.
- Features of portal hypertension.
- Spread beyond the abdomen – Uncommon.

Q. 8. What are the investigations done in a case of HCC?

1. **Ultrasound** is the **first line** of investigation. **Small tumours** are typically **hypoechoic** but as **they enlarge** they become **hyperechoic.** Hence **mixed echogenicity** is a **common finding**. Presence of a **hyperechoic rim (capsule)** is noted in **some** of these **cases. Invasion** of the **portal vein** by the **tumour** can be **distinguished** from a **thrombus** by colour **Doppler** examination. The **former** shows **pulsatile blood flow.** More significantly the **echogenic status** of the **remaining liver tissue** will show the **extent of cirrhosis. Intraoperative US** is extremely **useful** during **hepatic resections**.

   Splenomegaly and other **features** of **portal hypertension** will be seen in patients with **cirrhosis.**

2. **CECT** is the **standard investigation**. The **results** are **based** on the **fact** that the **blood supply** to the **tumour** is mainly via the **hepatic artery** and **not** the **portal vein.** **HCCs** therefore **enhance early** during **the arterial phase (20 to 40 sec.),** but the **parenchyma** of the **rest of the liver enhances** during the **portal venous phase (50 to 90 sec.).** In addition, the **contrast is washed out** during the **venous phase from** the **tumour.** This **triphasic appearance** is **diagnostic** of HCC. Presence of **enlarged nodes** at the **porta hepatis** and the **hepato-duodenal (HD) ligament** are **detected. Extrahepatic spread** to the adjacent structures like the **diaphragm** is made out by **CT.** But the limitation is that **small tumours** may be **missed** following a **CECT.** There is a significant percentage of **false negative** results **following CT.**

3. **MRI angiography** is used as the primary investigation in many institutions. The **morphological differences** between the **tumour** and the **rest of the liver** are **made out** clearly by **MRI**. The **increased blood flow** during the **arterial phase** and the **washout** at the **venous phase** is the **same** as seen with **CECT**.

4. **Tumour markers. Serum AFP** levels of more than **400 ng** are helpful in the **diagnosis**. But **normal values** do **not rule out HCC**. This **investigation** is more important in **assessing** the **response** to **treatment**.

5. **LFT—ALT and AST** levels are usually **raised** but are **nonspecific. Child Pugh's Classification** of the **status** of the liver is **vital** both in the **treatment** and **prognosis.**

6. **Liver biopsy. FNAC is diagnostic. Tumours** located in **difficult areas** (**close** to **important vessels**) are **biopsied** with the help of **US or CT**. The **cells** usually are **arranged** in a **trabecular pattern** with **increased nuclear** to **cytoplasmic ratio** and **abnormal nuclei**.

As an **exception**, a **small group of patients** with **HCC** are **treated without** a **pathological diagnosis**. If a **curative resection** is **planned**, the **typical CECT findings** along with **AFP levels** of **more than 500 ng** are considered **adequate** for a **diagnosis** and a **FNAC** is **not performed**. The **rationale behind** this **decision** is the **risk of bleeding,** which is real in a **cirrhotic patient,** and the **risk of tumour seeding** along the **needle track following a FNAC,** which has been **proved** by **retrospective studies.**

Occasionally **biopsy** of the **nonmalignant area** is done to **assess** the **presence** and **extent of cirrhosis.**

Box 10.4: Points regarding investigations

- US – Mixed echogenicity – Hyperechoic rim – Small tumours.
  - Doppler – Involvement of the portal vein.
- CECT – Standard investigations – Diagnostic.
- Arterial phase – Enhancement – Venous phase – Wash out.
- Enlarged nodes along the porta hepatis and HD ligament.
- MRI – Morphological difference between tumour and rest of liver better made out.
- AFP – More than 400 ng – Helpful in diagnosis – Assessing response to treatment.
- LIVER BIOPSY – In curative resections LIVER BIOPSY NOT DONE.
- LFT – Limited use – Useful in cirrhotics.

Q. 9. Describe the applied surgical anatomy of the liver.

A study of the **surgical anatomy** is **absolutely essential** to understand the **principles** of the various types of **liver resections** done for HCC. In the past the **falciform ligament** was used to divide the liver into **two anatomical lobes,** namely, the **right and left lobes.**

The **Couinaud's classification** forms a rational basis for HCC. The **principal plane of Cantlie,** running from the **gall bladder bed** anteriorly to the **groove for the inferior vena cava** posteriorly, divides the liver into the **right and left surgical lobes.** The **hepatic artery and the portal vein** divide **into two branches** at the **hilum** of the liver to **join the right and left lobes. Further division** takes place inside the liver to supply **individual segments. Every segment** receives a **branch of the hepatic artery and portal vein. Bile from each segment** is drained by a **tributary** of the **bile duct.** These **join together** to form the **right** and **left hepatic ducts.** They join at **the hilum** to form the **common hepatic duct.** But the **venous drainage is more complex.** The **right and left hepatic veins** drain their **respective lobes.** In addition,

the **middle hepatic vein** drains certain **segments of both these lobes.** Their **extrahepatic course** is **very short** before they **join the inferior vena cava (IVC)** just **below the diaphragm.**

Segmental anatomy of the liver.

Segment 1 - caudate lobe of the liver.

Segments 2, 3, and 4A and 4B constitute the **left surgical lobe.**

Right surgical lobe consists of segments **5, 6, 7 and 8.**

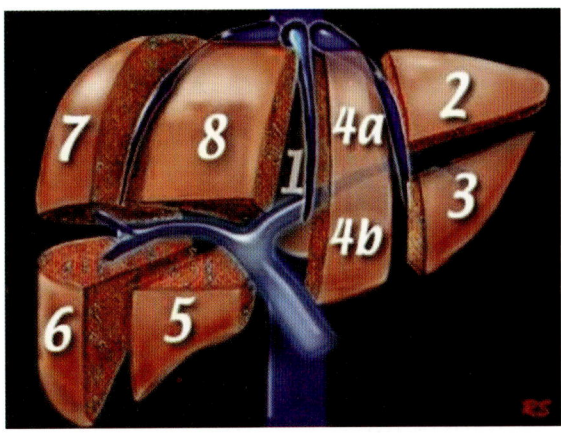

Fig. 10.1: Segmental anatomy of the liver.

The segments are named as follows.

1. **Caudate lobe.** It is **located posteriorly** and **separated** from the rest of the **liver** by the **fissure for the ligament venosum.**

2. **Left superior lateral segment.**

3. **Left inferior lateral segment.**

4A. Left superior medial segment.

4B. Left inferior medial segment.

5. Right inferior anterior segment.

6. Right inferior posterior segment.

7. Right superior posterior segment.

8. Right superior anterior segment.

Q. 10. Describe liver resections for HCC.

Surgery offers the **best outcome** for patients with **HCC**. But the **limiting factor** is the **status of the liver**. Since **majority** of **cancers** arise in a **cirrhotic liver**, **resections rates** are in general **very low**. Again it is known that when a **cancer develops** in this **group**, it could be **multicentric.** In addition to the **extent of** the **tumour** in the liver, the **functional status** of the **remnant** is equally **important**. Otherwise patients will **die** of **acute hepatocellular failure** in the **postoperative period.** Among all the vital organs in the body, the liver is unique in its ability to regenerate following resection. In a **noncirrhotic** liver a **remnant of 25%** is adequate to **sustain life.** But in **cirrhotics** the figure is **higher at 40%. Regeneration following**

a resection usually takes place over a period of **several months**.

Many of our patients at the **time of admission** have **extensive involvement** of the **liver** that **precludes resections**. The **presence** of a **liver disease directs** even an **educated person** towards **alternative systems of medicine**. Hence there is **considerable delay** before they are **properly investigated**. Thus even in the **noncirrhotic group,** the **resection rates** in general are **low.**

Hepatic resections. This is the **ideal treatment** for **noncirrhotic patients**. The indications are as follows.

1. **Single tumour less** than **5 cm** in size.

2. **No evidence** of **vascular invasion.**

3. **No evidence** of **extrahepatic spread**.

4. **Rest of the liver** is **healthy** or patients belonging to **Child Pugh class A** with **no evidence** of **portal hypertension.**

5. A **2-cm margin** of **healthy parenchyma** at the **edge of the tumour** should be available for a **R0 resection**.

The **procedure** may be a **right or left hemihepatectomy** (excision of the right or left surgical lobe) or **selective single** or **multiple** segmentectomy. The **operative mortality** is between **2% and 5%.** The **five-year disease-free interval** is **60%. Local recurrence** is **frequent** despite **R0 resections.**

Q. 11. **What is the role of liver transplantation in HCC?**

Ideally this is the **best option for HCC, especially in the presence of cirrhosis.** It **eliminates** the chances of **local recurrence** and the **development** of **cancer de novo** in the **liver remnant.** It also **reduces** the **complications** associated with **portal hypertension.** In addition, the **functional status** of the **liver remnant** does **not influence** the **outcome. Hepatic function** is restored to **normal levels.**

Q. 12. **What are the indications for this procedure?**

1. **Tumour less than 5 cm in size.**

2. If **multiple tumours** are present they should be **less than 3** in number and **3 cm in size**.

3. **No evidence of extrahepatic spread.**

4. **No evidence of vascular invasion**

5. The **waiting period** should be preferably **less than 6 months**.

Disadvantages: The most important **limiting factor** is **availability. Organ donation** has **not yet** caught the **imagination of the public** in this country. Despite having the **highest incidence of road accidents** in the world, with a **significant number** of the cases being declared **brain dead**, the **percentage of organ donation** is **miniscule. Religious and social factors** also work **against this type of donation. Centres** performing **liver transplants** are **increasing** especially in **the metros** of our **country.** But **affordability** becomes an **important issue.** For many patients, the **waiting period** is too long and either **they die** or **become inoperable** before an **organ becomes available**.

Living donor transplantation is an attractive **alternative,** but has several **inherent problems**. The incidence **of donor mortality** in the best of **centres is about 1%. Transplantation** is associated with a **mortality of 15%** in the **first year**. Transplant patients need to take **immunosuppressive therapy** for the **rest of their life.** But the **five-year** survival rate is **80%** in properly selected cases.

Box 10.5:	Points regarding liver resections for HCC

- Functional capacity of the remnant – 25% Noncirrhotics – 40% cirrhotics.
- Right or left hemihepatectomy – Segmental resections – Surgical mortality 2%-5%.
- Single lesion > 5 cm – No extrahepatic spread – No vascular invasion.
- 2-cm margin – R0 resection.
- local recurrence are known to occur ever after R0 resections.

Box 10.6:	Points regarding transplantation

- Ideal for cirrhotics. Tumour > 5 cm – 3 lesions less than 3 cm.
- No vascular invasion – No extrahepatic spread.
- Waiting time less than 6 months.
- No local recurrence – Function of the remnant-not relevant.
- Availability – Cost of treatment – Lifelong immune suppression.
- Living donor – Not popular – Donor mortality - Availability.

Q. 13. What are the types of ablative therapy available for HCC?

Most of **our patients** are **not suitable for resections** and transplantation is not a **practical solution. Ablation** of the tumour is a **good option** under these circumstances. **Radio frequency (RF) ablation** under **US guidance** gives **considerable relief.** When an **alternating current** is passed through a **RF probe,** the **resulting heat (nearly 100° C.)** leads to **coagulative necrosis** of the tumour. The effect is **distributed** to an area **about 5 cm. all round the probe.** In **tumours less than 2 cm** in size, the **results** are almost **equal** to that of **surgery.**

Intratumoural injection of **absolute alcohol under US guidance** also leads to **ablation** of the tumour. The advantage is that it can be **repeated** if needed in **tumours larger than 5 cm.**

Transarterial Chemoembolisation.(TACE)

The **procedure** depends on the fact that the **tumour derives** its **blood supply** from the **branches of the hepatic artery,** whereas the **surrounding liver** receives both **portal and arterial blood.** Initially a **selective arteriogram** is performed after **catheterising** the **branch of the hepatic artery** supplying the **tumou**r. An **emulsion** of a **cytotoxic drug** like **Doxorubicin or Cisplatin** with **lipiodol** (iodine in poppy seed oil) is **injected into the tumour.** **Lipiodol** has been found to **retain the drug** in **contact with tumour** for a **longer period of time enhancing its effects.** It also **confirms** the proper **localisation of the drug** in relation to **the tumour.** It is **followed** by **embolisation** of the **feeding artery** with **gel foam** or other methods. **Extensive tumour necrosis** occurs in more than **80%** of patients. The procedure is **contraindicated** when there is **diffuse involvement** of the liver, in the presence **of liver failure** (**Child Pugh class C**) and in cases of **portal venous thrombosis.** It can be used to **control the tumour** during the **waiting period for transplantation.**

Box 10.7: Points regarding ablative therapy

- RF probe – US guidance – Heat (100°C) – Coagulative necrosis-tumour size 2 cm or less – Good results.
- Intratumour absolute alcohol – Repeated for large tumours.
- TACE – Blood supply – Arterial-selective angiogram – Inj. Doxorubicin with lipiodol.
- Prolonged contact – Localisation.
- Embolisation of feeding artery by gel foam.

Q. 14. Describe the roles of chemotherapy and monoclonal antibody in HCC.

Chemotherapy: It is usually a **palliative** line of **treatment**. Many drugs have been tried, but the **results are disappointing**. The **quality of life** also may **not improve due to drug toxicity.**

Monoclonal antibody (mAb). Sorafenib is an mAb that has been shown to be effective in the treatment of **advanced HCC**. It is used **orally** and acts as a **multi–tyrosine kinase inhibitor. Cost and availability** are two limiting factors that affect its use in our patients.

Unfortunately, **most of our HCC patients** present with either **advanced cirrhosis** or **multiple large tumours**. In this group only **palliative symptomatic treatment** is possible and the prognosis is very poor. Mean **survival time** is **6 to 20 months.**

Q. 15. What are the general features of metastatic liver disease?

Liver is a **common site** for **metastases** from **many cancers**. Almost **all malignancies** have been reported with **liver metastases**. Till recently these were considered to **be more frequent than HCC**. But the present incidence is said to be about **20% of all liver cancers**. **GI tract** malignancies are responsible for **most** of these lesions, since the **liver acts as a primary filter**. **Carcinomas** of the **breast and thyroid** (follicular type) as well as **malignant melanoma** contribute a significant number to this group.

Most patients with **secondaries in the liver** are at an **advanced stage** with **disseminated disease** in other parts of the body. The **peritoneal cavity, lungs and bones** are the **common sites** for these metastases. Hence these patients **do not need any specific treatment** for the liver metastases. Only **palliative symptomatic** treatment is needed. The **common cause** of **death** in this group is **liver cell failure** due to **extensive infiltration** of the organ.

Box 10.8:	Points regarding the features of metastatic liver disease

- 20% of liver cancers.
- GI tract – Most common primary – Liver is the primary filter.
- Breast, thyroid and melanoma.
- Widespread disease – Palliative symptomatic treatment.
- Death – Liver cell failure.

However, there are **exceptions** to the statements made above. Secondaries from carcinoma of the **colorectum** and **neuroendocrine tumours** of the **GI tract** behave in a **different way** and hence demand a detailed study. Their **biological behaviour** sets them **apart from other tumours** and makes them **amenable for effective treatment.**

Q. 16. Describe the special features of colorectal cancer with liver metastases.

Most of them are **metachronous** in nature. They appear **several months** or **years** after the **primary tumour** has been **treated. Majority** of these occur **within two years**. A **small number** of patients present with the **primary tumour** as well as **synchronous secondaries** in the liver. The clinical picture is of **an enlarged liver** with **nodules**. The nodules are **firm-to-hard in consistency. Umbilication** due to **central necrosis** is an **unreliable sign**. Unfortunately, only in about **10% of** cases, the **metastases** are **confined to the liver, while the** rest have **enlarged lymph nodes or ascites. CT is necessary to** confirm that the **disease** is **confined** to the **liver.** A **diagnostic laparoscopy** rules out **surface lesions in the liver** and **peritoneum.** The **CT** also helps to take a decision regarding **resectability. A single lesion less than 5 cm** is **ideal for resection.** But **multiple secondaries** depending on their **number and location** can be treated by **segmentectomies.** The **five-year disease-free interval** in this group is between **50% and 60%.** Thus it is logical to keep patients operated on for colorectal cancer on **surveillance before clinical manifestations** of liver metastases appear. It includes estimating the levels of **CEA a**nd US **examination** of the abdomen at periodic intervals.

Box 10.9:	Points regarding liver metastases from colorectal cancers

- 10% metastases only in the liver.
- Single lesion less than 5 cm or multiple lesions suitable for resection.
- CECT - Selection of patients.
- Hemihepatectomy or multiple segmental resections.
- 5-year DFS 60%.
- Regular surveillance - CEA levels and abdomen US.

Q. 17. What are the special features of secondaries in liver from GI neuroendocrine tumours?

Apart from the lung, the **small intestine** is a frequent site for these tumours. They arise from **enterochromaffin cells** present in the **wall of the intestine**. They were called as **carcinoid tumours** in the past. Though their **neural origin** has been **disproved**, the **nomenclature** has been **retained**. The cells contain **chromaffin granules** demonstrable by **special staining**. Again like the colorectal group, the **number of patients** with **isolated hepatic secondaries** is **low.** Clinically they present with **enlarged nodular livers.** But their **biological behaviour** makes them **suitable for aggressive treatment.**

Tumour markers like estimation of **cgA (chromogranin A)** and urinary hydroxyl indole acetic acid (**HIAA**) are useful in the **diagnosis. CECT scans** pick up lesions **more than 3 cm** in size**. Somatostatin receptor scintigraphy** and **Gallium-68 receptor scan** are sophisticated investigations performed in specialised centres. **Surgical resection** when feasible offers the best outcome. It may mean a **surgical lobectomy or segmentectomy. Nonsurgical** treatments are still in an experimental stage. Peptide receptor nuclide therapy (**PRNT**) given intravenously is being tried with **fairly satisfactory** results. But many are prone to develop **local recurrences** with a **poor prognosis.**

Box 10.10:	Points regarding secondaries from GI neuroendocrine tumours

- Small number has isolated secondaries in liver only.
- cgA and HIAA – Useful.
- CECT – secondaries > 3 cm.
- Somatostatin receptor scintigraphy and gallium 68 receptor scan.
- Resection – Best results – Surgical lobectomy or multiple segmentectomies.
- Nonsurgical – PRNT.
- Recurrence rate – High.

Q. 18. Describe the general characteristics of hydatid cyst of the liver.

Hydatid disease is a **parasitic disease** caused by the **Echinococcus** group. *Echinococcus granulosus* is the **common type** responsible in most of the patients. **Hydatid cyst** is common in **certain parts of the world,** especially the **sheep rearing areas.** It is more prevalent in the **states of Andhra Pradesh and Tamil Nadu** in our country. More than **70% of these cysts** occur in the **liver**, followed by occurrences in the **lungs** and other organs. Since the **lesions** are **discovered** only when they reach a **large size,** they can **cause severe morbidity.**

Q. 19. Describe the life cycle of *E. granulosus.*

The **canine species** is the **definitive host.** The **adult tape worm *E. granulosus*** measuring **6 to 7 mm** resides in the **small intestine** of these **animals.** The **eggs** or **ova** are **passed in the stools.** These are ingested by sheep or cattle, which form the **intermediate host.** A **human being** becomes an **accidental intermediate host** when the person **comes in contact with the eggs.** This can happen due to **direct contact with dogs** or **ingesting food or water contaminated** with these **eggs.**

Once the **eggs** are **ingested** they **release larvae** in the **duodenum.** The **larvae migrate** through the **duodenal wall** and gain **access to** **the mesenteric vessels**, reaching the **liver** where **most are trapped**. Thus the **liver** becomes the **most common organ** to be affected in the **human body.** The **larvae develop** into **small cysts** surrounded by a **fibrous capsule.** The **cyst grows** at a rate of **1 to 3 cm in a year.** Thus until they grow into a **large size** they are **not detected.** An **adult primary cyst** is composed of **three layers.** The adventitia or the **pericyst** comprises of **compressed liver and fibrous tissues.** The **ectocyst** is a **laminated membrane**, which appears as an **elastic white covering** easily **separable** from the **pericyst** in **uncomplicated cases.** The **germinal epithelium** or **endocyst** is a **single layer of cells** lining the **inner wall of the cyst.** This is the only **living component** of the cyst being **responsible** for the formation of other **layers and hydatid fluid.** The **cyst produces brood capsules** containing **many scolices.** Some of **these daughter cysts separate** from the **cyst wall** to **float freely** in the **hydatid fluid. Scolices** are seen as **hydatid sand.** Each of these **particles** contains as many as **800,000 eggs.**

Box 10.11:	Points regarding the life cycle of E. granulosus

- Dog – Definitive host – Sheep or cattle – Intermediate host.
- Humans – Accidental intermediate host – Contact with dog.
- Ingestion of eggs by contaminated food or water.
- Egg – Larva in the duodenum – Penetration – Mesenteric vein.
- Trapped in liver – Cyst – Growth very slow.
- Pericyst – Compressed liver tissue with fibrosis.
- Ectocyst – White laminated membrane – Easily separated from ectocyst.
- Endocyst – Single layer of cells – Hydatid fluid – Daughter cysts and scolices.
- Free floating cysts – Scolex – 800,000 eggs.

Q. 20. What are the clinical features of hydatid cyst of the liver?

1. **Mass in the right upper quadrant** of the abdomen of **several years** duration is the chief complaint.

2. Some may have **dull dragging pain** in this region.

3. The **liver** is found to be **enlarged**. The surface is **smooth**. It is **nontender**. The consistency is **soft or firm**. **Hydatid thrill** when present **confirms the diagnosis**. The physical explanation for this sign is as follows. When a **mother cyst** packed with **unruptured daughter cysts** is **percussed**, the **vibrations** of the **fluid inside**

the **daughter cysts** are felt by the **adjacent fingers**. The availability of various **imaging modalities** has made this sign **redundant.**

4. **Jaundice** is present only in the presence of **complications.**

Box 10.12:	Points regarding clinical features

- Mass right side abdomen – Several years – Dragging pain.
- Liver enlarged – Smooth – Nontender – Soft or firm.
- Hydatid thrill.
- Jaundice – Complications.

Q. 21. What are the complications?

1. **Rupture** into the **peritoneal cavity** manifests as an **acute abdomen**. It can cause a **life-threatening anaphylactic reaction.** A picture simulating **peritonitis** is also possible.

2. A **minor continuous leak** can lead to **dissemination of the daughter cysts** into the **peritoneum.** The associated **fibrosis** results in **adhesive obstruction**. It is associated with **severe morbidity and mortality**.

3. **Rupture** into the **biliary tract produces jaundice**. Again **spread** along the **biliary tree** causes **difficult management problems**. It also leads to **secondary cholangitis.**

4. **Infection.** The clinical presentation may be like a

liver abscess. Patients have **pain in the right upper abdomen** with **fever**. The **liver is enlarged** and **tender**.

5. **Calcification** is the result of **necrosis** and indicates usually an **inactive cyst**.

Box 10.13:	Points regarding complications

- Rupture – Anaphylactic reaction – Peritonitis.
- Minor continuous leak – Daughter cysts in peritoneal cavity – Adhesive obstruction.
- Rupture into biliary tree – Difficult to manage.
- Infection.
- Calcification.

Q. 22. What are the investigations done in these cases?

An **US study** is diagnostic in most patients. The **Gharbi classification** is as follows.

1. **Pure fluid** collection.
2. **Fluid collection** with a **split wall**
3. **Fluid collection with septa**.
4. **Heterogeneous echogenic** pattern.
5. **Cyst with reflecting thick walls** due to **calcification.**

CT abdomen is needed when the US findings are **inadequate.**

Plain X-ray. Calcified cysts show a **thin margin of calcification** at the **periphery.**

Serologic tests. **Haemoagglutination** is the **only test** per-formed in the diagnosis of hyda-tid disease.

LFT is usually within normal limits.

Box 10.14:	Points regarding investigations

- US – Diagnostic – Gharbi classification.
- CT – If needed.
- Plain X-ray – Calcification.
- Haemoagglutination.
- LFT.

Q. 23. Describe the surgical treatment of hydatid cyst of the liver.

The **abdomen** is opened with an **upper midline incision**. **Coloured packs** soaked with either **20% hypertonic saline** or **0.5% cetrimide** are used to **isolate** the **operative area** and to **identify and destroy daughter cysts** that might **spill over** during **surgery**. The contents of the cyst are **aspirated** again taking care to **avoid spillage**. A **scolicidal agent** such as **20% hypertonic saline or 0.5% cetrimide** is **injected** into the **cyst cavity. Formalin and silver nitrate** are **no longer used**. Enough **time** is given for **destroying the contents** which is then **re-aspirated**. The **collapsed** cyst is **excised** by developing a **plane between the ectocyst and pericyst**. The cavity is **irrigated** with a **0.5% solution** of **povidone iodine**. The **operation** can also be performed **laparoscopically.**

Percutaneous Aspiration Injection Re-aspiration (PAIR). This novel technique is an alternative line of treatment where laparotomy is avoided. It consists of **percutaneous aspiration** of the cyst contents **under US guidance,** followed by **injection of a scolicidal agent**. The **sterile contents** are **re-aspirated** resulting in **collapse** of the **cyst**. But **recurrences are common** and the treatment is not **universally accepted.**

Q. 24. What is the medical treatment?

Albendazole is an **antihelminthic** agent. The dosage is **10 to 15 mg per kg** body weight to be given for **several months** separated by **14 days intervals** to reduce the **toxic effects** such as **hepatic enzyme elevation** and **neutropenia.** The drug has been used in the **preoperative period** to reduce the risk of **complications due to spillage.**

Box 10.15:	Points regarding the treatment

- Surgical – Isolation – Aspiration – Scolicidal drug injection.
- Re-aspiration – Excision.
- Laparoscopic route.
- PAIR – Avoids laparotomy – Recurrence common.
- Drug – Albendazole – Several months – Preoperative.

Q. 25. What are the features of a congenital nonparasitic cyst of the liver?

Congenital **nonparasitic cyst** of the liver is a **rare** condition. Often it is **discovered incidentally** during **imaging studies** of the abdomen. These cysts are said to be the result of an **aberration during the development of the biliary duct system**. The presence of **cuboidal epithelium** in the **lining** of the **cyst wall** supports this theory. The disease may be **associated** with **polycystic** disease of the **kidney** and occasionally of the **pancreas**, suggesting a **common genetic origin.**

Box 10.16:	Points regarding congenital nonparasitic cyst

- Rare condition – Incidental finding on imaging.
- Aberration of development of biliary duct system.
- Associated cysts in kidney and pancreas – Genetic origin.

Q. 26. What are the clinical features?

1. **Age**. Common in the **fifth decade**.
2. **Gender**. More common in **females**.
3. **Symptoms** appear only when the **cyst assumes a large size**. **Dull dragging pain** or a **mass in the upper part of the right side of the abdomen** are the presenting features.

4. On **examination,** the **liver** is found to be **enlarged**. It is **nontender**. The surface is **smooth** and the consistency, **soft. Fluid thrill** may be elicited in **large superficial cysts.**

Complications like **jaundice** (**extraneous pressure** on a major **bile duct**), **rupture, infection and bleeding** have described, but are **very rare.**

Box 10.17: Points regarding clinical features

- Fifth decade.
- More common in women.
- Asymptomatic hepatomegaly – Smooth – Soft – Fluid thrill
- Jaundice – Pressure on a major bile duct.
- Complications – Rupture, infection – Bleed – Very rare.

Q. 27. What are the investigations needed in such cases?

US is **diagnostic**. A **unilocular cyst** with a **smooth wall** clearly **separating** it from the **rest of the liver is seen.**

It also **rules out** associated **cysts** in the **kidney and pancreas**.

CT abdomen is needed only if **US is not confirmatory** of the diagnosis.

LFT is normal

Q. 28. How are these cysts treated?

Small asymptomatic cysts do **not need any treatment. Large cysts are de-roofed** after **emptying the cyst** by **aspiration.**

A **large residual cavity** may be **packed** with **greater omentum**. A **cystojejunostomy** with a **Roux-en-Y loop** of **jejunum** is needed if the contents are **bile stained. Hepatic resections** though described appear to be **too radical a procedure** for such an essentially **benign condition.**

Box 10.18: Points regarding treatment

- Small cysts – Observation.
- Large cysts – Aspiration – De-roofing – Pack with greater omentum.
- Bile as content – Cystojejunostomy with a Roux-en-Y loop of jejunum.
- Resections – Too radical.

Q. 29. Describe the features and management of haemangioma of the liver.

The topic is being discussed for the sake of **differential diagnosis**. Most of them are **asymptomatic** and do **not need any treatment**. Though the **capillary type** is **more common,** they are usually **small and insignificant**. The **cavernous type** tends to become **large** and **produce symptoms**. A **lesion of more than 4 cm** in size is referred as a **giant haemangioma. Pain and a mass** in the **right hypochondrium** are the common **clinical features,** both being **nonspecific** in nature. The **diagnosis** can only be made with the help of **imaging studies. US is confirmatory** in most cases. It shows an area of **hyperechogenicity** with **well-delineated margins**. **Colour Doppler does not show increased vascularity**. **CT** is advised if **US findings** are **doubtful**. On CT the lesion appears as an **area of hypo-attenuation**. **CECT** shows **filling** of the **contrast** at the **periphery initially** and **spreading centripetally** inside the **lesion**. **Complications** like **rupture** and **bleeding** are very rare. **Most** of these lesions do **not need specific treatment**. **Hepatic resections** are planned for **huge haemangiomas**.

Multiple Choice Questions

1. The most appropriate investigation to diagnose HCC is
   (*a*) Ultrasound abdomen.
   (*b*) FNAC of a nodule.
   (*c*) Raised AFP levels.
   (*d*) Triphasic CECT scan.
   Answer (*d*).

2. The following are the aetiological factors for HCC EXCEPT
   (*a*) Hepatitis A virus infection.
   (*b*) Hepatitis B virus infection.
   (*c*) Hepatitis C virus infection.
   (*d*) Haemochromatosis.
   Answer (*a*).

3. Child Pugh classification for liver disease includes all of the following EXCEPT

   (*a*) Serum bilirubin.
   (*b*) Prothrombin time.
   (*c*) Jaundice.
   (*d*) Encephalopathy.
   Answer (*c*).

4. Which of the following is NOT INDICATED in hydatid cyst of the liver?
   (*a*) ELISA.
   (*b*) FNAC.
   (*c*) US abdomen.
   (*d*) CECT abdomen.
   Answer (*b*).

5. In the surgical treatment of hydatid cyst of the liver, the plane of dissection is between the
   (*a*) Ectocyst and endocyst.
   (*b*) Ectocyst and pericyst.
   (*c*) Endocyst and pericyst.
   (*d*) Outside the pericyst.
   Answer (*b*).

6. In the treatment of hydatid cyst of the liver, PAIR is
   (*a*) Puncture Aspiration Injection Re-aspiration.
   (*b*) Percutaneous Aspiration Injection Re-aspiration.
   (*c*) Percutaneous aspiration Incision Re-aspiration.
   (*d*) Percutaneous Antihelminthic Injection Re-aspiration.
   Answer (*b*).

■ ■ ■

Carcinoma of the Female Breast

11

A CASE OF CANCER BREAST

Setting

- Surgical OPD.

Chief Complaint

Swelling in the **right breast** of **eight months** duration.

History of Present Illness

A **38-year-old lady** came to the surgical OPD with the complaint of a **swelling** in the **right breast** of **eight months duration**. It was **small** in size at onset and there were **no other complaints**. Over the last **few months** the swelling had been **rapidly increasing** in size and hence the patient came to the hospital. She had not noticed any **swellings in the axilla.**

- There was **no** history of **pain**.
- Patient did not give any history of **discharge from the nipple**.

- There was no history of **fever**.
- There was no history of **abdominal distension** or **chronic cough** or **low back pain**.
- The patient did not give any history of **trauma.**

Past History

The patient did not have any **major illness** in the past. She did not suffer from any **breast disease** in the **past.**

Family History

No member in the family had similar problems.

Obstetric History

She had **2 children**. Both were **normal deliveries** and both children were **breast fed**. She had undergone tubectomy nine years ago after the birth of the second child.

Menstrual History

The patient had attained **menarche** at the age of **12** and was having regular periods. The last menstrual period (LMP) was 22 days ago.

Treatment History

The patient had consulted a **lady medical practitioner** who advised her to attend a tertiary **hospital**.

General Physical Examination

The patient was **well built and nourished**. There was no **pallor, jaundice or pedal oedema.**

Examination of Right Breast

Inspection

The patient was made to **sit** with the **arms by the side** and the entire chest was exposed for **examination. A swelling was seen** in the **upper part** of the **right breast**. The **margins** were ill defined.

- The **size** was 6 cm by 4 cm. The **shape** was irregular.
- The **skin** over the swelling was **stretched. Peau d'orange** appearance was seen in the upper half of the breast. No **dimpling** or **puckering** was seen.
- **Dilated veins** were seen over the breast.
- Both the **nipples** were at the **same** level. The right **nipple** was **retracted** and the **areola** appeared **normal.**
- No obvious **oedema** could be made out in the **right upper limb**.

- The patient was made to **stand up** and **raise** both **upper limbs above** the **head**. The level of the **right nipple** was found to be at a **higher level**.

Palpation of the Right Breast

- Patient in **supine position**.
- The lump was **warm** to touch but was **not tender**.
- The **lump** was occupying the **upper half** of the **right breast** including the **subareolar region** and extending into the **lower outer quadrant**. The **borders** were **well defined**.
- The **size** was 11 cm by 5 cm. The **shape** was irregular.
- The **consistency** was **hard.**
- The **skin** was **adherent** to the lump over an area of **2 cm²** at the **summit** of the **lump.** It was **fixed** to the **breast tissue**. It was **not fixed** to the **pectoralis major** muscle or the **chest wall.**
- There was **no other palpable lump** in the right breast.
- There was no **discharge** from the **nipple** during **palpation** of the breast.

Palpation of the Right Axilla

- **Patient in sitting position**.
- There were **multiple lymph nodes** palpable in the **right axilla**. They belonged to the **anterior** and **central** groups. The size varied from **1 cm to 3 cm**. They were **hard**

in consistency. The nodes were **discrete**, **mobile** and **nontender.**

- **No lymph nodes** were **palpable** in the **right supraclavicular** region.

Box 11.1:	Points to be noted in history

- Lump – Few months duration – Rate of growth.
- Pain late symptom.
- Ulceration.
- Discharge from the nipple – Bloodstained.
- Symptoms due to secondaries.
- Breathlessness, cough, haemoptysis.
- Distension of abdomen, jaundice.
- Bone pains - Low back pain.

Box 11.2:	Points to be noted on inspection

- Lump or change in contour. Visible lump – Site, size and shape. Margins.
- Skin changes – dimpling, puckering, redness. Peau d'orange, skin nodules and ulceration.
- Nipple – Retraction. Paget's disease (ulceration).
- Areola – Puckering with pigmentation – Enlargement.
- Lymphoedema of the upper limb.

Box 11.3:	Points to be noted on palpation of the breast and nodes

- Lump – Site(in relation to quadrants), size, shape and borders.
- Lump – Consistency – Hard or variable.
- Anatomical plane. Fixity to skin, breast tissue, pectoralis major and chest wall
- Additional lumps in the breast.
- Discharge from the nipple.
- Palpation of the axillary nodes – Anterior and central groups.
- Supraclavicular nodes.

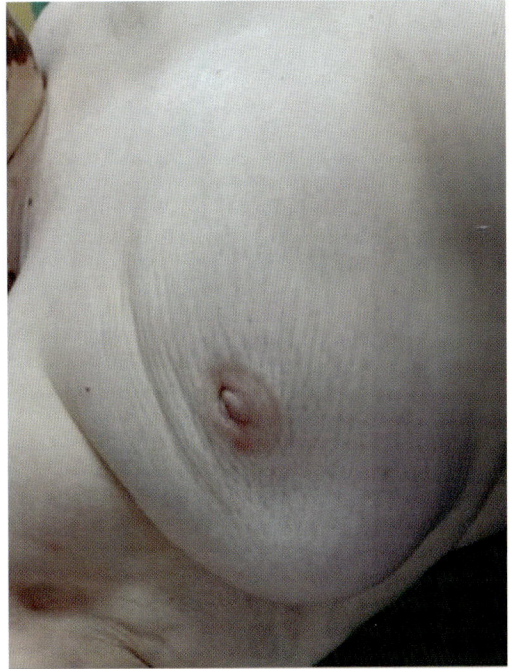

Fig. 11.1: Diffuse swelling of the breast with peau d'orange and retraction of the nipple.

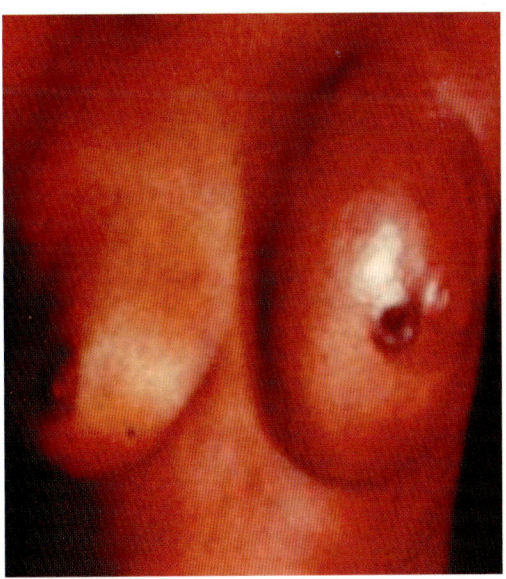

Fig. 11.2: Inflammatory carcinoma of the breast with erythema of the skin.

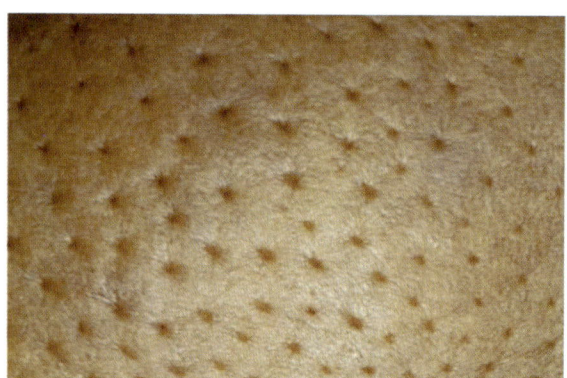

Fig. 11.3: Peau d'orange appearance
of the skin.

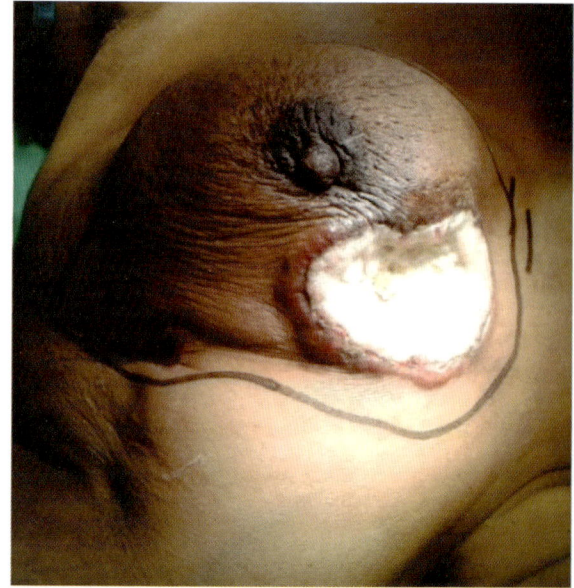

Fig. 11.5: Ulcerated carcinoma of the breast with
peau d'orange and distortion.

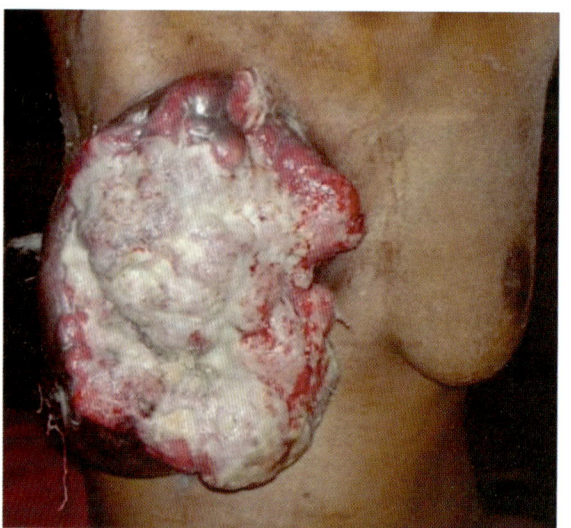

Fig. 11.4: Large fungating carcinoma fixed to the
chest wall.

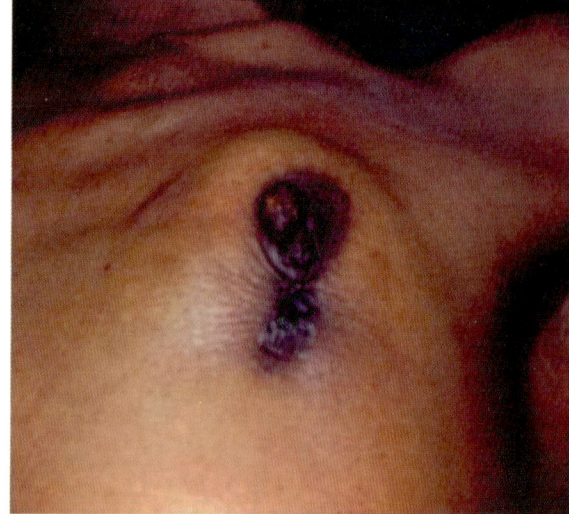

Fig. 11.6: Subareolar tumour with puckering and
pigmentation.

- Examination of the **left breast** did **not** reveal any **lump.**

- **No nodes** were palpable in the **left axilla**.

- The **left supraclavicular** region showed **no nodes**.

Examination of other System

- **Liver** was not palpable.

- There was no **free fluid**.

- No **masses** were felt in the **lower abdomen**.

- **Examination** of the **chest** was normal.

- There were no areas of **bony tenderness**.

- **Pelvic and rectal examinations** did not reveal any abnormality.

Box 11.4:	Points regarding rest of the clinical examination

- Left breast – Lump fixed to breast tissue diagnostic of malignancy.
- Left axilla and supraclavicular region – Lymph nodes.
- Abdomen – Liver Free fluid – Krukenberg tumours.
- Chest – Pleural effusion - Consolidation.
- Skeletal system – Tenderness – Lumbar spine.
- Pelvic and rectal examination.

Q. 1. What was the clinical diagnosis?

The diagnosis was a **carcinoma** of the **right breast**. The findings were **typical** of **malignancy**. No other clinical condition could be considered in the differential diagnosis. A **hard lump** of **few months** duration with **fixity** to the **breast tissue** and **skin** with **enlarged hard nodes** in the **axilla** supports only **one diagnosis**.

Q. 2. What is the clinical stage?

The clinical stage is **Stage III (T4B, N2 and Mx)**

It can also be classified as **locally advanced breast cancer (LABC)**

Q. 3. What were the investigations carried out in this patient?

1. **Core needle biopsy (CNB)** was **preferred** to **FNAC,** since **tissue** was needed for **receptor studies**.

2. **Chest X-ray** was normal.

3. **US abdomen. Liver** was normal. There was no **free fluid**. No **other masses** were seen.

4. **Technitium 99 bone scan**. The scan did not show any **secondary deposits**.

5. **Receptor studies**. The tumour was both **ER and PR positive**. It was **negative** for **Her2 neu** receptor.

Setting: A week later**. CNB** report was an infiltrating duct carcinoma.

Q. 4. What was the treatment strategies planned for this patient?

Since the patient had **LABC** the following were the **broad outlines** of the **treatment**.

The treatment was to **start** with **neoadjuvant chemotherapy** to **down-stage** the tumour. The drugs to be used were **Adriamycin, 5 fluorouracil (FU) and Cyclophosphamide**.

If the tumour showed **response** after **two cycles** of **chemotherapy**, a **modified radical mastectomy** (**MRM**) was planned.

Postoperatively the patient was to continue with **chemotherapy** with the addition of external beam radiation therapy (**EBRT**).

At the time of **discharge**, the patient was to be put on **tamoxifen** for a period of **five years**.

Q. 5.   Describe in detail the treatment given to the patient.

The patient was started on **chemotherapy**. The drugs given were **Adriamycin, 5FU** and **Cyclophosphamide**. After an interval of **21 days** the **course** was **repeated. Three weeks** after the second course the **patient** was **reassessed. The size** of the **tumour** was **reduced** by about **50%** and the **lymph nodes** had become **smaller.** These findings indicated a **partial response** of the tumour to **chemotherapy**.

The patient then underwent MRM. An **elliptical incision** which included the **involved** skin and the **nipple areola** complex was made. The **skin flaps** were raised and the entire **breast** was **removed** with the **fascia** exposing the **pectoralis major** muscle. The **dissection** was continued to the **axilla,** and **level I and II nodes** with the surrounding **fat** were removed along with the **breast specimen**. **Closure** with a **suction drain** completed the operation. Ten days later the sutures were removed. The incision had healed well.

The **histopathology** showed a **ductal carcinoma**. All the **margins** were **free** of the tumour. All the **axillary lymph nodes** showed **metastatic deposits.**

Setting: Patient readmitted after three weeks**.**

The patient was **readmitted** to the hospital for **continuation of treatment**. She underwent **concurrent chemoradiation. Six** more **cycles** of **chemotherapy** was given at **intervals** of **21 days**. Simultaneously, she had EBRT. The total dose was **60 Gy** given in **fractions** over a period of **six weeks**.

At the time of discharge, she was prescribed **10 mg Tamoxifen tablets** to be taken **twice daily** for a period of **five years**. She was also advised to attend the OPD for regular follow-up.

Q. 6. What is the incidence of cancer breast in our country?

Carcinoma of the breast is the **second most common malignancy** in women in our country. But it is likely to **overtake carcinoma** of the **cervix,** and occupy the **first place** in the near future. Though **genetic factors** are important, **changes** in **life style** are probably responsible for this **marked increase** in the incidence.

Q. 7. What are the important points in the history in a patient with breast cancer?

1. **Age:** Basically a disease of the **middle age,** it is being seen **more frequently** in the **young.** It can also occur in the **elderly.**

2. A **painless lump** is the most common **mode of presentation.** This is most **unfortunate,** since **painless lesions** in general are **neglected** by **our patients.** An **innate shyness** on the part of our **women** to get **examined** even by **lady doctors** causes **further delay.** The **duration of the lump** is usually of several months. A **rapid increase** in size over a **short period** of time often **brings** the patient to the **hospital.** By the time they reach the hospital, **most** of our patients have lumps of more than **3 cm** in size.

3. **Pain** is a **late symptom.** It may be described as **dragging** or **pricking** type by the patient.

4. **Discharge** from the **nipple** is an **uncommon symptom.** The discharge may be **serosanguinous** or **bright red** in colour.

5. Some of our **patients** have an **ulcer** in the breast at the **time of admission.** Though the main reason is **infiltration by the tumour,** occasionally it is due to the **local** application of **counter-irritants.**

6. A **small group of patients** present with **symptoms** due to **metastatic disease.** One example would be a patient having an **axillary mass** in the **absence** of a **lump** in the **breast. Symptomatic secondaries** are more often **seen** after the **primary** has been **treated.** The **time interval** may vary from **several months** to **years.** The **clinical presentation** at that stage depends on the **system** that is **involved.**

   (*a*) **Respiratory system: Breathlessness** due to a **pleural effusion** is the most frequent symptom. When the **lungs** are involved, the patient will have **cough, chest pain and haemoptysis.**

(*b*) **Abdomen**: **Ascites** presents as an **increasing distension** of the **abdomen. Massive ascites** can cause **respiratory embarrassment. Jaundice** will develop when there is extensive involvement of the liver. Multiple **peritoneal secondaries** can induce **mechanical** small bowel **obstruction** due to **adhesions**.

(*c*) **Skeletal system**: The **lumbar vertebrae** are a **common site** for metastases. As a result, the patient has **low back pain** aggravated by **movement**s. The pain may radiate down the lower limbs. **Compression** of the **spinal cord** or the **nerves** will manifest with **neurological deficit**. Secondary deposits in **other bones** present as **painless swellings increasing rapidly** in **size** over a **short period** of time.

(*d*) **Secondaries** in the **brain** act as **space occupying** **lesions (SOL)** and manifest with **headache** and **vomiting.**

Box 11.5:	Points regarding history

- Painless lump – Increasing in size – Pain at a late stage.
- Skin changes – Ulceration.
- Discharge from the nipple.
- Metastases – Chest – Breathlessness – Cough – Haemoptysis.
- Abdomen – Distension – Jaundice – Lower abdomen mass.
- Skeletal – Low back pain – Lumbar vertebra.
- CNS (SOL) – Headache and vomiting.

Q. 8. What is the importance of obstetrical history in these cases?

The **risk** of malignancy is **higher** in **nulliparous** women. **Early pregnancy**, having **a larger number of children** and **breast feeding** the children are all **protective factors** against breast cancer. The **hormonal balance** is maintained in a **better manner** in these women.

Q. 9. Why is menstrual history important?

The patients are divided into **premenopausal** and **postmenopausal** groups for purposes of **hormonal manipulation**. Usually, the ovarian function persists for about **six months** after the **last menstrual period.**

Q. 10. Describe the steps of local examination of the breast.

Inspection:

The patient is made to **sit** with the **arms by the side.** The **entire chest** should be **exposed** so that **comparisons** can be made between the **two sides.**

For **examination purposes**, the breast is **divided** into **four quadrants** by **two lines** passing through the **center of the nipple**, at **right angles** to each other. The **upper outer quadrant** is most **frequently** involved.

The first step is to study the **contour** and the **shape** of the breast, as **compared** to the **opposite side.** If the appearance is **normal**, the patient is made to **raise the arms** well **above the head**, whereby **subtle variations** may now become **manifest.** Further if needed, the patient is asked to **bend well forwards.** The **diseased breast** may not be **falling forward** to the same **degree** as the **normal side.** **Subtle changes** in the **contour** as well as the **position** may be **detected** at this stage. The **level** of the **nipples** may get **altered** by these manoeuvers. **Fullness** is the term used when the **contour** is **altered** but the **borders** are **not well defined.** But many of our patients have a **visible lump.**

In this **group** the additional **tests** described above **may not** be **needed.**

Once a **lump** is seen, the **inspection** proceeds in the **following manner.**

(*a*) **Site,** with reference to the **quadrant** of the breast.

(*b*) **Size.** The average size of the lump is **3 cm**. But it is not **uncommon** to see women from the **rural areas** presenting with **large ulcerated tumours.**

(*c*) **Margins** are **well defined** in breasts with **minimal fat.**

(*d*) The **shape** is usually **irregular.**

(*e*) The **skin** over the swelling may be **normal** or show the following changes.

1. Due to the **rapid rate** of **increase** in the **size** of the tumour, the overlying **skin** becomes **stretched** and **shiny.**

2. **Erythema** of the skin indicates that **ulceration** will occur within a **short period**. This finding is also seen in **inflammatory carcinoma.**

3. **Dimpling** of the **skin** is due to **infiltration** of a **ligament of Cooper** which **extends** from the **pectoral fascia to the skin.**

4. **Puckering** of the **skin** is the result of **infiltration of several ligaments of Cooper.**

5. **Peau d'orange.** The **skin** over the **breast** comes to **resemble** an **orange peel.** When the **dermal lymphatics** are **blocked by malignant cells**, there is **lymphoedema**. But at **sites** where the **sweat ducts open** and the **hair follicles** are **attached,** the **skin is depressed**, giving rise to this **appearance**.

6. **Skin nodules.** This is a **late manifestation** and results from **retrograde spread** of **malignant cells** from the **blocked dermal lymphatics.**

7. **Ulceration** is a **common finding,** as mentioned earlier. The **shape** is **irregular** and the **margins** are **discrete.** The **floor** is comprised of **reddish granulation**-like **tumour tissue.** There is a **foul smelling discharge.** Quite often it is **blood stained.** The **surrounding skin** may show **pigmentation**.

Examination of the nipple and areola. Retraction of the **nipple** is the most significant finding. It occurs due to **infiltration** of the **periductal lymphatics** by **malignancy. Congenital retraction** can be **distinguished** by its **long duration** and **bilateral nature.** Hence **unilateral retraction** of **recent origin** is **sinister.**

The **nipple** is **destroyed** and **replaced** by a **malignant ulcer** in **Paget's disease**.

The **areola** may be **puckered** and **irregular** in shape with **hyperpigmentation** in some cases. The areola may be **stretched** by a rapidly growing **subareolar tumour.**

Inspection of the upper limb. Lymphoedema is present if the metastatic **axillary nodes** have **blocked** the **lymphatic vessels** draining the **limb.** But this is most often seen **after surgery** or **radiotherapy** for the **primary tumour.**

Box 11.6: Points regarding inspection
• Patient sitting – Arms by the side – Both sides exposed.
• Fullness or a lump – Site – Quadrant – Size – Shape – Margin.
• Skin – Stretched – Erythema, dimpling ,puckering peau d'orange – Nodules – Dilated veins.
• Ulcer – Site – Size – Margin – Floor – Surrounding area.
• Nipple – Retraction - Ulceration (Paget's disease) – Floor – Margin – Surrounding area.
• Areola – Puckering – Enlargement – Pigmentation.

Q. 11. What are the findings on palpation?

Palpation of the **breast** is done in general with the patient in **supine** position.

1. **Warmth** is felt in **inflammatory carcinomas**.

2. **Tenderness** is absent, unless **infection** complicates an **ulcerated tumour**.

3. The **size and the extent** are **more accurately** defined by **palpation.** In many instances, the **size** is much **larger** than what was suspected at **inspection.** This is especially true in **fatty breasts**. The **borders** are usually very **distinct.**

4. Most of the **lumps** are **firm-to-hard** in **consistency.** Areas of **softening** indicate **necrosis** of the tumour. But **medullary carcinoma** produces a **soft tumour.**

5. **Anatomical plane and mobility.** This part of the examination is very important for a proper diagnosis.

   (*a*) **Skin** The skin is **free** of the tumour in the **early stages** of the disease. But at a **later** period, **skin fixity** can occur over a **small area** (**summit** of the swelling) or a **wider extent**. This factor assumes **significance** during **surgery** for the **primary tumour**. These **cases** if **untreated** go on to the stage of **ulceration**. The **ulcer** has raised and **everted edges**. The **base** is formed by the **underlying tumour** and feels **indurated. Induration** may extend **beyond** the **edges** of the **ulcer** and defines the **real size** of the tumour.

   (*b*) **Breast tissue.** The **mobility** of the **lump** is **examined while fixing the breast** with one hand**. Malignant tumours move** with the breast because of **infiltration** into the surrounding **breast parenchyma**. This **sign** is very **significant** in the diagnosis of **early malignancy**. A **benign** lesion such as **fibroadenoma** is **mobile** within the **breast tissue** because of **encapsulation.**

   (*c*) **Pectoralis major muscle.** If the **mobility of the lump** is **restricted** on contracting this **muscle** against resistance, it suggests **spread** of the tumour into the **deeper planes.**

(*d*) **Totally immobile lumps** indicate fixity to the **chest wall.**

Palpation of the breast for **additional lumps. Fibrocystic disease** and **lobular carcinoma** (**multicentricity**) produce **more than one palpable lump** in the breast.

Discharge from the nipple. Occasionally during palpation, there may be a **serosanguinous discharge** from the nipple.

Box 11.7:	Points regarding palpation

- Patient supine, arms by the side – Warmth and tenderness.
- Site and extent – Lump larger and extensions to other quadrants.
- Surface – Nodular or irregular. Consistency – Hard – Variable.
- Fixity to skin – Over the summit or larger area.
- FIXED TO BREAST TISSUE.
- Fixity to pectoralis major and chest wall – Late stages.
- Additional lump – Fibrocystic disease – Lobular carcinoma.
- Discharge from the nipple during palpation – Uncommon.

Q. 12. How is palpation of the axilla for enlarged lymph nodes performed?

This part of the **clinical examination** is **difficult** because the **shape** of the **axilla** is like a **cone,** and the **contents** are **covered by a tough fascia.** The **apex** of the **axilla** is **narrow** and **deeply placed** and **nodes** belonging to this **group** are not **clinically palpable.**

The **patient** is made to **sit** and **hyperabduct** the limb **to** palpate the contents of the axilla. The **right axilla** is **palpated** with the **left hand** and **vice versa.** The **fingers** of the **examiner** are **inserted** as **deep** into the **axilla** as possible and the **limb** is brought **down** to **rest** on the **forearm** of the **examiner** to **adduct the shoulder** and **relax** the **axillary fascia.** In general nodes belonging to the **pectoral** and **central group,** when enlarged, are **palpable.** They are **firm or hard** in **consistency.** Once **extracapsular spread** takes place, the **nodes** are **adherent** to **each other.** They may also get **fixed** to the chest wall.

Palpation of the supraclavicular region.

This is carried out with the **patient sitting** and the **examiner standing behind. Lymph nodes** may be **palpable** in this region due to **malignant** cells travelling along **lymphatics** from the **apical node** in the axilla.

Q. 13. What are the reasons for palpating the opposite breast, axilla and the supraclavicular fossa?

Opposite breast: A **lump** may be palpable in the **opposite breast** under the following circumstances. The patient may have **bilateral synchronous primary** tumours. This is a **rare phenomenon** and is to be proved by **pathological examination.** But **metastatic spread** from the **diseased breast** is more **common.** Since **lymphatics** draining the **skin** over the **breast communicate** with **each other,** **tumour cells** can **spread** to the **opposite side** by this route. But it must be **remembered** that **lymphatics** draining the **breast parenchyma do not have** this type of **communication.**

Opposite axilla: Enlarged nodes at this site result from **spread** from the lesion in the **breast** or retrograde spread from the **internal mammary (thoracic) nodes.** These **nodes communicate** with **each other** across the **midline.**

Supraclavicular nodes become **palpable** because of **lymphatic spread** from the **axillary nodes.**

Q. 14. Describe the steps of clinical examination for metastatic disease.

Chest: There may be evidence of **pleural effusion** or consolidation. **Pleural effusion,** which is more **common,** may be seen even on the **opposite side,** since the **spread** occurs via the **subpleural lymphatics,** which communicate freely between the **two sides.** Clinical evidence of **consolidation** may also be detected.

Abdomen: Secondary **metastases** in the **liver.** The **tumour cells reach the liver** by **two routes. Blood spread** can occur like in many other malignant tumours. But a **lymphatic** spread along a **transcoelomic** route has also been described. The **lymphatic vessels** draining the **lower inner quadrant communicate** with those under the **anterior rectus sheath.** These are **connected** to the **subdiaphragmatic lymph plexus.** Once **malignant cells** reach this **site** they can **drop down transcoelomically** to the **liver** and the **peritoneal cavity.** These **metastases** produce a **hard** and **nodular liver. Umbilication** said to be present in **secondary deposits** is a very **unreliable sign.** It is the **result** of **central necrosis.**

Peritoneal deposits lead to **ascites,** which can be **massive** causing **respiratory distress.**

Large secondary deposits in the **ovary (Krukenberg tumour)** may be **palpable** in the **lower abdomen.** These are seen **exclusively** in the **premenopausal group.**

Skeletal system: Blood spread to the **bones** is **common** in this malignancy. **Bones** having a **red marrow** are more frequently involved. The **lumbar vertebrae** may show evidence of **metastatic disease** by presence of **tenderness. Compression** of **neurological structures** leads to **nerve deficit.**

Metastases in other bones such as the **pelvis, skull, ribs** and **upper ends** of femora and **humeri** present as **hard irregular swellings.**

Pelvic and **rectal examinations** are performed to detect **secondaries** in the **rectouterine pouch** of **Douglas** and also small Krukenberg tumours.

Box 11.8:	Points regarding rest of the clinical examination

- Ipsilateral axilla and supraclavicular region – Nodes
- Opposite Breast – Lump – Spread via cutaneous lymphatics - Metastases.
- Bilateral Synchronous carcinoma – Rare.
- Opposite axilla and supraclavicular fossa – Nodes.
- Abdomen – Hepatomegaly – Free fluid – Krukenberg tumour.
- Chest – Pleural effusion – Consolidation.
- Spine – Lumbar – Tenderness.
- PR and pelvic exam – Secondaries in rectovesical pouch.

Q. 15. What are the investigations needed in a case of breast cancer?

Since many of **our patients** present **late** in the **course of the disease**, with a **hard lump**, **fixed** to the **skin** and associated often with **ulceration** and **hard nodes** in the **axilla**, the diagnosis is **easy.** It is hoped that with **improvement** in **educational standards** especially in **women** and better **health facilities**, our patients will seek **medical help** at an **earlier stage. Early cases** pose more **problems** and **investigations** are needed for the **diagnosis.** These are also **necessary** for **proper staging** that forms the **basis** for a **rational treatment.** In the developed countries, many **patients** are **diagnosed before** the **clinical symptoms** and **signs** appear, with the help of various **investigations.** This has made a **huge difference** in the **prognosis** of breast cancer.

The advent of various **imaging modalities** as well as the availability of **cytological examinations** has made the **diagnosis** of this disease at a **very early stage** simple even when **symptoms and signs** are **minimal,** thus helping to **improve the prognosis.**

Mammography: Mammography is a **specialized X-ray** examination. It plays an **important** role in **imaging** of the breast. A **malignant lesion** is detected as early as **four years** before it **manifests** itself **clinically**.

Routine evaluation includes obtaining **two views** (craniocaudal and mediolateral oblique) of each breast.

Screening mammogram is used in **asymptomatic women** to detect **very early cancer**. But in India **logistical** problems **restrict** the use of this **investigation** to **high risk women only**. **Diagnostic mammogram** is performed in **women** who present with **breast complaints** or have **abnormal clinical findings**.

The **advantages** are as follows:

1. Gives a **good overview** of **both the breasts** and allows for **comparison** of the two sides for **better appreciation** of **subtle abnormality**.

2. **Increased breast density.** Unfortunately, this **anatomical fact increases** the **risk** of breast cancer, but **decreases** the **sensitivity** of **mammography** to detect **small lesions**. Hence mammography is **more useful** in **fatty breasts**.

3. **Abnormalities** detected on mammography include **masses, calcifications, architectural distortion or asymmetry.**

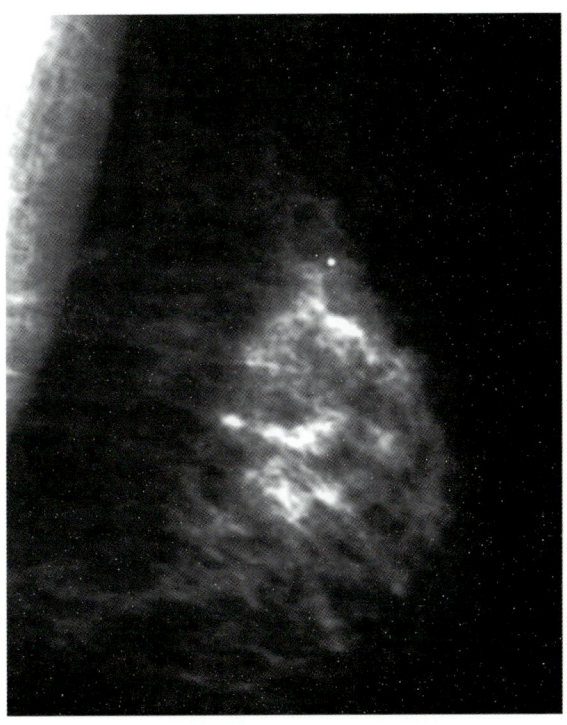

Fig. 11.7: Mammogram showing distorted architecture, spiculation and microcalcification.

4. **Digital mammography** offers **lower radiation dose** for the same image quality and causes **less distress** to the **patient.**

The **Breast Imaging Reporting and Data System (BI-RADS)** standardises the reporting of **mammographic findings** and helps in **decision making**. A **negative mammogram** should not deter further intervention if there is clinical suspicion of **malignancy**. Presence of

microcalcification, spiculation and **architectural distortion** are diagnostic of **malignancy**.

In patients with a **lump** proved as malignant, mammography is performed if **breast conservation surgery** is being planned. This is to rule out **multicentricity,** which is an **absolute contraindication** for **breast conservation**. Mammography of the **opposite breast** is performed in some patients to rule out the presence of **nonpalpable secondaries.**

Ultrasound:

Linear high-resolution probe 5-12 MHz is used to evaluate the **breast and axilla**.

1. The **primary role** of US is in the **diagnostic follow-up** of an **abnormality** detected in the **mammogram**, particularly in many **benign conditions**. It is used to further **evaluate masses** or asymmetries, and can very reliably differentiate a **solid mass** from a **cyst**.

2. But it is **less useful** in **asymptomatic patients**. However, if patient has a specific **complaint** (**lump, pain, discharge etc.**), US can be focused on that **particular area** and the necessary data **may be obtained**. Hence it is a very **good adjunct to mammogram**.

3. It can evaluate the **axilla that** is **clinically negative** for **enlarged nodes.**

4. It is the **first line** of imaging in a pregnant woman or in one who is below 30 years of age, so that unnecessary irradiation may be avoided.

5. It is also used to provide **guidance** for **biopsies** and other interventions.

Tissue diagnosis:

In a patient with a **suspicious mammographic abnormality** or a **palpable breast mass**, the obligatory diagnostic technique is **biopsy.** A preoperative **cytological diagnosis of malignancy** is **mandatory** before the **management strategies** are **planned.**

Fine needle aspiration cytology (FNAC). FNAC has been used for **years** to evaluate **breast lesions**. The usual report in a **malignant lump** is an **infiltrating duct carcinoma.**

Advantages:

1. It can be **easily performed** and **quicker interpretation** of the results is possible as compared with a **core needle biopsy**.

2. **US-guided FNA** helps in **accurate placement** of the needle.

3. With reference to **axillary lymph nodes**, the procedure is **less painful and safer**.

Disadvantages:

1. The **inability** to **distinguish** between **in situ** and **invasive cancer.**

2. Significant rate of **nondiagnostic** samples and **false negative** results in **inexperienced hands**.

Core needle biopsy (CNB):

Image-guided CNB can be performed using **mammographic** or **US guidance**.

Advantages:

1. **CNB** offers a more definitive **histologic diagnosis, avoids inadequate samples** and may permit the **distinction** between **invasive** versus **in situ cancers.**

2. Provides **enough tissue** for **hormonal** and **tumour marker study**.

Hence in most centers, **CNB** is the most common initial biopsy method for **nonpalpable mammographic abnormalities**.

Incision and **excision biopsies** are **no longer performed** as a **diagnostic tool** in the **management** of **breast cancer**.

Edge biopsy. Ulcerated tumours are diagnosed by an **edge biopsy** of the **ulcer.**

FNAC of the axillary nodes. This procedure is **not commonly performed, although it may be needed in patients who have palpable suspicious nodes** in the axilla but no **lump** in the breast. But this mode of **presentation** is **rare.** The procedure is **technically difficult** and is performed under **US** guidance. But **FNAC** of the **nodes** in the **opposite axilla** is **needed** in some cases for **accurate staging** of the disease.

Receptor Studies:

Most cancers of the breast are **hormone-dependent tumours**. The **tissue** obtained either by CNB or surgical resection is tested for **ER, PR and Her2 neu status**. **ER and PR positivity** indicate a **better prognosis** because such tumours are **amenable** for **hormonal manipulation. Her2 neu** is an **oncogene** present in about **20%** of patients with breast cancer. A **higher level** of this **tumour marker** is suggestive of an **aggressive cancer**.

Genetic Studies. If facilities are available, studies for **amplification** or **overexpression of BRCA gene 1 and 2** in the **patient** as well as in first degree relatives are performed. **Lumpectomy** as we learn later is **contraindicated** in patients with this **genetic abnormality**.

As is well known, the **risk** of malignancy is much **higher** in **siblings** carrying this **genetic defect.**

Box 11.9:	Points regarding investigations

- Mammography – Screening – Healthy women.
- Diagnostic – Symptomatic – Microcalcification, spiculation and altered architecture.
- US - Complementary to mammography – Useful in benign disease.
- FNAC – Diagnostic – Infiltrating duct carcinoma.
- CNB – Preferred-distinction between in situ carcinoma and invasive cancer.
- Tissue adequate for receptor studies – LABC – Neoadjuvant chemotherapy.
- Ulcerated tumours – Edge biopsy.
- ER, PR and Her2 neu receptor studies – Genetic studies.

Q. 16. What are the investigations done in these cases?

(*a*) **Chest X-ray:** The findings could be as follows:

1. **Pleural effusion.**

2. **Multiple secondaries** in the **lung produce round shadows** (**cannon balls**). The **globular shape** of these lesions is due to the **uniform lack** of **resistance** by the **lung parenchyma**, allowing the **cells** to **grow equally** in **all directions**. A **solitary circular deposit** is called as a **coin shadow.**

3. **Multiple fine granular deposits**, producing a **snowstorm** appearance.

(*b*) **CT chest** is ordered only when the **chest X-ray** shows **doubtful lesions**. CT will detect **tiny deposits** and **internal mammary nodes** more often than a routine X-ray.

(*c*) **US abdomen:** The findings are mentioned below:

1. **Secondary deposits** in the **liver**.

2. **Minimal free fluid** not detected by clinical examination.

3. **Ovarian secondaries**.

4. **Peritoneal secondaries**.

(*d*) **Bone scan: Technitium 99** is the **radio isotope** used for this investigation. It is **injected intravenously** and a **scintiscan** of the **whole body** is performed. Since the **metastases** take up **more of the isotope,** they appear as **hot spots** in the scan. All patients with **T3** and **T4** stage disease need this **scan** before **treatment is started.**

(*e*) **Plain X-ray** is performed in the presence of **clinically** identified **secondary deposits** in **bones**. They are most often **osteolytic** in nature. But occasionally

osteosclerotic lesions have also been described.

(*f*) **MRI scan:** This investigation is needed when a patient presents with **vertebral** (usually lumbar) **deposits** with **neurological deficit**. It demonstrates the **nature and degree** of compression of the **nerves,** often **needing** an **urgent decompression**.

(*g*) **Sentinel node biopsy**. The rationale behind this procedure is to **avoid** the **morbidity** of **lymphoedema** associated with an **axillary lymph dissection**. It is **indicated** in patients with the diagnosis of **TI and TII, N0 disease** where the **primary** lesion has been **proved** to be malignant by cytological examination. It is based on the **principle** that these are the **first group** of nodes to be involved and if they **show evidence** of the disease, an **axillary clearance** is indicated. The technique makes use of both a **radio isotope** and a **dye** to identify the **sentinel node**. The **isotope** used is **radioactive technetium sulphur colloid** and the **dye, vital blue.** These are **injected in and around the tumour**. The **axilla** is then **scanned** with a hand-held **gamma camera**. An area of **high intensity** suggests the presence of a **node** that has **taken up** the **isotope**. An **incision** is made at that **site.** One or more **blue coloured nodes** are now **visualised**. These are **excised** and sent for **frozen section examination**. If they show **metastatic disease**, an **axillary clearance** is **performed**. A **negative biopsy** avoids an **unnecessary dissection**.

Box 11.10:	Points regarding investigations for metastases

- Chest X-ray – Pleural effusion – Cannon balls – Coin shadow – Snowstorm appearance.
- Abdomen US – Metastases. In liver – Minimal free fluid – Krukenberg tumours.
- Bone scan – Stage III and IV – Technitium 99 – Hot spots.
- MRI – Secondaries in lumbar vertebrae with nerve deficit.
- Sentinel node biopsy – N0 – avoids axillary clearance – if negative.

Q. 17. How are breast cancers staged?

The **treatment** and the **prognosis** depend on the **stage of the disease. Clinical staging** is the **first step** towards the treatment. But the **treatment** schedule is **finalised** only after the **results** of the various **investigations** mentioned above are available.

The standard **TNM** classification is as follows.

Primary tumour. (T)

Tx. The primary tumour cannot be **assessed** (usually cases **treated earlier** and presenting **with inadequate information**).

T0. No palpable tumour. These are **picked up** as a result of **investigations** like **mammogram.**

T1. Primary tumour **2 cm or less in size.**

T2. Tumours between **2 cm and 5 cm in size.**

T3. Tumours **more than 5 cm** in size.

T4. Tumour has infiltrated the **adjacent structures.** The group is further subdivided into four subtypes.

T4A. Tumour adherent to the **deeper structures** like **chest wall.**

T4B. Involvement of the **skin** as shown by **skin fixity, peau d'orange, skin nodules** and **ulceration.**

T4C. Combination of both **T4A** and **T4B.**

T4D. Inflammatory carcinoma of the breast.

Status of ipsilateral axillary and supraclavicular lymph nodes. (N)

There is some variability in classifying the metastatic nodes.

A practical classification is described below.

Nx. Nodal status **cannot be assessed.**

N0. No palpable nodes in the axilla.

N1. 1 to 3 nodes in the axilla **less than 3 cm** in size.

N2. Nodes more than **4** in number, or **bigger than 3 cm** in size. Nodes **fixed** to **each other** or to the **chest wall.**

N3. Palpable supraclavicular nodes.

Distant metastases (M)

M1. Metastatic disease. It may be located in the **opposite breast, opposite axilla, lungs, bones, liver or brain.**

The **TNM classification** can be simplified into the following **four clinical stages.**

Stage I. T0 to T2, N0, M0.

Stage II. T0 to T2, N1, M0

StageIII. T0 to T4, N2 and N3, M0

Stage IV. Any T, any N, M1

But the most **pragmatic** and **practical classification** is as follows. This has become **more relevant** with the advent of **breast conservation surgery** as well as the **concept** of **neoadjuvant chemotherapy.**

1. **Early breast cancer (EBC).**

2. **Locally advanced breast cancer (LABC).**

3. **Metastatic breast cancer.**

Q. 18. What are the basic principles of treatment of cancer breast?

Carcinoma of the **breast** is an excellent example of a **cancer** where **rational treatment** can be given only if the **biological behaviour** of the tumour is **clearly understood. Halstead's radical mastectomy** was the **gold standard** as a **curative treatment** for several decades. **Halstead** proposed that these **cancers followed three stages** during their **evolution.** A **local disease** to begin with, the tumour then **spread** to the **regional nodes** in the axilla, and still **later spreads** via the **blood stream** to produce **distant metastases.** All **other types** of treatment were **compared** against this **operation.** It afforded **excellent locoregional control** but patients were **dying of distant metastases** leading to a poor outcomes. Large retrospective studies led by Bernard Fisher have identified a **fundamental error** in this **theory—Malignant cells** do **not follow rules** of **cell division and function.** The **three stages** described by Halstead may **not occur** in such an **orderly fashion.** It is possible that at an **early stage of the** **cancer, cells** may migrate via the **blood stream** to produce **distant metastases.** Hence a radical change has occurred in the **understanding** and **treatment** of **this cancer.** The extensive **research** that is being done **world over** at the **genetic level** may result in further **modifications** in treatment **protocols** in the **future.** Thus we can conclude that the **management strategies** are still **evolving.**

The **following principles** underline the **treatment of breast cancer** at the **present time.**

1. **Breast cancer** is a **systemic disease** from the onset, because it tends to **metastasise** at an **early stage** both via the **lymphatics** and the **blood stream.** Thus **distant metastases** may occur **at any stage** of the disease. Since these **distant metastases** cannot be **detected** by the **investigations** presently **available,** they have been termed as **micrometastases.** As the **disease progresses** the **risk** of these metastases **increases exponentially.** Hence depending on the **biological aggressiveness** of the tumour, a **small size tumour** with a short history

may have a **worse prognosis** as compared with a **bulky one** of a **long duration.**

2. **Multiple specialties** are involved in the **treatment** of the disease. The team consists of a **surgeon,** a **radiotherapist,** a **medical oncologist** and an **endocrinologist**. The **ancillary staff** include **psychological counsellors** and **specially trained nurses**. Most hospitals have a **Tumour Board** consisting of all these **experts,** and the **treatment** schedule is **planned by this team**.

3. The **treatment** of the **primary** tumour has a **limited objective** of **ADEQUATE LOCAL CONTROL**. The purpose is to **minimise** the incidence of **local recurrence**, which unfortunately is associated with a **poor prognosis.**

4. The presence of **metastatic nodes** in the axilla is taken **as PRESUMPTIVE EVIDENCE** of **MICROMETASTASES** in the body since **none of the investiga-tions** presently available are **helpful.** Hence the disease is presumed to be a **systemic one** and demands

SYSTEMIC TREATMENT, namely **chemotherapy.**

If in patients with T3 and T4 disease the bone scan is positive, it indicates metastatic disease with palliative treatment.

5. **EBRT** is needed to improve the **prognosis** under **certain circumstances**.

6. **Hormonal manipulation** and **monoclonal antibodies** are used under **specific situations**.

Box 11.11:	Points regarding the basic strategies of treatment

- Primary tumour – Obtain adequate local control.
- Axillary clearance for evidence of micrometastases.
- Positive nodes – Presumptive evidence of micrometastases – Systemic disease-Indication for systemic treatment – Chemotherapy.
- External radiation – Specific indications.
- Hormonal manipulation – Specific indications.
- Monoclonal antibodies.

Q. 19. What are the principles of treatment of EBC?

These are patients belonging to **T0 or T1 and N0** in most instances. Occasionally a patient with **T2, N0** disease may **be** suitable for breast conservation surgery. The basic aim is cosmetic and **psychosocial,** with **conservation** of the **breast.** It provides the patient with an **aesthetically acceptable breast.** But the **size** and **location** of the tumour has to be considered in **relation** to the **size** and **contour** of the **breast as a whole,** before planning this operation. **Peripherally** placed tumours, often confined to **one quadrant,** offer the **best chance.** In patients with **BRCA gene mutation,** breast **conservation** is **contraindicated** since the incidence of **local recurrence** is **high.**

Lumpectomy is the surgery performed in this group. It consists of **excising the lump** with a **surrounding margin** of **1 cm of normal breast tissue.** In the case of a **nonpalpable** tumour diagnosed by **mammography,** the radiologist places a **wire** at the site of **microcalcification** under **stereotactic control.** The **tissue surrounding** the wire is excised by the **surgeon** with a **similar margin** of **normal breast** tissue. A **repeat mammogram** is performed to ascertain that the **suspicious lesion** has been **completely excised.**

The **lumpectomy specimen** is then sent for frozen section examination. A **positive margin** detected by the **pathologist** indicates a need for **mastectomy.** If the **margins are free,** the patient needs a **course** of **radiotherapy** to the **breast** to reduce the **incidence** of local recurrence. **Radiotherapy** is given **after** the **incision** has **healed.** The **dose** is rather **small,** being in the range of **30 Gy** given over a period of **three to four weeks.** This dose causes **minimal disturbance** to the **breast.**

Patients **not suitable** for **lumpectomy** are treated by **Modified Radical Mastectomy (MRM).** This is the **most frequent operation** for **breast cancer** in **our country.** In the **developed countries,** the **number** of patients undergoing **breast conservation** surgery is **quite high.**

Q. 20. How are axillary nodes treated in this group of patients?

A **sentinel node biopsy** is performed. It is undertaken **along** with the **lumpectomy.** **Frozen section reports** are necessary. If there is no evidence of **malignancy,** the patient is kept under **surveillance.** If the report is **positive,** an **axillary clearance** is undertaken. In this operation, **level I** nodes (**below** the **pectoralis minor** muscle) and **level II** nodes (**behind the muscle**) are removed along with the **axillary fat.** If **more** than **4 nodes** show evidence of **malignancy,** the patient is **presumed** to have a **systemic disease** with **micrometastases.**

Such patients **are given** the benefit of **chemotherapy.** This treatment is started after a period of **3 to 4 weeks,** by which time the **surgical incisions** have healed completely. The regime consists of **6 to 8 cycles** of **combination chemotherapy,** given at intervals of **three weeks.** The drugs used are **Adriamycin, 5 FU and Cyclophosphamide. Taxane** group is added as the **first line** of treatment more frequently at present, since it **improves the outlook.**

Box 11.12:	Points regarding treatment of EBC, usually stage I

- Aim – Breast conservation – Psychosocial advantage.
- TI N0 and selective TII cases – Size and location of lump in relation to size of breast – Postop – Aesthetically acceptable breast.
- Lumpectomy – Excision with 1 cm normal tissue margin.
- Lump detected by mammogram – Wire placed at site – Excision around the wire – Confirmation – Repeat mammogram.
- Frozen section report – No tumour at margin – No further surgery.
- Postop short course of radiation 30 Gy to reduce local recurrence.
- Frozen Section positive – Mastectomy.

Box 11.13:	Points regarding additional measures of treatment for EBC

- Sentinel node biopsy – Along with lumpectomy.
- Report – Positive – Axillary clearance – Level I and II nodes removed.
- If mastectomy is performed, axillary clearance added.
- More than 4 nodes positive – Presumptive systemic disease – Chemotherapy.
- Hormonal manipulation and MAB – Receptor status – Only after completion of chemo regime.

Q. 21. How are patients with stage 2 (T1, T2, N1) disease treated?

These patients are treated by an **MRM.** The basic **steps** of the operation are as follows. A **transverse elliptical incision** is made over the breast **including the areola and nipple** (the **subareolar plexus of Sappey** drains the **lymph** from the **entire breast parenchyma**). The area of **skin** to be **removed** depends on the **extent** of its **involvement.** The **entire breast** is removed along with **axillary clearance.** During **dissection** of the **axilla,** care is taken to **conserve** the **nerves** to **serratus anterior** and the **latissimus dorsi muscles.**

If the patient is concerned about the **aesthetic appearance,** an **immediate reconstruction** is performed. Either a **latissimus dorsi myocutaneous flap** or a **TRAM flap** (**rectus abdominus muscle** and the **abdominal** skin) is used for **reconstruction.** Plastic surgical expertise is available to **reconstruct the areola and nipple** as well.

Chemotherapy:

Depending on the histopathological report on the **nodal status** these patients are given **chemotherapy.** The **N status** may get **upgraded** after this report has been received. Once the **surgical incisions** have **healed,** the chemo regime is given in the same fashion as described earlier.

Hormonal manipulation:

Additional treatment depends on the **ER, PR and Her2 neu** status. This **treatment** is started only after **chemotherapy is completed.** Patients with **ER** and **PR positive** tumours are given **Tamoxifen.** It is a **selective oestrogen receptor modulator (SERM).** It selectively **binds** to the **oestrogen receptors** on the **cell wall, preventing** the action of the **hormone,** which acts as a **stimulator** of the **malignant cells.** Hence its **main action** is as an **antagonist,** but **occasionally** it acts like an **agonist** making **matters worse (oestrogen flare). Aromatase inhibitors** like **Letrozole or Anastrozole** have the **advantage** that they **prevent** the **production** of **oestrogen.** These drugs are usually given for a **period of 5 years.** The **response** rate is **better** in **postmenopausal women,** since the **hormone burden** is much **less** in this group. Those who are **Her2 neu positive** are administered a course of **Trastuzumab (Herceptin),** which is a **monoclonal antibody.** Unfortunately, **cost** is a **limiting factor** for many of our **patients.**

Box 11.14:	Points regarding treatment of stage II

- MRM – Standard operation – Removal of the breast, variable area of skin, nipple areolar complex (subareolar plexus of Sappey), pectoral fascia and axillary clearance – Reconstruction if requested – LD or TRAM flaps.
- Axillary nodes positive – Chemotherapy.
- More than 4 positive nodes – EBRT.
- Hormonal manipulation and MAB – Receptor status.

Q. 22. What is the treatment of LABC (usually stage 3 - T3 or T4, N2 or N3)?

A **vast majority** of **our patients** fall into this **group** at the time of **admission.** They are **presumed** to have **micrometastases,** suggesting a **systemic disease,** and therefore need **systemic treatment.** Hence there is a **significant change** in the treatment schedule.

1. **Neoadjuvant chemotherapy** is the **first line** of treatment. The **rationale** behind this regime is as follows.

(*a*) The **micrometastases** are controlled by the **drugs**, **reducing** the **systemic component** of the disease.

(*b*) **Down-staging** of the tumour occurs due to **chemotherapy**, making **surgery easier**.

The treatment consists of **two or three cycles** of **drugs** mentioned above at an **interval of three weeks**. As a result the **tumour** may show **complete or partial regression**. But in some patients, the tumour does **not show any change (stable disease)** or even **worse**, can **progress further**.

Surgical Treatment:

Patients who have shown a **partial or complete response** undergo **MRM**.

Chemotherapy: Once the **surgical incision** has **healed**, the **chemo regime** is continued for **six more cycles**.

Hormonal manipulation:

The regime is the same as **described** for **T0 to T2 cancers**.

EBRT:

To **reduce the risk** of **locoregional recurrences**, the following **groups** of patients need **EBRT**. **Unfortunately, most of the patients** presenting in **our hospitals** fall into these **groups.**

(*a*) **Primary** tumour belonging to **T III and T IV.**

(*b*) Presence of more than **four positive nodes** in the axilla on **histopathology**.

(*c*) Evidence of lymphovascular invasion-high grade tumor.

(*d*) Many of the **younger patients** usually have an **aggressive disease.**

The **EBRT dose** is **50 to 60 Gy** given over a period of **five to six weeks**. The **areas** that are **irradiated** include the **chest wall**, the **internal mammary region** and the **supraclavicular fossa**. Since axillary clearance has already **been done, radiotherapy** is not given to the **axilla. Irradiation** of an **operated axilla** results in **severe refractory lymphoedema.**

Box 11.15:	Points regarding management of LABC
• Neoadjuvant chemotherapy – Controls micrometastases – Down-stages primary tumour.	
• Assessment after 2 or 3 cycles – Complete or partial response – MRM.	
• Continue chemotherapy – 4 to 6 cycles.	
• EBRT – Either concurrent or after chemotherapy.	
• Hormonal manipulation and MAB – Receptor status.	

Q. 23. What is the treatment of metastatic breast cancer?

The **common pattern** in this disease is that despite adequate **locoregional control achieved** by the **treatment modalities** described **earlier,** patients **return** to the hospital **later** with **metastatic disease**. The term "**cured**" is not used in the management of **cancer breast** since **metastases** can develop at any **time** ranging from a **few months** to **several years.** However, a **small number** of our patients have **metastatic disease** at the time of **presentation.**

The **treatment** of metastatic breast cancer is **basically palliative. Chemotherapy** is the **primary** line of **treatment.** Usually **second line** of drugs such as the **Taxane** group is used at this stage. **EBRT** is given depending upon the **location** of the **secondary deposits**. A **local recurrence** may be treated by **irradiating the chest wall**. In a **small number** of patients with **metastatic disease**, a **palliative mastectomy** is performed if there is a large fungating and bleeding **tumour** to improve the **quality of life.** The **outlook is very poor**.

Box 11.16:	Points regarding treatment of metastatic cancers

- Usually metachronous – Months or years after treatment of primary.
- Palliative – Chemotherapy – Mainline – Liver secondaries – Problematic – Most drugs metabolised in liver.
- EBRT – Bony secondaries and local recurrence.
- Ulcerated and bleeding primary present (uncommon) – Mastectomy.
- Prognosis – Poor.

Box 11.17:	Points regarding chemotherapy

- Drugs – Adriamycin, 5 FU and cyclophosphamide. Taxanes.
- Three settings – Adjuvant in stage I and II – Positive nodes in axilla following lumpectomy or mastectomy.
- Neoadjuvant – LABC – Reduce tumour burden – Down-stage primary.
- Palliative – Metastatic cancer.

Box 11.18:	Points regarding EBRT

- Rationale – To reduce local recurrence post surgery.
- Post lumpectomy – Short course to breast 30 Gy.
- Post mastectomy – 50 to 60 Gy given over 5 to 6 weeks – Chest wall, internal mammary and supraclavicular regions. Axilla not included.
- Indications – Tumour more than 4 cm, more than 4 positive nodes in axilla, evidence of lymphovascular invasion on HP (high grade malignancy) and young patients who usually have aggressive tumours.
- Palliative – Local recurrence and bony secondaries.

Box 11.19:	Points regarding hormonal manipulation and MAB

- ER and PR positive patients – Good prognostic factor – Tamoxifen (SERM) for five years.
- Better results in postmenopausal group.
- Aromatase inhibitors – Superior – Block production of oestrogen.
- Anastrozole and Letrozole.
- Her 2 neu positive – Poor prognosis – Trastuzumab (Herceptin).
- Treatment given only after chemoradiation.

Q. 24. What are the important prognostic factors?

1. **Stage** of the **primary** tumour. In the **developed countries**, a **large number** of patients are identified at **T0 stage**. They have an **excellent prognosis**. Unfortunately, most of **our patients** present at **stage III**. The outlook is **much worse** in this group.

2. **Status of the axillary lymph node** on histopathology. Presence of **metastases** is associated with a **poorer prognosis**.

3. **Age** of the patient. **Younger patients** tend to have an **aggressive** tumour and a **poor prognosis**.

4. **Histological type and grade.** A **papillary or tubular** type of carcinoma has a **favorable** outlook. **Lymphovascular invasion** is an indicator of a **worse prognosis**.

5. **Response to treatment.** Response to **neoadjuvant chemotherapy** decides the **outcome** in LABCs.

6. **Hormone receptor status.** ER and PR **positivity** especially in **postmenopausal** women is a sign of **good prognosis**.

7. **Her2 neu status. Overexpression** of this **gene** is associated with a **poor outcome.**

Box 11.20:	Points regarding the prognostic factors

- Stage of the disease – T0 Excellent outcome – Later stages poorer outcome.
- Status of axillary nodes – Positive – Systemic disease – Poor.
- Age – Younger patients – Aggressive disease.
- Histology – Tubular and papillary – Better.
- Lymphovascular invasion – Poor.
- Response to treatment – LABC – Neoadjuvant chemo - Complete response - Good prognosis.
- Receptor status – ER and PR positive – Good outcome.
- Her 2 neu positive – Poor.

Q. 25. What are the five-year survival rates in breast cancer?

Stage 0 100%

Stage I 100%

Stage II 90%

Stage III 70%

Stage IV 20%

The figures quoted above show us that with **better understanding** of the disease, the **outlook for the patients** has shown a **significant improvement**. It would be **ideal to identify the disease** at an **early stage,** preferably **before a lump becomes palpable** in the breast, which is impractical in our country. Even a simple **examination of the breast** by the **patient herself** has been shown to **improve** the long-term results.

Q. 26. What are the differential diagnoses of a lump in the breast?

It is often taught that **any lump** in the breast is **considered** to be **malignant until proved otherwise**. But this **should not** lead to an impression that **cancers** are the **most common lumps**. This **statement** has been made so that a **high degree of suspicion is always present** in the **clinician's mind.** The following are the other conditions that produce palpable lumps in the breast.

Benign breast disease. Although **fibrocystic disease** and **fibroadenoma** are discussed under **dlargeferent heads**, they are presently **grouped together** as **ANDI (Aberration or Anomaly of Normal Development and Involution**).This group is responsible for nearly **90%** of all palpable **lumps** in the breast. Though the **exact aetiology** is not known **disturbances** in the **hypothalamus-pituitary-gonadal axis** leading to **increased hormonal levels** is probably the **main cause**. In addition, **stress** and **diet rich in saturated fatty acids** causing **supersensitivity** to the **normal levels** of the **hormone** are also blamed. The basic **classification of ANDI** runs as follows.

(*a*) Disorders of development.

1. **Fibroadenoma including Phyllodes tumour**.
2. **Adolescent hypertrophy**.

(*b*) **Disorders of cyclical changes**.

Cyclical mastalgia and nodularity.

(*c*) **Disorders of involution**.

1. **Fibrocystic disease**.
2. **Cysts in the breast**.
3. **Sclerosing adenosis**.

FIBROCYSTIC DISEASE is the **most common** cause for a **lump** in the breast. The presentation is that of a **lump** associated with **pain,** most often felt in the **premenstrual period**. The lump is **single** when only **one lobule** is affected, but **frequently multiple lumps** are palpable. The condition can be **bilateral.** The lump is **firm** with a **nodular**

surface. **Tenderness** is often present. **US and mammography** are helpful in the **diagnosis.** If the suspicion of **malignancy** is **high,** an **FNAC** is performed. The treatment is **essentially conservative.**

FIBROADENOMA: It was considered to be a **benign tumour** in the past. **Two** different **types** have been described, but there may be some **overlapping** and **one type** may **morph** into **another** over a **period of time.** The only complaint is a **painless lump** of **several months** duration.

HARD FIBROADENOMA is a disease of the **young.** The **size** is usually **small** and the consistency **firm.** Because the tumour is **encapsulated,** it **is freely mobile** within the **breast tissue.** A **small tumour** in **comparison** with the **size of the breast** is referred as a **breast mouse. Enucleation is** the treatment of choice. But these patients are **prone** to develop **similar tumours** at a **later date** on the **same or opposite side.**

SOFT FIBROADENOMA tends to occur at **middle age.** The rate of **growth is faster** and it can assume a **large size.** A **hard** variety may turn into **this type** over a period of time. The consistency is **soft** and hence may be **missed** in a **fatty breast.**

Both **US and mammograms** are **diagnostic. Enucleation** can easily be performed usually via an **inframammary incision.** M**astectomy** may be indicated in a small number of **elderly patients** who have a **large tumour** occupying the **entire breast.**

GIANT SOFT FIBROADENOMA is a **variety** of **soft fibroadenoma.** It varies from **5 to 10 cm** in size. These are also known as **Phyllodes tumours** because the **cut section macroscopically** resembles a **leaf.** The **specific feature** of this tumour is its **propensity for ulceration.** This is due to the **pressure necrosis** of the **overlying skin,** resulting from a **rapidly enlarging tumour.** It must be stressed that this tumour is a **rare example** of a **benign lesion** undergoing **ulceration.** Most **large tumours,** especially when associated with **ulceration,** end up with a **mastectomy.**

The risk of **malignant transformation** is **highest** in this group. It is the **stromal** and **not the epithelial element** of the tumour that turns **malignant** and hence the result is a **sarcoma.** These are very **aggressive tumours** spreading via the **bloodstream. Secondaries** occur most often in the **lungs. CT**

imaging is needed to determine the stage of the disease. If **resectable,** an **extended mastectomy** is performed. The **breast** along with the **involved adjacent structures** is removed. **Postoperative radiotherapy** is given to reduce the chances of **local recurrence.** But the **outlook** is universally **poor.**

CYSTS in the breast. A **common condition**, it is seen in the age group of **35 to 50 years**. The **size** is **variable**. They are **fluid-filled sacs** in the **breast tissue**. Depending on the **tension** of the **fluid** within, they may **feel soft or firm**. Both **US and mammography** are useful in the diagnosis. The **treatment is** to **aspirate the cyst** preferably under **US guidance**. The fluid is always examined **cytologically** to rule out **malignancy.**

ANTIBIOMA: The abundant **fat** in the breast makes it **vulnerable** for **infection.** The common result is an **abscess,** which is **drained** under **antimicrobial** cover. But **occasionally** the contents are **sterlised** by the **antimicrobials.** Thus a **cavity** lined by **granulation tissue** containing **sterile fluid develops** in the breast. As the **inflammation resolves**, the wall is **replaced** by **thick fibrous tissue**. At this stage, it presents as a **lump** firm or **hard**

in consistency and **fixed** to the **breast tissue.** To confuse matters further, **enlarged lymph nodes** may be palpable in the **axilla.** The advent of **imaging and FNA** has **modified** the **treatment** to a large extent. These **lumps** can safely be kept under **surveillance** with **repeated US** studies. A **small** number of **persisting antibiomas** may need **excision.**

TRAUMATIC FAT NECROSIS: This is an **uncommon condition**, resulting from **minor trauma.** **Rupture** of the **interlobular fat cells** induces an **aseptic inflammation**, giving rise to a **palpable mass,** which is **fixed** to the breast tissue. In some of these patients, a history of **trauma** may **not be available**. Thus **clinically** it is **indistinguishable** from **early malignancy.** It is necessary to **remember** that a **history of trauma** does **not rule out malignancy**. It may bring the **attention** of the **patient** to a **pre-existing tumour. US** confirms the diagnosis and is **repeated** to study the **resolution** of the disease. Hence the **treatment** is **conservative.**

TUBERCULOSIS OF THE BREAST: Tuberculous bacteria reach the breast by **retrograde spread** from the **axillary lymph nodes**. **Chronic inflammation** leads to **fibrosis a**nd the formation of a **firm lump**, **fixed** to the **breast tissue. Matted lymph nodes** are palpable in the **axilla.** Once complications like a **cold abscess** or **sinuses** develop, the diagnosis is **easy. FNA** proves the diagnosis. **Chest X-ray** is usually **normal. ATT is** the main line of treatment. **Surgical intervention** is indicated only in the presence of **complications.**

Box 11.21:	Points about other lumps

- Fibrocystic disease.
- Fibroadenoma – Hard, soft and Phyllodes tumour.
- Cysts.
- Antibioma
- Traumatic fat necrosis.
- Tuberculosis of the breast.

Q. 27. What is the incidence and the aetiological factors of male breast cancer?

Male breast cancer is an **uncommon** disease. It constitutes only **1%** of all **breast cancers.** The common age is **after 60 years**. Hormonal imbalance is probably the most important aetiological factor. **Increase** in the **oestrogen levels** (secreted by the adrenals) is probably **responsible** for the development of malignancy.

Q. 28. What are the differences in the clinical presentation and the behaviour of these cancers?

The male breast consists of a **set of ducts** without any lobular structures. Hence **lobular carcinoma** does **not occur** in a male.

Lack of fat makes make these cancers **spread early** into the **deeper structures** like the **pectoralis major** muscle and the **chest wall.** Even **lymphatic spread** to the **axillary nodes** is seen **more frequently.**

The presentation is of a **hard lump** in the **subareolar region**. The lump is **fixed** to the **breast tissue.** In **most instances** the tumour is **adherent** to the **overlying skin** and the **deeper structures.**

Absence of pain delays the patient from seeking **medical advice**.

Blood-stained or less commonly serous discharge from the **nipple** is an alarming symptom. The **nipple** may be **retracted** or **ulcerated.**

Most patients have **palpable nodes** at the time of diagnosis.

Q. 29. What are the investigations?

They are **similar** to cancers in the female. **CNB** helps in the **diagnosis,** and supplies **adequate tissue** for **receptor studies**.

Q. 30. How are these patients treated?

A majority of our patients belong to the **LABC group**. Hence **neoadjuvant chemotherapy** is the initial treatment. Once the tumour is **down staged**, an **extended mastectomy** is performed. It may mean **removal** of the involved structure such as the **pectoralis major muscle**. **Postoperatively,** they are treated by **chemoradiation. Response** to **tamoxifen or aromatase inhibitors** is equal to that seen in the **postmenopausal group** in women. **Orchidectomy** is **no longer performed.** The **same result** can be obtained by **injections** of **leutinising hormone releasing hormone (LHRH) antagonists**. Since these patients often belong to either **stage III or IV group**, the **outlook** in general is **poor.**

■■■

The Circulatory and Lymphatic Systems

12

PERIPHERAL ARTERIAL OCCLUSIVE DISEASE PART 1

A CASE OF THROMBO ANGIITIS OBLITERANS (BUERGER'S DISEASE)

Setting

- Surgical OPD.

Chief Complaint

- **Blackish discolouration** of the **left great toe** along with **pain** of **one month duration**.

History of Present Illness

A **25-year-old man** came to the OPD with a history of **blackish discolouration** of the **left great toe** along with **severe pain** of **one month** duration. The **patient** was getting cramp-like pain in the **left calf** for the **last six months**. The **pain** used to appear on **walking a distance** of about 2 km. At that stage, the **pain** was **relieved** on **further walking**. But within a **couple of months** the **pain** became so **severe** that he had to **take rest** for **relief of pain**.

For the last **one month** the patient was experiencing **rest pain**. It was **continuous** and **very severe** in intensity. The pain was **disturbing his sleep**. The pain was localised to the **foot** and the **toes.**

About a **month ago** he noticed that the **tip** of the **left great toe** was **dusky** and the **pain** had become **worse**. Slowly over the **next four weeks** the **entire toe** had **turned black** in colour.

- The patient did **not** have any **pain** in the **right lower limb**.
- The patient did **not** give any history of **chest pain** or **breathlessness.**
- He did **not** complain of **syncopal attacks** or **problems** with **vision.** `

Past History

There was **no** history of either **hypertension or diabetes**. He had not suffered from any major illness in the past.

- **Family history** was **noncontributory**. He was not married.

Personal History

He was a **beedi smoker** for the past **10 years**. He used to smoke about **2 packs of beedi** every day. He was **not consuming alcohol** or **chewing paan**.

Treatment History

He had consulted **several doctors** before reaching the hospital. All of them had advised him **to stop smoking**. **Various drugs** had been prescribed but with **no relief**. He **confessed** that he had **continued to smoke beedis despite doctors' advice.**

General physical examination showed a patient who appeared in **distress** because of **pain.**

Local Examination

Inspection of the Left Lower Limb

There was **dry gangrene** of the **great toe.** There was a **line of demarcation** at the **base of the toe**. Hyperpigmentation was seen on the **dorsum** of the **foot.**

- There was **pitting oedema** of the foot.
- The **skin** over the lower part of the limb was **shiny and showed absence of hair.** The **remaining toes** showed **flattening** at the **pulp.**

The **nails** had **ridges** and appeared **irregular in shape**.

- The **saphenous vein** was not **visible** in the **standing position**.
- There was evidence of **muscular wasting** below the knee.

Palpation

- The **left foot** was **cooler** as compared to the opposite side.
- The area **around the great toe** was **very tender**. An area of **paraesthesia** was present **proximal** to the **gangrenous toe.**
- **Muscular wasting** was confirmed by **measurement** of the **girth** of the **limb** below the **knee joint.**

Pulsations

- The **dorsalis pedis, posterior tibial and popliteal artery** pulsations were **absent**. The **common femoral pulsations** were **weaker** as compared to the right side.
- There was **no evidence** of **sensory or motor deficit.**
- Multiple enlarged **lymph nodes** were palpable in the **inguinal region**. They were **small** in size, **soft, mobile and nontender**.
- **External iliac nodes** were **not palpable**.
- **Examination of the right lower limb** did not reveal any abnormality.
- Pulsations of the **abdominal aorta** and both the **radials** and **carotids**

as well as **superficial temporal arteries** were **normal.** There was **no thickening** of the **arterial wall.**

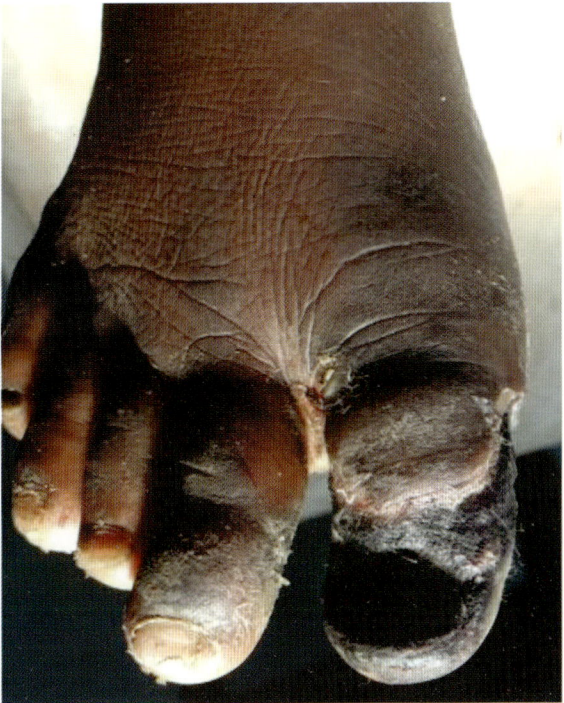

Fig. 12.1: Dry gangrene of the great toe with a line of demarcation.

Examination of the CVS

No abnormality was detected. The **pulse rate** was **78** per minute and **regular**. The **BP** was **128 by 82** mm of Hg.

Other systems were clinically normal.

Q. 1. **What was the diagnosis?**

A **peripheral arterial occlusive disease** probably due to **TAO.**

The **first part** of the **diagnosis** was **easily made**. The patient had **severe rest pain** with a

gangrenous toe. In addition, **signs of ischaemia** like **shiny skin, loss of hair, ridged nails** and **muscular wasting** were **present** in the limb. Since the peripheral **arterial pulsations** were **absent, arterial occlusion** was **identified.**

The **following factors** were taken as **circumstantial evidence** to suggest that the **cause** was **TAO.** The patient was a **25-year-old male**, a **beedi smoker** and the disease was affecting the **lower limb**. The most **important clinical finding** was **involvement** of the **medium-sized arteries** of the lower limb.

Q. 2. **What were investigations done in this patient?**

Fasting and post prandial (PP) blood sugar levels were within normal limits.

Serum lipid levels were normal.

ECG was normal.

Duplex US study of the left lower limb. The **dorsalis pedis** and the **posterior tibial** arteries were **completely blocked**. There was a **90% block** in the popliteal artery.

The **common and superficial femoral arteries** showed a **50% block**.

Examination of the vascular system in the **right lower limb** was essentially normal.

Q. 3. What was the treatment strategies planned for this patient?

The **nature** of the **disease** and the need for **total abstinence from smoking** was explained to the **patient and his relatives**. In order to emphasise the dangers associated with smoking, **a video** was shown to the group depicting all the **side effects** of smoking. A **diligent search for beedis** was conducted **daily** since the commodity was **freely available** with **other patients**, **conniving staff** and the **nearby shops**. The **hidden places** included the **bed** and the **pillow**. He was told that an **operation** would be **performed** to **improve the blood flow** to the **limb**. The **nature** of the **operation** was explained in **detail**. The **need for amputation** of the **gangrenous toe** was also made clear to him. He was **reassured** that with **customised footwear** he would be able to go back and **work** like a **normal person.**

Setting: A week passes.

During this week the patient was prescribed **pentoxyphylline** tablets along with **analgesics**. He also needed **sedatives** at night to get **relief** from **pain.**

Q. 4. What was the operation performed on this patient?

The patient underwent a **transfer** of the **greater omentum** to the **left lower limb** in the form of a long pedicle **based** on the **left gastroepiploic artery. The rest pain disappeared** within a **couple of days.** The **limb** showed evidence of **oedema. This** was **controlled** with an **elastic stockinet.**

The **patient** underwent an **amputation** of the **great toe a week later. The omental transfer** had helped in **improving blood flow** to the **limb.** The **wound edges were left open.** He was advised to attend the OPD for **dressings daily** at the **local hospital.**

Q. 5. How was the patient managed postoperatively?

He **returned** to the **hospital after six weeks.** His **rest pain** had **disappeared completely.** The **wound** at the site of **amputation had healed.** But his **pain-free walking distance** had **remained** the **same.** He was **warned** that if **he started smoking again,** the **disease** could **recur** in the **same or opposite limb** and that **even the upper limbs** could be **affected. Convinced** about the **dire consequences,** he **promised not to smoke again.** He was sent to the **Prosthetic Department** with a **request** for **customised footwear.**

Q. 6. What is the definition of TAO?

TAO is a **peripheral arterial occlusive disease** seen exclusively in **users of tobacco, and** has been defined as **a segmental vascular inflammation** with **vaso-occlusive phenomenon** involving the **small- and medium-sized arteries and veins** of the **lower** and less commonly the **upper limbs.**

Q. 7. What are the general features of TAO?

TAO is a disease **more frequently** seen in the **lower strata of society**. **Bidi smokers** have a much **higher incidence** compared to those **smoking cigarettes**. It is **more prevalent** in those areas where **bidi production** is a **cottage industry**; The **raw materials** are **supplied** at **home** and the **bidis are made** at the **same place**. The **habit** is almost **universal**. The **average age** when a person **starts smoking** is found to be about **10 to 12 years**. At the **global level**, the condition is more **prevalent** in the **Indian Subcontinent, Korea, Japan and Israel**. Though described by **von Winiwarter in Germany in 1879**, it was **Buerger of New York**, USA, who described the **disease** in great detail, **nearly a quarter century later**. But recently there **seems** to be a **decrease** in the **incidence** of the **disease.**

Q. 8. What are the aetiological factors of TAO?

An **immunologic basis** for the **causation** of the disease is now **established. Tobacco** as the **primary aetiological factor** has been **proved.** These patients show **hypersensitivity** to **intradermal injection** of **tobacco extract**, with **increased titers** of **serum antiendothelial cell antibodies**. They also have **impaired peripheral vascular endothelium dependent vasorelaxation**. In addition a **genetic component** has also been implicated. **Depletion of HLAB antigen** is said to lead to a **genetic modification,** but **without** a causative **genetic mutation**. There are a **large numbers** of **families** where **each member** is a **heavy smoker,** but the **disease is seen** in only **one or two** who are **probably hypersensitive**. Further it is **not dose related**. This is mentioned to **support** the **immunological concept**.

In addition **nicotine** is a known **vasoconstrictor** and may play an **aetiological role. Elevated levels** of **carbon monoxide** in the **blood stream** have been shown in this group, leading to **further depletion** of **oxygen supply** to the **tissues.**

Box 12.1:	Points regarding the aetiology of TAO

- Seen only in smokers – Beedi in our country.
- Hypersensitivity to tobacco – Intradermal injection of tobacco.
- Elevated levels of serum antiendothelial cell antibodies.
- Impairment of vascular endothelium – dependent vasorelaxation.
- Genetic factors.
- Nicotine – Vasoconstriction.
- Raised levels of carbon monoxide – Poor oxygenation of ischaemic tissues.

Q. 9. **Describe the clinical features of TAO.**

It is **important** to understand that there are **no specific features** due to the **disease** and the **entire clinical spectrum** is the **result of ischaemia**.

Sex: The disease is seen **almost exclusively in males**, though if one looks at the **total figures all over the world,** the **number** of **ladies who smoke** is **more than men**. It could be due to the **geographical distribution** of this condition, where **smoking** is a **habit** seen in **men.**

Age is very significant. It is most frequently seen between the ages of **20** and **45.**

Pain is the cardinal symptom. **Ischaemic pain** is one of the most **severe** type of **pain** experienced by a **human being**. It may result from **ischaemia** of the **heart, bowel** or the **extremities.**

Intermittent claudication. In the **initial stages** of **TAO,** the **pain** is in the nature of **intermittent claudication**. To **claudicate** would mean to **limp**. There are several **theories** as to the **etymology** of this word. **Claudius**, a **Roman god,** had his **upper part** of the **body** shaped like a **human being,** but the **lower half** resembled that of a **horse.** The **gait,** where the **heel is raised off** the ground while **walking,** is **comparable** to that of a **horse,** and is called **limping**. **Claudication** is described as a **cramp-like** and **agonizing pain** in the **calf muscles** during **walking.** It is due to the **accumulation** of **factors P** (probably **lactic acid** and **other metabolites**) following **muscular activity.** In a **normal person**, during **this phase,** there is **profound arterial dilatation**, bringing in more **blood** into the **muscles. The extra blood** is removed by a **competent venous system**. The increase in blood flow results from **decreased sympathetic vasoconstrictor activity (neurogenic**) and the **metabolites** acting directly on the **vessels** causing **vasodilatation**

(humoral). Due to **occlusion** of **arteries**, this **increase does not occur** in **ischaemic limbs,** thus allowing the **P factors** to **accumulate.** These **stimulate** the **sensory nerve endings** in the **muscles** resulting in **pain.**

Over a period of time, it became clear that **similar episodes** of **pain** can involve **other groups of muscles** like the **small muscles** of the **foot, gluteal muscles** and those of the **upper limb**. But the **term** has been **retained** though **one cannot limp** with **one's hand**. When a patient has an **ischaemic foot**, the **pain** may be **mistaken** for an **orthopaedic problem.**

What are the grades of intermittent claudication?

Grade 1: The patient after **walking a certain distance** experiences claudication type of **pain,** which **surprisingly disappears** as he **continues** to **walk further**. At this **stage** of the disease, the **collateral vessels** are **healthy** and they undergo **dilatation** in the manner described above and the **P factors are washed away** by the **improved circulation**. Unfortunately, **very few patients** reach the **hospital** during this **stage,** since the **relief of pain** makes them **believe** that the **disease** is not a **serious** one.

Grade 2: The **pain** is so **severe** that he is **forced** to take **rest** for the **relief of pain**. Many of these patients can be seen **sitting** and **massaging** the **calf muscles**. At this **stage** most of the **collateral vessels** are also **involved** and the **P factors remain at the site**. Once the **patient stops walking**, the **depleted circulation** washes away the **collected metabolites** and the **pain** gradually **disappears.**

Q. 10. Describe rest pain in detail.

Rest pain is classified as grade 3 of **claudication.** Rest pain suggests **gross impairment of blood flow** to the limb with **danger** to the **viability of the limb**. The **pain** is due to **severe ischaemia** of **all tissues** including **nerves**. It can **aptly** be **compared** to **anginal pain** at **rest**. The **intensity of pain** is more severe because of the **involvement of nerves** in **TAO.** Often these **patients** present with either **impending** or **frank gangrene** or **painful nonhealing ulcers**. **Claudication pain** may continue for **several months without progression** of the disease, but once **rest pain** develops, things take a turn for the **worse** rather **quickly.** This stage has been aptly described as **critical limb ischaemia.**

Recently, the term **claudication distance** has been replaced by **two new terms**.

(*a*) **Maximum Walking Distance** which is much **longer** than the **claudication distance. It is comparable to grade 1 of intermittent claudication.**

(*b*) **Pain-Free Walking Distance:** This is the **distance a patient** is able to walk **before** the **onset of pain** and this equals the **claudication distance (grade 2).**

These **distances** are **important** because they provide an **indirect clinical parameter** for the **effectiveness** of the **treatment. Improvement** in the **maximum or pain-free walking distance** is an indicator of **increased blood flow**.

Box 12.2:	Points regarding the symptoms of ischaemia

- Males between 20 and 40 years.
- Intermittent claudication – Agonizing cramp-like pain in a group of muscles during muscular activity.
- **Grade 1:** Pain walking a certain distance – Disappears on further walking – Dilated collaterals.
- **Grade 2:** Pain on walking – Takes rest – P factor removed – Pain disappears.
- **Grade 3:** Rest pain – Critical limb ischemia – Loss of tissue or parts of limb.

Q. 11. **What are the special points to look for in general physical examination?**

The only **significant finding** to look for is **pallor.** Presence of **anaemia aggravates** the condition because the **tissue perfusion** becomes **worse** due to the **poor quality of blood** in a **limb** where the **quantity** has already been **reduced** by the **occlusive disease**.

Q. 12. **Define gangrene and describe the types.**

Gangrene is defined as **macroscopic death of tissue** due to **loss of blood supply** with **putrefaction. Putrefaction** is the **result** of **invasion of dead tissues** by **saprophytes**. It is one of the **easiest clinical conditions** to **identify.** The following are the **classical manifestations** of gangrene.

(*a*) **Loss of pulsations** due to occlusion of the lumen of the artery.

(*b*) **Loss of sensation** resulting from death of sensory nerves.

(*c*) **Loss of temperature:** A normal limb is warm due to circulating blood and hence the gangrenous area is cool.

(*d*) **Loss of function:** The dead muscles or tendons cannot act and hence the part loses its function.

(*e*) **Loss of colour:** The area of gangrene is **black** because of the colour of the **degraded products of haemoglobin.**

Two types of gangrene are seen in clinical practice. **Dry gangrene** occurs when there is a **gradual occlusion** of the **arteries** as in **TAO and atherosclerosis.** The part involved is **dry and shriveled,** and best described as **mummified.** The **gangrenous process** spreads **proximally** over a **period of weeks** until a **line of demarcation is seen.**

In **wet gangrene**, there is a **sudden occlusion** of an **artery** as in **thrombosis** or **embolism. Sudden occlusion** of a **vein** can also cause **wet gangrene.** The area is **swollen** and associated with a **large quantity of discharge,** which is **foul smelling** and **blood stained.** The **gangrenous areas** are **patchy** and **spread** across the **limb** in a **proximal direction** within a **very short period** with **no line of demarcation. Wet gangrene** is associated with **extreme toxaemia** and a **high** degree of **morbidity** and **mortality,** and is considered to be a **life-threatening emergency.**

Line of demarcation. In the case of **dry gangrene,** the **zone** between the **dead and living** tissues is known as a **line of demarcation.** It is to be considered as a **three-dimensional** one comprising of **granulation tissue.** This **terminology** is used because on **inspection,** it appears like **red line** between the **two areas.** During the **progression** of **dry gangrene,** the **line of demarcation** will **appear** only when the **process** is **completely evolved.** Therefore this sign is **not seen** in **every case** of **dry gangrene.**

Box 12.3:	Points regarding gangrene

- Definition – Types – Dry and wet.
- Dry – Gradual occlusion of an artery – Atherosclerosis, TAO.
- Wet – Sudden occlusion of an artery – Thrombosis or embolism.
- Sudden occlusion of a vein – DVT uncommon

Q. 13. What are the signs of an ischaemic limb?

Gangrene indicates a **state of irreversible damage.** It is necessary to **identify** the **ischaemic process** before **gangrene develops.** In **chronic occlusions** like TAO the **gangrene** is of the **dry variety.** The **following signs** are significant:

(*a*) **Skin changes:** The skin will be **thinned out** and **shiny. Loss of hair** is frequently seen.

Colour changes associated with change of posture as described by Buerger are difficult to demonstrate in our patients since we are basically a dark-skinned race.

(b) Ulceration: Delay in treatment or failed amputations lead to the development of ulcers. Classically, an ischaemic ulcer is seen in the dorsum of the foot or at the amputation stump. The margins may show a blackish rim. It is very tender. A zone of paraesthesia is seen around the ulcer. The edges are punched out and the floor is pale. The base is formed more often by the underlying bone. The picture of a person sitting on his bed looking miserable, holding on to his ulcerated painful foot, will leave behind an indelible impression in a clinician's mind.

(c) Nails: The nails appear to have transverse ridges and are also brittle. The capillary filling time in the nails is a reliable indicator of the disease in the upper limb. In this test, pressure is applied on the nail bed by compressing it against the nail. The nail now appears pale. The time taken for the nail to regain its original pink colour once the pressure is released is known as capillary filling time. In the presence of ischaemia, the capillary filling time is prolonged. This test has a limited value because most patients with TAO have lower limb disease, with deformed and discoloured nails.

(d) Muscles: There is obvious muscular wasting.

(e) Superficial veins show poor filling even when the patient is made to stand. If the patient has superficial thrombophlebitis, seen in TAO occasionally, the veins are tender and firm and do not empty on pressure. A red streak is seen in the overlying skin in fair individuals.

(f) Peripheral pulsations: This is the most critical finding in occlusive arterial diseases. But there is a caveat. Though an absent pulse is an important clinical sign of an occlusive disease, it does not always indicate a total occlusion of the vessel. It only suggests absence of a pulsatile flow. If the vessel wall is thickened, or there is significant narrowing of the

lumen, pulsations will be **absent**. So the **level of block** in the arterial system cannot be **ascertained accurately** by **clinical examination** alone.

With a **clear knowledge** of the **anatomy** of the arterial system, a **careful examination** of all the **important arteries** is carried out. An **isolated absent dorsalis pedis pulse** could be due to a **congenital abnormality**, where in the **blood supply to the foot** is taken over by an **abnormal peroneal artery**, felt **behind the lateral malleolus**. If the **common femoral pulsations** are **weak**, **auscultation** at the mid-inguinal point may reveal a **bruit.**

Box 12.4:	Points regarding signs of ischaemia

- Gangrene – Late irreversible stage.
- Skin – Shiny and thin.
- Ulcer – Very tender, punched out edges and pale granulation tissue.
- Muscles – Wasting.
- Superficial veins – Poor filling.
- Arterial pulsations – Weak or absent.
- Bruit.

Q. 14. What is the indication for examination of CVS in a case of dry gangrene?

The abnormality to look for is **mitral stenosis**. In this condition, **eddying** and **pooling** of the **retained blood** in the **left atrium** produces a **mural thrombus**.

An attack of **atrial fibrillation** may cause a portion of this **thrombus** to get **dislodged,** and the **embolus** thus formed enters the **systemic circulation**. If these microemboli were to **block the digital arteries**, **gangrene** would follow. Anatomically, these vessels are **end arteries**. But in general, **most emboli** get into the **carotid system** resulting in episodes of transient ischaemic attacks (**TIA**).

Q. 15. How is TAO diagnosed clinically?

As **most of the patients** present rather **late to the hospital**, at the end of a **good history** and a **careful clinical examination**, one can most often come to **clinical diagnosis** of a **peripheral arterial occlusive disease**. But to **prove** that this **occlusion** is the **result of TAO** is much **more difficult**. One is forced to look for **circumstantial evidence** at this stage. **Essentially, TAO** is a **diagnosis** made by **excluding** other **vascular conditions** with the help of **various investigations**.

Based on the following **clinical criteria**, a **provisional diagnosis of TAO** can be made.

(*a*) **Male sex**

(*b*) **Age between 20 and 45 years.**

(*c*) Always a **smoker**, more often in this part of the world the **bidi** is the culprit.

(*d*) Involvement of the **lower limbs**. **One side** may show evidence of a **more advanced disease**. At a **later stage** the disease can spread to the **upper limbs** also.

(*e*) **Occlusion** of the **small and medium-sized arteries** is the **key** to the **clinical diagnosis**. In the lower limb the **dorsalis pedis**, the **posterior tibial** and the **popliteal arteries** are affected. **Superficial femoral** (between the origin of the profunda branch and the adductor foramen) and the **common** femoral arteries are **less frequently** involved. In the **upper limb**, the affected vessels are the **radial, ulnar and the brachial**. The **proximal arterial system** is always **normal.**

(*f*) **Gangrene** when present is of the **dry variety. Great toe** is most often involved. If the **heel** is the **primary site** of gangrene, it suggests a **significant decrease in blood supply** and the need for a **major amputation** becomes **higher**.

(*g*) Prolonged regular follow-up manifests the episodic nature of TAO. The condition passes through **periods of activity** lasting for **weeks or months** followed by an **equal period** of quiescence, the reasons for which are unclear.

Q. 16. What are the investigations done in these patients?

As mentioned earlier, the **diagnosis** is arrived at more by a process of **exclusion**. Therefore the investigations can be broadly divided into two groups.

Group 1: These are performed to **rule out other causes** of **vascular occlusion**. They include the following:

(*a*) **Urine** and **blood sugar** studies to rule out **diabetes.**

(*b*) **Serum lipid profile** to rule out **atherosclerosis.**

(*c*) **Immunological studies** to rule out **connective tissue disorders**.

(*d*) In the past, **tertiary syphilis** was to be ruled out by **specific tests**, since **endarteritis obliterans** resulted in **digital gangrene.**

Group 2: These tests are more important since they **demonstrate** the **vascular status** of the **limb accurately**. As already mentioned, **clinical examination** gives **inadequate information** regarding the **level** and the **degree of block**. In addition, the **state of the collateral circulation** cannot be determined **without the help** of **investigations.**

Q. 17. What are the specific investigations performed in patients with occlusive disease?

Ankle–brachial index (ABI): It is the **ratio** of the **systolic BP** measurement of the **posterior tibial artery** at the **ankle** to that of the **brachial artery**. A **normal ABI** should be **1.1.** An index **less than 0.9** is indicative of **occlusive disease**. An **ABI** of **less than 0.5** is suggestive of **severe ischaemia**. A figure of **less than 0.3** indicates **limb-threatening ischaemia**. A **test** conducted **after 5 minutes** of **exercise** is **more reliable.**

Limitations: Patients with **calcified medial wall** have **noncompressible arteries.** Hence the test **cannot be done** in such cases. If both the **brachial** and the **posterior tibial** arteries are **stenosed,** the values will **not be accurate**.

Toe pressure measurement: **Medial sclerosis** does **not** affect the **digital arteries.** Hence the **toe artery pressure** can be used to **measure** the index. Normally, the **toe pressure is 60%** of the **ankle pressure**. Both **these tests** are being used in the developed countries **to screen** the **high risk group** (elderly with hypertension).

Segmental arterial pressure: **Arterial pressure** can be measured at **different levels** in the **limb.** The figures can be **compared** with that of the **opposite limb**. A **difference** of more than **20 mmHg** is **significant.**

Duplex US study: It combines **gray-scale imaging** with **colour Doppler studies**. A triphasic wave indicates a normal flow. It indicates the **site** as well as the **degree** of **stenosis**. A **two-fold** increase in **peak systolic velocity** indicates **50% or more stenosis**. A **three-fold increase** suggests a **stenosis** of **more than 75%.** The **advantages** of this study are as follows. It is **noninvasive** and hence can be **repeated** as and when necessary. This becomes important after **direct arterial interventions** have been performed to **assess** the **patency** of the **graft or the stent**. It **eliminates** the need for **invasive procedures** in a group of patients who do **not** have **good distal run-off.**

The **disadvantages** are as follows. Like all US studies it is **operator dependent.** A **dedicated specialist** is an asset. The **state** of the **collateral circulation** may **not** be **accurately identified** by this investigation.

CT angiography: If **direct arterial intervention** is being planned, the patient needs **CT angiography.** It helps to **accurately define** the **site, extent** and the **morphology (calcification and thrombus)** of the **lesion** in the **arterial system**. **Segmental blocks** are detected. The **collaterals** are clearly **visualized.**

MRI angiography: It is noninvasive. It can visualize the **most distal parts** of the **arterial system** using **gadolinium-enhanced contrast**. Both **specificity** and **sensitivity** are above **90%**. In **many centers** it has **replaced CT** angiography as the **investigation of choice. MRI is superior** to CT in visualizing the **intima–media thickness** which is important in certain **types** of arterial diseases.

Box 12.5:	Points regarding specific investigations

- AB index – 1.1: normal – Less than 0.9: occlusive disease – Less than 0.7: severe – Less than 0.3: limb viability doubtful. Toe arterial pressure – Alternate to ABI.
- Duplex US – Noninvasive – Site and degree of block – Collaterals not identified.
- CT angiogram - Direct arterial intervention – Site, degree and morphology – Thrombus.
- MRI angiogram – Gadolinium-enhanced – Distal vessels well defined.

It **needs to be stressed** that neither **CT nor MRI angiograms** are **routinely performed** in this group of patients because the **distal run-off** is **very poor,** indicating the **absence of a patent distal vessel** suitable for **direct arterial intervention.**

Q. 18. **What is the role of arterial biopsy in the diagnosis of TAO?**

In **most surgical situations,** **cytological** or **histological proof** is needed **before treatment is started. TAO is an exception** to this rule **for two reasons.** The **symptoms and signs** are the result of **ischaemia** and the **focus of treatment** is to **improve the blood flow.** Further, **there are no specific measures** to treat the cause, except **cessation of smoking.** In addition, obtaining **material for biopsy** demands an **invasive approach,** which can lead to **more complications** in a **limb** that is **already ischaemic.** Hence these studies are **confined** to only **academic centres** for **research purposes.**

Q. 19. **What are the histopathological findings in a case of TAO?**

Blood vessels dissected from **amputated limbs** offer the **best material**. **Arterial biopsies** are never performed. The **basic pathology** is one of **panarteritis. Three distinct pathological phases** are described during the course of the disease.

1. **Acute phase**, demonstrated by a **highly cellular segmental occlusive thrombus** with **minimal inflammation**. **Neutrophil cellular aggregate** with **microabscesses** and **multinucleated giant cells** are seen **microscopically (thrombosis).**

2. **Subacute phase** is characterised by the **inflammatory thrombi** progressing to **organisaton,** but **attempts at recanalisation** (unlike the veins) are not seen **(angiitis).**

3. **Late phase** shows a completely **organised thrombus** with **fibrosis** leading to **obliteration of the lumen**. The **fibrous reaction** extends to involve the **neighbouring veins** and **nerves (obliterans).**

4. The most **significant microscopic finding** that distinguishes this condition from all **other occlusive diseases** is the presence of an **intact internal elastic lamina**. This is considered to be **diagnostic of TAO.**

Box 12.6:	Points regarding the pathology of TAO

- Acute phase – Highly cellular segmental thrombus – Minimal inflammation.
- Subacute phase – Inflammation involving all the layers of the arterial wall – No attempt at recanalisation.
- Late phase – Fibrosis – Occlusion of the lumen.
- Involvement of the contiguous vein and nerve.
- Intact internal elastic lamina – Diagnostic.

Q. 20. Discuss the treatment strategies in TAO.

There is **no specific treatment** for this disease. Since its relation to the use of tobacco is well established, **CESSATION OF SMOKING** is the only measure to **prevent further progression** of the disease. Unfortunately, **majority of patients** do **not comply,** and hence **failure of treatment** is **very common**, leading on to **major amputations.**

Measures to improve the blood flow.

Direct procedures on the arteries.

As mentioned earlier, **TAO involves** the **small and the medium-sized arteries**. **Obliteration of the lumen by fibrosis** is reflected in the total

absence of an **adequate distal run-off** in **imaging studies.** Again the **collateral vessels** are seen to have **dilated to the highest** extent. Therefore, **direct interventional procedures** such as **bypass surgery** or **endovascular stenting** are **not possible** in the treatment of this disease.

Indirect methods of improving the blood flow.

Various **drugs** and **procedures** are available to **improve the blood supply** in TAO. They include the following.

1. **Drugs:**

   (*a*) **Pentoxyphylline** is a drug that enhances the blood supply by **altering the shape of the RBC** and **reducing** the **viscosity of blood. Intravenous pentoxyphylline** is seen to **reverse impending gangrene** in some cases. **Hypotension** can be an **undesirable side effect**. **Oral tablets** of **400 mg bd** are given over long periods of time to **prevent** further **deterioration** in the **vascular status**.

   (*b*) Cilostazol acts by preventing **platelet aggregation** as well as facilitating **vascular**

dilatation, especially of the **collateral vessels**. Hence it is very useful at the stage of **intermittent claudication. Maximum walking distance** has been reported to **increase by 50%** following the use of this drug. The standard dose is **100 mg bd.** The commonest **side effect is headache.**

   (*c*) **Intravenous Iloprost**, a **prostaglandin analogue,** is said to have **beneficiary effects** but is **not yet available** in this **country.**

Box 12.7:	Points regarding medical treatment

- CESSATION OF SMOKING.
- Pentoxyphylline.
- Cilostazol.
- Intravenous iloprost – Not available.
- Systemic vasodilators contraindicated.

2. **Surgical procedures:**

Many **operations** have been **performed** for **this condition.** But **none** have given **consistently good results. Unfortunately, most patients end up** with a **minor or a major amputation.**

Lumbar sympathectomy was a very **popular operation** in the **past.** It was based on the **presumption** that **removal** of the **sympathetic**

vasoconstrictor tone would dilate the collateral vessels, thus improving the blood flow. But imaging studies like CT angiography have shown grossly dilated collateral arteries. Thus the operation has now fallen into disrepute.

Pedicled omental transfer to the limb.

The principle behind this operation is the fact that the proximal arteries are never involved in TAO. The greater omentum derives its blood supply from the gastroepiploic arteries. It is mobilised and brought down to the lower limb in the form of a long pedicle to improve the blood flow. This procedure gives good results in some patients.

ILIZAROV'S operation. An operation described originally for nonunion of fractures or for limb lengthening, this has also been employed to improve the blood supply to the lower limb. The procedure induces intentional bone distraction, resulting in neovasculogenesis. The hazards associated with this extensive and invasive procedure in an ischaemic limb have not made this a popular operation.

Electrical manipulation of the pain-carrying fibres of the spinal cord for the relief of rest pain is still not well established.

Box 12.8:	Points regarding surgical treatment

- Sympathectomy - Operation of the past.
- Omental transfer to the lower limb.
- Ilizarov's operation – Invasive in an ischaemic limb – Not popular.
- Electric manipulation for relief of pain – Symptomatic.

Q. 21. What are the indications for amputations in TAO?

The presence of gangrene is an absolute indication for an amputation. But several patients who suffer from severe rest pain associated with nonhealing ulcers will also need an amputation if all other treatment measures have failed. Most patients belonging to this group would have started smoking again.

Q. 22. What are the amputations performed for these patients?

The level of amputation is never decided on clinical grounds alone. Duplex US, CT angiogram, ankle brachial index as well as the calf muscle systolic pressure as measured with Doppler, are the factors that are taken into consideration. The

key to a **successful procedure** is the **status of the popliteal artery.**

A **local amputation** at the level of a **well-defined and complete** line of **demarcation** often succeeds, if the **vascularity of the limb** has been **improved** by the procedures mentioned above. It may **mean disarticulation** of **one or more number of toes** at the **metatarsophalangeal joint** along with excision of the **cartilaginous cap** at the **articular head** of the **metatarsal bone.** This step is **imperative** because the **cartilage is avascular** and the **risk of sepsis** is **high.** Again once the **cap is removed**, the **cancellous marrow,** being more **vascular,** will help in the **growth of granulation tissue,** hastening the **process of healing. Primary closure** of these incisions is **never performed** in an **ischaemic limb.**

The **problem** becomes **more complex** when the **local amputations fail.** These **patients** are often a picture of **misery,** with **extremely painful nonhealing ulcers** at the **site of the amputation** stump with either a zone of **hyperaesthesia** or a **blackish rim** around the ulcer, indicating a **likely progression of dry gangrene. Amputations** at the level of the **ankle** like **Syme's** are **absolutely contraindicated**, since the **dorsalis pedis and the posterior tibial arteries** are always totally **obliterated.** A **below-knee amputation** should always be considered, since the **knee joint** plays an **important part** of the **social habits** of people of this **country.** If the **popliteal artery** is shown to have **adequate flow** by the **investigations,** or if the **Doppler calf muscle pressure** is above **70 mm** Hg, an **amputation below the knee joint** will **succeed.** A **small number** of patients will end up with an **above-knee amputation.** Stem cell therapy is a new method that is being tried.

Box 12.9:	Points regarding surgical treatment

- Sympathectomy - Operation of the past.
- Omental transfer to the lower limb.
- Ilizarov's operation – Invasive in an ischaemic limb – Not popular.
- Electric manipulation for relief of pain – Symptomatic.

Q. 23. Describe the postoperative management.

Care of the **feet.** The **patient** must be **advised** to wear **customised footwear.** The **feet** must be kept **clean** and **exposure** to **extremes** of **temperatures** must be **avoided.** The **correct way** of **cutting nails** should be **taught** to the **patient.** Even **minor injuries** must be **reported** to the doctor immediately. A **trivial looking paronychia** may be a **heralding sign** of **ischaemia.** The **intensity of pain** is **out of proportion** to the **clinical signs** in this **situation.**

Rehabilitation is often **neglected** or **inadequately done.** The purpose is to make the **patient fully functional** and **economically viable,** since the **disease** involves **men** at the **most productive period** of their **lives. Physiotherapy** along with good **psychological counseling** is an **integral part** of the treatment. **Efficient prosthetic limbs** are now **available** and are supplied **free of cost** for **poor patients.** Even for patients with an **above-knee amputation, prosthetic limbs** are available with some degree of **function at the knee joint.** The patient may have to **adjust his lifestyle** or **occupation** so that **he limits** his **walking** to **within the pain-free walking distance. All these measures** will **work only** if **the patient** continues to **TOTALLY ABSTAIN FROM SMOKING.**

PERIPHERAL ARTERIAL OCCLUSIVE DISEASE PART 2

ATHEROSCLEROSIS

Setting

- Surgical OPD.

Chief Complaint

- **Blackish discolouration** of the **right heel** with **pain** of **3 weeks duration.**

History of Present Illness

A **65-year-old man** came to the OPD with complaining of **blackish discoloration of the heel** of the **right foot** along with **severe pain** of **3 weeks** duration. The patient was having **pain** in his **right leg** on **walking** to his place of **work** for the previous **8 months.** Initially the **pain** was **mild** and he was able to **start work** soon after **reaching the place.** Later the **pain** became **severe** and he had to **rest** for **some time** before he **started working.** For the **last three months** he had to **sit down** in between for **relief of pain. Pain at rest** appeared about **3 weeks** ago. At that stage he noticed a **blackish area** on the **heel** of the right foot. The area was **extremely painful.** He had **not** been going to **work** for the **last 3 weeks.** The **area** at the heel had been **rapidly increasing** in size with **increase** in the **intensity of pain.** He did **not** get any **sleep** at night because of pain. He **needed external help** to **walk inside** the house for his **daily activities.**

- He did not complain of **chest pain** or **breathlessness.**
- There was no history of **syncopial attacks** or **disturbances of vision.**

Past History

- He had been a **hypertensive** for the last **4 years.** He had been taking **treatment irregularly** from a **local doctor.** He was **not** a known **diabetic.** He did **not suffer** from any **other major illness** in the past.

Family History

- **Three of his brothers** were known **hypertensives.** There was **no history** of **diabetes** in the family.

Personal History

- He was a **smoker** for the last **40 years.** He used to smoke about **1 packet** of **cigarettes** daily. There was no history of consumption of alcohol or chewing paan.
- **General physical examination** did not show any abnormality.

Local Examination of Right Lower Limb

- Gait
- The patient was able to take a **few steps** with help. He was keeping his **heel** raised **off the ground.**

- An area of **dry gangrene** was present in the **right heel.** It was **circular** in shape and measured **4 cm in diameter**.
- There was **swelling** on the dorsum of the foot.
- All the **toes** were in a position of **flexion** at the metatarsophalangeal joint.
- The **pulp** of the **toes** was **flat** and the **nails** showed **transverse ridges.**
- The **skin** over the leg was **thin and shiny. No hairs** could be seen in this area.
- There was significant **muscular wasting** in the right lower limb.
- **Venous filling** was poor.

Palpation

- The limb was **cool** below the level of the **knee.**
- The **area around the gangrene** was very **tender. Hyperaesthesia** was also present.
- **Pitting oedema** was present on the dorsum of the foot.
- **Muscular wasting** was confirmed by **measurement** both in the thigh and leg segments. There was **no sensory deficit** in the limb.

Pulsations

- **All the pulsations** in the right lower limb starting from the **common femoral artery** were **absent.**

- **Enlarged lymph nodes** were palpable in the **right inguinal region**. They were soft in consistency and small in size.
- The **right external iliac artery** pulsations could **not be felt.**
- **Pulsations** in the **left lower limb** and **abdominal aorta** were normal.
- **Rest of all the pulsations** were felt normally.

Examination of CVS

- The **pulse rate** was **82** per minute and **regular.** The **arterial wall** appeared **thickened.** The **BP** was **170 by 100** mmHg.
- **Examination of the heart** was clinically normal.
- **Examination of other systems** did not show any abnormality.

Q. 1. What was the diagnosis?

A diagnosis of a **peripheral arterial occlusive disease** most probably due to **atherosclerosis** was made in this patient. The **diagnosis** of an **arterial occlusive disease** was made on the strength of the following **clinical findings**. Presence of **rest pain** along with **gangrene** and other findings like **skin changes**, **muscular wasting** and **absent pulsations confirmed** the diagnosis of an **occlusive disease.**

Atherosclerosis was considered because of the **following factors.**

The patient was a **65-year-old man**. He was a **smoker**. He also had **hypertension**. The **pulsations** of **proximal large arteries** such as the **external iliac** and **common femoral arteries** were absent. There was **thickening** of the **arterial wall**.

Q. 2. What were the investigations done in this patient?

Fasting and PP blood sugar levels were within normal limits.

Serum triglycerides and **LDL levels** were raised.

Blood urea and **creatinine** levels were normal.

The **ECG** and **echocardiograms** were normal.

The **ankle brachial index** was **0.7**.

Duplex ultrasound study. It showed a **90% block** of the **right external iliac artery**. There was **reduced flow** in the **arteries** of the **right lower limb**. There was **no** evidence of **calcification** of the arterial wall in the limb.

A **CT angiogram** showed the presence of a **severe stenosis** in the **right external iliac artery**. The **femoral** and the **distal arteries** showed partial filling by the **collaterals**. The **collateral vessels** were more **prominent** in the **thigh segment**.

Setting: One week passes. During this period the need to **abstain** from smoking permanently was explained to the patient. His **hypertension** was **controlled** with **drugs**.

Q. 3. What were the treatment strategies planned for this patient?

The **patient** had **reached** the **hospital late** in the course of the **disease.** He had **gangrene** of the **heel** with a **block** at the **external iliac artery.** To **increase** the **blood flow** to the **limb,** a **prosthetic aortoiliac bypass** was **planned.** Since **heel gangrene** indicated **severe impairment** of **blood flow** to the **distal part** of the **limb,** the chances of a **major amputation** was **explained** to the **relatives.**

Q. 4. What was the operation performed in this patient?

He underwent an aortoiliac bypass surgery with the placement of a prosthetic graft between the abdominal aorta and the right common femoral artery. His rest pain improved over a period of few days. The limb below the knee became warmer. The gangrene remained static but the hyperaesthesia was reduced to a large extent.

Q. 5. How was the patient managed postoperatively?

Antihypertensive drugs were **continued,** and he was also started on **statin group** of drugs as well as **antiplatelet drugs.** The **gangrenous region** was found **fixed** to the **calcaneum.** He was **advised** a **below-knee amputation. The patient was not willing** for the **same. Following repeated persuasion and visits by a couple of patients** who had **undergone** the **procedure earlier,** the **patient agreed to undergo** the **operation.**

A **below-knee amputation** was **performed. The incision** had **healed well** in about **10 days.** He was discharged with the **advice to continue** all the **drugs on a regular basis. Abstinence from smoking** was again **emphasised.** He was told to **attend** the **physiotherapy department daily.**

Q. 6. How was the patient rehabilitated after the amputation?

Regular **pressure bandage** was used to **reduce** the **bulky below knee stump to a cone shape** so that a **prosthesis** would be **fitted easily. Exercises** were **taught** to keep the **knee joint** in a **stable state. Most importantly** due to the **exercises, the muscles** of the **thigh would** also be **supple.** Thus the **patient** and the **stump** would be **ready to receive** an **artificial limb.**

Six weeks later the patient was **readmitted** for fitting the

artificial limb. A custom-made prosthesis was applied to the **stump.** The **physiotherapist was guiding the patient daily** about the **proper use** of the **prosthesis.** At the end of **10 days the patient** was able to **walk** with his **artificial limb.** At the time of **discharge, instructions were given to the patient** regarding the **care** of the **stump** as well as the **prosthesis. TO ABSTAIN FROM SMOKING WAS STRESSED SEVERAL TIMES** to the patient.

Q. 7. Describe the general features of peripheral arterial occlusive disease due to atherosclerosis.

Atherosclerosis is the most **common cause** for **peripheral arterial occlusive disease** seen in **clinical practice**. The **incidence** is **increasing** due to the **following factors:**

(*a*) **Increasing life expectancy** in the general population. As **age advances**, the **risk** becomes **higher.** Beyond **50 years**, it is **very common.**

(*b*) **Association with diabetes. India** being the **diabetic capital** of the **world, atherosclerosis** is also seen **more frequently**. In **diabetics**, the disease is seen at a **younger age.**

(*c*) There is a very **high incidence** in **smokers**.

(*d*) **Life style changes** such as **lack of regular exercise** along with **consumption of fatty diet** lead to **obesity**, which is a **recognised risk factor**. **Elevated levels** of low density lipoproteins (**LDL**) along with **decreased levels** of high density lipoproteins (**HDL**) are recognised **risk factors**.

(*e*) **Genetic predisposition.**

(*f*) Increased levels of **homocysteine** and **fibrinogen levels** are also considered to be additional **predisposing factors.**

(*g*) **Increased platelet reactivity** is also implicated in the aetiology.

Box 12.10:	Points regarding aetiology

- Most common cause for PAOD.
- Genetic disposition.
- Elderly men commonly affected.
- Diabetics – A decade younger.
- Smoking and obesity.
- Elevated levels of homocysteine and fibrinogen.

Q. 8. Describe the basic pathology of atherosclerosis.

A **clear understanding** of the **basic pathology** is needed to **identify** as well as **treat** the disease. **Atherosclerosis** results from an **excessive fibroproliferative response** to numerous **vascular insults**.

This leads to an alteration in the **homeostatic properties** of the **endothelium** with **increased permeability** to **lipoproteins**. It also causes **increased migration** of **leucocyte**s into the **arterial wall.** The **ultimate result** of these changes is to produce **focal necrosis**. An **atheroma** hence consists of a **core of lipid**, a **mixture of leucocytes** and **necrotic tissue**, covered by a **fibrous cap. Thinning** of this **fibrous cap** due to release of **metalloproteinases** and other **proteolytic enzymes** leads to **rupture** of the cap. **Ulceration, thrombosis and accelerated plaque growth** are the **sequences** of these changes.

Box 12.11:	Points regarding pathological changes

- Excessive fibroproliferative response to vascular insults.
- Increased permeability of the endothelium.
- Migration of lipoproteins and leucocytes – Focal necrosis.
- Atheroma – Core of lipid, mixture of leucocytes and necrotic tissue covered by a fibrous cap.
- Rupture of the cap – Ulceration, thrombosis and accelerated plaque growth.

Q. 9. What are the clinical features of PAOD?

It is important to remember that **atherosclerosis** is a **systemic disease** with **involvement of**

many arteries in the body including the **aorta.** The **coronary, carotid, renal and superior mesenteric** arteries are usually seen to be diseased. Hence when the **disease affects the vessels of the lower limb**, it is only a **part** of the **total clinical spectrum**. The status of the **vital organs supplied** by **these vessels** is more **important** than the **disease in the limbs**. Ultimately the **morbidity and mortality** figures are **directly related** to **these factors.**

Age: Classically described as a disease of the **elderly,** it is being recognised quite frequently in **younger patients** today. It is more common in **men.**

The disease is **more common in diabetics**.

There is a very high incidence in **smokers.**

Since the **symptoms** are due to **ischaemia, intermittent claudication** and **rest pain** are always seen. **Fontaine's classification** is more useful in this situation as compared to the **Boyd's.**

Grade I. Asymptomatic but with **investigative evidence** of **vascular occlusion**. This group **assumes significance** since **preventive steps** will **benefit these patients**. This stage is **unlikely to be seen** in **our patients** because **investigations** for **ischaemia** at **this stage** quite often **do not include** the **lower limb**.

Grade II: Mild to moderate intermittent claudication corresponding to **Boyd's grade I & II.**

Grade III: Severe intermittent claudication equal to **Boyd's grade II, late stages.**

Grade IV: Presence of rest pain. Same as **Boyd's grade III.**

Grade V: Evidence of ulceration and/or gangrene.

Symptoms due to involvement of other systems.

(*a*) **Cardiovascular system. Chest pain** indicative of cardiac disease.

(*b*) **Blurring of vision** or **syncopial attacks** due to **atherosclerosis** involving the **carotid arteries**.

(*c*) **Abdominal pain** becoming **worse** after **intake of food** may be suggestive of partial **occlusion** of the **superior mesenteric artery**.

Family history of **hypertension** or **diabetes** is often present.

Q. 10. What are the physical signs?

Both the **lower limbs** have to be **examined** even if the **symptoms** are **unilateral. Signs of ischaemia** have been described in detail in the previous chapter.

Absence of pulsations is significant.

Grading of pulsations.

III: Bounding pulse.

II: Normal pulse.

I: Weak pulse.

0: Absent pulsation.

It is to be **emphasised** that an **absent pulse** does **not** always indicate a **totally occluded artery**. A **grossly thickened** or a **calcified wall** along with a **markedly reduced blood flow** will **not** show a **pulsatile flow.**

The **abdominal aorta** and the **iliac arteries** need to be **palpated carefully**, since the **pathology** involves these **major arteries**. **Thickening** the **arterial wall** is an **important finding**. This is more **easily made out** by **palpating the radial artery**.

Ulceration and gangrene involving the toes or the **foot** are features of a **late disease.**

Other signs of ischaemia are seen in the limb.

Examination of CVS. Since atherosclerosis is a systemic disease, a careful **examination** of **this system is necessary**. Associated hypertension may lead to **left ventricular hypertrophy**. Later patients may develop **coronary artery disease** or **congestive cardiac failure**.

Q. 11. What are the investigations done in cases of atherosclerosis?

1. **Blood sugar** for detection of diabetes.

2. **Serum lipid profile**. An elevated level of LDL along with decreased high density lipoproteins is the usual finding.

3. **Increased levels of homo-cysteine** and **fibrinogen** levels are seen frequently.

4. **Specific investigations** to define accurately the **vascular status** of the **lower limb**. These will define the **presence of a block**. The **site** and the **degree of stenosis** can also be **identified**. The **state** of the **collateral circulation** is well **documented**. The investigations include **AB index, Duplex US, CT and MRI angiography.** Since most of the vessels involved are **large and proximal** and also the chances of a **good distal run-off** are much higher, **CT or MRI** angiography are **routinely performed**.

Presence of a **segmental block** and a **good distal run-off** are useful in planning the management. Unfortunately, the **collateral circulation** in the **lower limb** is **poorer** as compared to the **upper limb**.

This factor also **influences the treatment.**

Q. 12. Name the other investigations performed in these cases.

These are performed to **assess the function** of different organs such as the **heart and kidney** as these have a **direct influence** on the **treatment strategies** and the **total morbidity** and **mortality.**

Q. 13. How are these cases diagnosed?

As mentioned in the previous chapter, **recognition of ischaemia** due to **arterial occlusion** is **obvious** in most of these patients. Identifying the **cause** as **atherosclerosis** is much **easier** compared to TAO. The following factors are significant.

(*a*) **Age group:** Although considered to be a **disease of the elderly**, it is being seen in **younger patients** as well. But most are **above 40** years of age.

(*b*) **Sex. Increased** incidence is seen in **males.** Association of **diabetes** makes it frequent in **females** also.

(*c*) **Smoking.** History of smoking is available in **majority** of patients.

(*d*) **Absence of pulsations** in the **proximal arteries** and **thickening of the arterial wall** are specific features.

(*e*) **Associated hypertension.**

(*f*) **Presence** of **atherosclerosis** in **other systems.**

(*g*) **Imaging of the arteries** is most often **diagnostic.** This also has an important **role** in **planning the management. Duplex US** followed by **CT or MRI angiography** gives **adequate information** of the **status** of the **vascular tree.**

Q. 14. What are the treatment strategies for atherosclerosis?

It is important to remember that atherosclerosis is a **systemic disease,** and in a **majority of patients**, the **morbidity as well as the mortality** is influenced by the **cardiac and cerebral components** rather than **lower limb disease. Coronary artery disease** is seen in as many as **65%** of these patients and is the most **common cause of death.**

The **natural history of atherosclerosis** when the **lower limbs** are involved is as follows.

(*a*) **75%** have **stable intermittent claudication**, most often managed with conservative measures like **exercises** under **expert supervision.**

(*b*) In **16%** of patients **claudication progresses** to a more **severe state** demanding **active treatment.**

(*c*) **7%** need **direct arterial intervention** for **limb salvage.**

(*d*) **4%** end up with **minor or major amputations.**

These **percentages** described above are **not likely** to be applicable to **our patients as** most of them are seen in **grade IV or V** of the **Fontaine classification.** Therefore **tissue loss and gangrene** will be seen in many **more patients.** Correspondingly, the **percentage** of **patients needing** procedures for **limb salvage** will be **higher.** Even the **amputation figures** are likely to be much **higher than 4%.**

There are **four significant steps** in the treatment. They are as follows:

(*a*) **Risk factor modification. Absolute cessation of smoking** is vital. **Adequate control** of **diabetes, obesity** and **hypertension** is an integral part of the treatment. **Correction** of **hyperlipidaemia** and **hyperhomo-cysteinaemia is** essential.

(*b*) **Exercise** and **cardiovascular rehabilitation.** In patients with **claudication, exercise** has been shown to improve the **maximum walking distance** by about **73%** and the **pain-free walking distance** by about **71%.** But these **exercises** must be **supervised by experts.**

(*c*) **Drugs:** Antiplatelet therapy with **aspirin and clopidogrel** are routinely used. Both **pentoxyphyllin and cilostazol** are used to **increase the blood flow.** The latter drug is **more useful** at the **stage of claudication** and is **contraindicated** in patients with **congestive cardiac failure.**

(*d*) **Invasive strategies to improve the blood flow.** These measures are more **often possible** as compared to those with **TAO.** This is because of **two factors.**

1. **Proximal arterial disease** making interventions easier.

2. **Good distal run-off** as shown by the investigations.

Q. 15. Describe the endovascular procedures.

Modern technology has made **endovascular procedures** a very **attractive proposition** for many **patients.** They are **less invasive** and the **limb salvage rates** have **increased considerably** following the **introduction** of these **procedures.**

Balloon dilatation with placement of a **stent** can be used for **short segment stenoses. The results** are very **satisfactory** for **large vessels** like the **iliac arteries.** They may also **be used** in the **absence** of a **good run-off,** for **distal vessels,** though the **long-term patency rates** are rather **low.** But they **may be** the **only option** for **infrapopliteal disease. Atherectomy** is used in **iliac** and **common femoral artery disease.** In the case of the **common femoral artery,** it is usually **combined** with a **profundoplasty**

Q. 16. Describe the open surgical procedures.

These **operations** are **indicated** when **endovascular procedures** are **not feasible** or have **failed.** They are also **indicated** in the presence of **long segment narrowing or multiple blocks. Prosthetic grafts** are used for **aortoiliac** or **aortofemoral bypass operations.** An **autogenous saphenous vein graft** is used to create a **femoral popliteal bypass** for a **block** in the **superficial femoral artery.** An **axillary artery** to the **femoral artery bypass can be performed** if the **aorta is** found to be **not suitable** for the **procedure.**

Box 12.12:	Points regarding treatment strategies

- Modifications in lifestyle – Stop smoking – Control of diabetes and obesity.
- Exercises under supervision – Claudication stage – Good results.
- Drugs – Pentoxyphylline and Cilostazol.
- Endovascular procedures – Balloon dilatation – Stenting – Short segment stenosis – Infrapopliteal disease.
- Atherectomy – Profundoplasty.
- Open surgical procedures – Bypass – Aortoiliac or aortofemoral – Prosthetic grafts.
- Long segment or multiple blocks – Iliac or femoral artery disease.
- Saphenous vein graft for femoropopliteal block.

As a result of all the **measures described above,** the **blood flow** may **improve** as shown by **reduction of pain, healing of chronic ulcers** and **localisation** of the **area of gangrene.** But there **remains a large group** of patients with either **major tissue loss** or **established gangrene.** These patients **invariably need** an **amputation. Measurement** of **segmental arterial pressure** with Doppler is a **useful guide** to decide the **level** of **amputation.** If the **toe pressure** is **less than 20 mm Hg** or the **ankle pressure** is **less than 40 mm Hg, local amputations** are doomed to **fail.** Such **patients** need a **below-knee amputation.** An **above-knee amputation** is **indicated** if the **calf pressure** is **less than 70 mm Hg.**

As mentioned in the previous chapter, **rehabilitation of the patient** is of **paramount importance**. One must also **remember** that there is a **life time** risk of recurrence.

CT

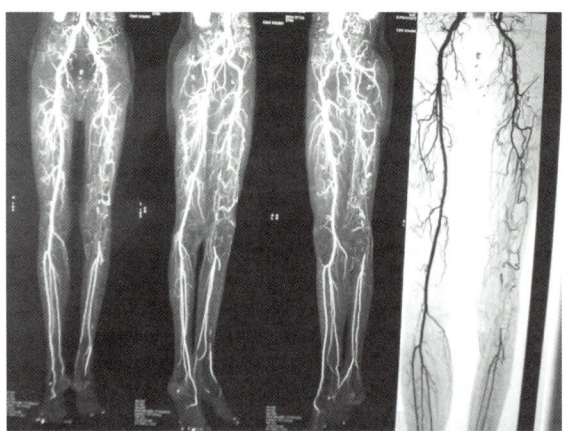

Fig. 12.2: CT angiogram showing a block in the superficial femoral artery extending to the proximal popliteal artery. Note the absence of collaterals below the knee.

Multiple Choice Questions

1. Duplex Ultrasound in vascular disease includes
   (a) Ultrasound with angiogram
   (b) Ultrasound with Doppler
   (c) Ultrasound with an MRI
   (d) Ultrasound with CT scan
   Answer (b)

2. Gangrene is defined as
   (a) Macroscopic death of tissue without putrefaction
   (b) Microscopic death of tissue without putrefaction
   (c) Macroscopic death of tissue with putrefaction
   (d) Microscopic death of tissue with putrefaction
   Answer (c)

3. In thrombo angiitis obliterans, there is
   (a) Inflammation of medium and large sized arteries
   (b) Inflammation of small and medium sized arteries and accompanying veins
   (c) Thrombosis with inflammation of medium and large sized arteries and accompanying veins
   (d) Thrombosis with inflammation of small and medium sized arteries and accompanying veins
   Answer (d)

4. In the stage of PREGANGRENE of an ischaemic limb, the patient usually complains of
   (a) Loss of sensation (Anaesthesia)
   (b) Increased sensation (Hyperaesthesia)
   (c) Normal sensation
   (d) Paraesthesia
   Answer (b)

5. In critical limb ischaemia the ankle brachial pressure index is
   (a) Less than 0.30
   (b) Between 0.30 and 0.65
   (c) Between 0.65 and 1
   (a) More than 1
   Answer (a)

A CASE OF TUBERCULOUS CERVICAL LYMPHADENITIS

Setting

- Surgical OPD.

Chief Complaint

- **Multiple swellings** on the **left side** of the **neck.**

History of Present Illness

- A **girl** aged **12** years was brought to the OPD with the complaint of **multiple swellings** on the **left side of the neck**. The mother had noticed a **peanut**-sized swelling in the **upper part of the neck six months** earlier. Over a period of time, **similar swellings** appeared all along the **left side of the neck**. The size of the swellings had **increased** to some extent over the last **six months**.

- The mother had **not** noticed **similar swellings** in any **other part of the body**.

- During the last **one month** the child was complaining of **mild pain.**

- The child had **intermittent low-grade fever** not associated with chills. There was **no** history of **night sweats.**

- The mother complained that the child was **not eating food** regularly and had **lost weight.**

- There was **no** history of **chronic cough.**

- **Past history** was insignificant.

Family History

- No member of the **family** was suffering from **chronic cough**.

Menstrual History

- The girl had not yet attained menarche.

Treatment History

- The child had been seen by **two doctors** earlier. Both had given **tablets** (?antimicrobials) for **one week** with **no relief**.

General Physical Examination

- The girl was moderately built and poorly nourished. **Pallor** was present. There was no jaundice or oedema at the ankles.

Local Examination

Inspection

- **Multiple swellings** were seen in the **left side of** the neck. The **vertical** extension was from the **lower border** of the **mandible** to about 2 cm above the **clavicle**. **Horizontally**, the swellings extended from the **anterior border** of the left **sternomastoid** to the the **trapezius**.

- The **borders** were **indistinct.**

- The **size** was about 10 cm by 6 cm.

- The **shape** was **irregular.**

- The **skin** over the swellings was **normal**.
- **No scars** were seen in the **surrounding area**.

Palpation

- The swellings were not **warm or tender**.
- The swellings comprised of **multiple lymph nodes** belonging to levels **II, III, IV and V**. The **size** of the nodes ranged from **2.5 cm to 1.5 cm**. The shape was **oval.**
- **Multiple** nodes belonging to **level IV and V** nodes were **matted. Single** nodes were palpable at level **II and III.**
- Most of the nodes were **firm** in consistency. Few nodes at level **IV** were **soft** and **fluctuant**.
- Level **II and III** nodes were deep to sternomastoid. The nodes were **not fixed** to the **skin.**
- There was **restricted** transverse **mobility.**
- **No l**ymph nodes were palpable on the **right side** of the neck.
- The **thyroid gland** was **not palpable**.
- **Intraoral examination** did **not** show any **abnormality.**
- **Examination** of the **chest** was **normal.**
- **Other groups** of **lymph nodes** were **not enlarged.**

Box 12.13:	Points to be noted during history

- Swellings – Site – Duration – Rate of growth.
- Pain – Fever.
- Chronic cough.
- Family history of chronic cough in the family.

Box 12.14:	Points to be noted during clinical examination

- Swellings in the neck – Site, size and shape.
- Levels of enlarged nodes.
- Consistency – Firm – Soft – Cold abscess.
- Mobility.
- Overlying skin.
- Thyroid examination.
- Oral cavity.
- Chest examination.
- Other groups of lymph nodes.

Q. 1. What was the clinical diagnosis?

(*a*) Chronic nonspecific lymphadenitis.

(*b*) Secondaries from a papillary carcinoma thyroid.

(*c*) Tuberculous lymphadenitis.

(*d*) Secondary nodes from a squamous cell carcinoma.

The correct answer is (*c*).

Chronic nonspecific lymphadenitis is very **common.** But it involves the **1b group** (submandibular) of lymph nodes. It is usually **single, firm** and **nontender**. It is associated with a **focus** of **infection** in the **oral cavity**. It remains **asymptomatic** for a **long time**.

Secondaries from a papillary carcinoma can manifest with enlarged lymph nodes without the thyroid being enlarged and palpable. But the nodes are soft and discrete. The disease is more common in women aged between 20 and 40 years, but can also be seen in children. There will be no history of fever.

Secondary nodes from a squamous cell carcinoma are hard and get fixed at an early stage. They may be present without an obvious primary (occult primary). The disease involves an older age group.

The clinical diagnosis in this case is tuberculous lymphadenitis. Matted nodes along with the presence of a cold abscess (fluctuant nodes) are helpful in the diagnosis.

Q.2. What were the investigations performed in this patient?

Chest X-ray was normal.

Blood - ESR was 72 mm. Rest of the blood tests were within normal limits.

FNAC: The smear showed epithelioid cells and a few acid fast bacilli confirming the diagnosis.

Setting: A week later. FNAC had confirmed the diagnosis.

Q.3. Describe the principles of treatment adopted for this patient.

Antituberculous treatment was started. A combination of Rifampicin, INAH and Ethambutol was the schedule used for this patient. The importance of continuing the drugs for 9 months was explained to the mother.

Cold abscesses were treated by aspiration. One of the abscesses needed a second aspiration.

The child was asked to come for review every six weeks. A physical examination revealed that the nodes were regressing in size. ESR values returned to normal at the end of 12 weeks.

At the end of 9 months the child had made a complete recovery.

Q.4. What are the clinical findings to suggest the anatomical nature as lymph nodes in the neck?

The sites of these swellings correspond with the areas where lymph nodes are commonly present. The supraclavicular region can be quoted as an example. Their size and shape are similar to that of enlarged lymph nodes.

Q.5. How are the cervical lymph nodes classified anatomically?

They are classified into 7 levels according to their location. The levels **extend from level I to VI** in the **neck** as per the figure shown below.

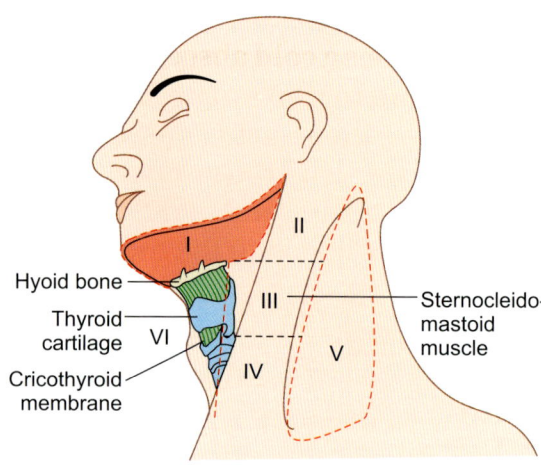

Fig. 12.3:

Level I: Below the **myelohyoid** muscle and **above** the **lower border** of the **hyoid bone** and occupy the **submandibular regions on either sides**.

Level I (A): (Submental nodes). These nodes are situated **between** the **anterior bellies** of the **digastric muscles below** the **lower border** of the **mandible.**

Level I (B): (Submandibular nodes). They are located **posterolateral** to the **anterior belly** of the **digastric muscles** on **either side.**

Level II: Internal jugular chain (Jugulodigastric).

These nodes extend from the **base of skull** to the **inferior border of the hyoid** bone vertically. The horizontal

extension is from the **posterior border** of the **sternomastoid muscles** to the **posterior border** of the **submandibular** glands.

Level III: Internal jugular chain (Jugulo-omohyoid).

The extension is from the **lower margin** of the **hyoid bone** to the **lower border** of the **cricoid cartilage** and from **the anterior to the posterior** borders of the **sternomastoid muscles.**

Level IV: Internal jugular chain in the **lower part** of **the neck**.

These nodes extend from the **lower border of the cricoid cartilage** to the **clavicle** vertically. Horizontally, they occupy an area **anteromedial** to an **oblique line** drawn from the **posterior margin of the sternomastoid** to the **posterior edge** of the **scalenus anterior** muscle.

Level V: (Posterior cervical). They are felt in the **posterior triangle** of the neck overlying the **trapezius muscle.**

Level VI: (Prelaryngeal and pretracheal nodes).

The position of these nodes is from the **inferior margin** of the **cricoid** to the **manubrium sterni.** They are present **within the pretracheal fascia** in the **central compartment** in the neck. These are **difficult** to **feel** since the space contains plenty of **fat.**

Level VII: Not shown in the picture (**Superior mediastinal nodes**). These nodes are **not** detected clinically.

Q. 6. How does the tubercle bacillus reach the cervical lymph nodes?

The **inhaled bacteria** are **trapped** by the **lymphoid tissue** forming the **Waldeyer's inner ring**. The **bacteria** then travel along the **lymphatics** to reach the **lymph nodes**. Hence level **II** and **III** are the **common groups** involved.

Q. 7. What causes matting of tuberculous nodes?

Matting is a sign **diagnostic** of **tuberculosis**. When **multiple nodes** are enlarged, they get **adherent to each other**. This is known as **matting** and is due to **periadenitis.** Periadenitis means **inflammation of the capsule** covering the lymph node. The capsule is involved in the disease process as the **afferent lymphatic** vessels carrying the **bacteria** drain into a lake of lymph called as the **subcapsular sinus, which is present under the capsule. Tuberculosis** induces **chronic inflammation** resulting in **fibrosis.** Hence, when **contiguous nodes** are involved, the **fibrosis binds** these nodes **together**, manifested as **matting clinically**. It must

be stressed that in **malignant nodes**, **extracapsular spread** can also produce a **similar clinical picture.**

Q. 8. How does a cold abscess develop in a tuberculous node?

Coagulative type of liquefaction necrosis leads to a thick **cheesy** material in the node. Clinically the **consistency** becomes **soft and fluctuant**. This is identified as a **cold abscess**.

Q. 9. Why is the term "cold abscess" used to describe these lesions?

The **classical signs** of **inflammation** like **warmth, redness and tenderness** are **absent.** Hence these are known as cold abscesses.

Q. 10. What is a collar stud abscess and what is its importance?

Most of the lymph **nodes** are present **deep** to the **investing layer** of the cervical **fascia**. A **cold abscess** tracks through a **small defect** in the **fascia** to form a large **subcutaneous collection** in the loose areolar tissue. Thus the **cold abscess** has **two components**, one **superficial** and another **deep** to the **fascia,** connected to each other by a **narrow channel resembling** a **collar stud.** Unless both of these are **drained completely,** the **collar stud abscess** will **not heal.**

Q. 11. **How is a tuberculous sinus formed in relation to a lymph node and what are its characteristics?**

When a **cold abscess** works its way **through the skin** it results in the formation of a **sinus.** Thus a **sinus** is always **connected** to an **underlying node.** The sinus has a **bluish rim** of epithelium at the **margin**. The **edges** are **undermined** and the **floor** is composed of **pale granulation tissue**. The **discharge** is **watery**.

Q. 12. **What is the finding that is diagnostic of tuberculosis on microscopy?**

Epithelioid cells are the cells that are **diagnostic** of the disease. These are **tissue macrophages,** which **resemble** the **epithelial cells** due to the **waxy coat** of the **tuberculous bacillus** being distributed in the cytoplasm, pushing the **nucleus** to the periphery. When the **bacilli** are digested by the **macrophages,** the **outer covering** (that makes the cell acid fast) is **distributed** in the **cytoplasm**.

Q. 13. **Describe the typical microscopic appearance of a tubercle.**

There is a **central area** of **caseation** due to **coagulative necrosis**.

It is surrounded by **Langerhans type of giant cells**. These are **foreign body** type of **giant cells** formed by **fusion** of **macrophages.** The **nuclei** of these cells are present in the **periphery** in a **horseshoe** pattern. These are **nonspecific** and can be seen in other **granulomatous** lesions as well. **Epithelioid** cells described above are also seen. The **periphery** is formed by many **lymphocytes.** A **fibrous capsule** forms the **outermost boundary**.

Q. 14. **What is the staining method employed to demonstrate acid fast bacilli?**

Ziehl Neelsen method of staining is employed for demonstrating these bacilli. These being **acid fast**, retain the **red Carbol Fuchsin stain** because of the **waxy outer layer**.

Q. 15. **What are the basic strategies in the treatment?**

(*a*) **General specific treatment:** It consists of administration of **ATT** drugs for a period of **six to nine months** depending upon the **response** of the **patient.**

(*b*) **Local treatment:** It is usually needed in the presence of **complications.**

An **early diagnosis** with **adequate medical treatment** ensures a **cure** in most patients.

Q. 16. What are the indications for surgical intervention in cervical tuberculous lymphadenitis?

The indications are:

(*a*) **Cold abscess** including the **collar stud** variety.

(*b*) **Tuberculous sinus.**

(*c*) **Group of nodes persisting** after **adequate ATT** treatment (uncommon).

Q. 17. What is the treatment of a cold abscess?

The **treatment** is always performed after a course of **ATT** has been given for at least a period of **six to eight weeks**.

Aspiration of the cold abscess is the **first line** of treatment. While aspirating, the **following precautions** are to be taken, basically to **reduce** the **risk of sinus** formation.

1. A **wide bore needle** is required to drain the **thick caseous** material.

2. The **approach** should always be through an area of **healthy skin**.

3. A **nondependent site** is chosen for aspiration.

4. A **fold of skin** is **lifted** before introducing the needle to produce a **zigzag track** for its passage.

Q. 18. What is the treatment for a recurring cold abscess?

A **repeat aspiration** can be tried. But most often, a **recurring one** indicates a **collar stud** abscess. Since a collar stud abscess has **two components**, it needs a more **elaborate procedure** for proper drainage. Under anaesthesia, an **incision** is made and the **subcutaneous collection** is **drained and curetted**. The **opening** in the **investing layer** of the deep fascia is then **enlarged** exposing the **cold abscess** adequately. All the **caseous material and the avascular tissues** are **curetted** till the area shows **fresh bleeding**. If the **culpable node** is away from important structures, it can be **excised**. In contra-distinction to that of a **pyogenic abscess,** which is incised and drained leaving the **incision open**, a **primary suturing** of the incision is performed in these cases. It not only **prevents sinus** formation, but also does **not allow secondary infection** from outside to enter the wound.

Q. 19. What is the treatment of a tuberculous sinus?

Many of these **sinuses** may **heal with ATT** treatment **without** needing any **intervention**. A sinus that persists usually has a **deep** seated **node** draining pus via this route. Since the **natural drainage is inadequate**, the sinus **does not heal**. The **sinus track** along with the underlying **lymph node i**s excised. **Primary suturing** completes the operation.

Q. 20. What is the indication for excision of a group of lymph nodes?

A **small section** of patients may have a group of **nodes persisting** even after **adequate ATT. Excision of these nodes** is necessary under these circumstances. But this indication has become very **uncommon** at the **present time.**

Multiple Choice Questions

1. The correct sequential method of Zeihl Neelsen staining for Acid Fast Bacilli is

   (*a*) Carbol Fuchsin , 20% Sulfuric Acid, Methylene Blue

   (*b*) Carbol Fuchsin, 5% Sulfuric Acid, Methylene Blue

   (*c*) Methylene Blue, 20% Sulfuric Acid, Carbol Fuchsin

   (*d*) Methylene Blue, 5% Sulfuric Acid, Carbol Fuchsin

   Answer (*a*)

2. In Tuberculous involvement of cervical lymph nodes what is the correct sequence?

   (*a*) Periadenitis, Lymphadenitis, Cold Abscess, Collar Stud Abscess

   (*b*) Lymphadenitis, Periadenitis, Collar Stud Abscess, Cold Abscess

   (*c*) Lymphadenitis, Periadenitis, Cold Abscess, Collar Stud Abscess

   (*d*) Periadenitis, Collar Stud Abscess, Lymphadenitis, Cold Abscess

   Answer (*b*)

3. The Most important side effect of Isoniazid is

   (*a*) Hepatotoxicity

   (*b*) Colour Blindness

   (*c*) Acute Gastritis

   (*d*) Peripheral Neuritis

   Answer (*c*)

4. Isoniazid is usually given in the dose of

   (*a*) 5 – 10 mg/Kg

   (*b*) 10 – 15 mg/Kg

   (*c*) 15 – 20 mg/Kg

   (*d*) 20 – 25 mg/Kg

   Answer (*a*)

5. Level V group of cervical lymph nodes are bounded by

   (a) Clavicle, Sternomastoid, Midline

   (b) Mandible, Anterior belly of digastric, Midline

   (c) Clavicle, Sternomastoid, Trapezius

   (d) Mandible, Anterior belly of digastric, Mylohyoid

   Answer (c)

6. The edge of a Tuberculous sinus is

   (a) Raised and everted

   (b) Undermined

   (c) Sloping

   (d) Raised and Inverted

   Answer (b)

7. Level II, III and IV cervical lymph nodes are closely related to

   (a) Anterior belly of Digastric and External Jugular vein

   (b) Sternomastoid and Internal Jugular vein

   (c) Inferior belly of Omohyoid and Common Carotid artery

   (d) Posterior belly of Digastric and Internal Carotid artery

   Answer (b)

A CASE OF HODGKIN'S LYMPHOMA

Setting

- Surgical OPD.

Chief Complaint

- **Swelling** in the **left side of the neck** of **three months** duration.
- An **eight-year-old boy** was brought to the surgical OPD with the complaint a **swelling** in the left side of the **neck** of **three months** duration. The swelling was noted in the **lower part of the neck** and was **small** in size. Since then it has been **rapidly increasing in size**.
- The parents had **not** noticed **similar swellings** in any **other part** of the **body**.
- The child did not complain of any **pain**.
- There was a history of **intermittent fever** not associated with chills or rigors.
- The parents felt that the boy had **lost weight** during the last **one month.** The child also complained of **fatigue** during this period.
- **Past, family and personal histories** were insignificant.

Treatment History

- The parents had taken the boy to a local hospital where an **FNAC** was done. After receiving the **report,** the parents were advised to attend a tertiary **hospital** for further treatment.

- **General physical examination** revealed a **sick child**. He appeared to be **febrile**. **Pallor** was present. There was no jaundice or ankle oedema.

Local Examination

Inspection

- A **large swelling** was seen in the **left side of the neck**. It extended from about **2 cm below** the lower border of the **mandible** to the level of the **clavicle**. The horizontal extension was from **2 cm** from the **midline** anteriorly to about **4 cm** from the **midline** posteriorly.
- The **margins** were ill defined.
- The **size** was 12 cm by 10 cm. The **shape** was irregular.
- The **surface** appeared **nodular.**
- The **skin** over the swelling was **stretched and shiny**.
- The **surrounding area** appeared normal.

Palpation

- The swelling was **warm** but **not tender**.
- It comprised of **multiple lymph nodes**. The enlarged nodes belonged to level **III, IV and V on** the **left side**. In addition, nodes belonging to levels **1A, 1B and II** were palpable on the **left side.**

- The nodes were of the **same size** measuring about **2 cm** in diameter. They were **soft** in consistency, **and discrete** with **restricted mobility**.
- The overlying **skin** was **free.**
- Examination of the **right side of the neck** showed **enlarged level IV** and **V** nodes. The features were **similar** to the nodes on the left side.

Oral Cavity

- No abnormality was detected.

Examination of Left Axilla

- **Multiple nodes** belonging to the **central group** were palpable. They were **soft and discrete**. The size varied from **1 cm to 1.5 cm**. They were **nontender.**
- **No other group of lymph nodes** was enlarged.

Abdomen

- **Liver and spleen** were not palpable. **No lymph node mass** could be felt.

Chest

- There was no **mediastinal dullness**. The **respiratory system** was clinically **normal.**

Box 12.16: Points to be noted on inspection

- Swelling – Site and extent – Margins.
- Size and shape.
- Surface – Skin over the swelling.
- Surrounding area.

Box 12.17: Points to be noted on palpation

- Swelling – Warmth and tenderness.
- Swelling – Comprising of lymph nodes. Groups enlarged – Levels.
- Size – Variable – Within a group – Size – Same.
- Consistency – Soft and rubbery – Discrete – Mobile.
- Opposite side of the neck – Enlarged nodes.
- Oral cavity.
- Other groups of lymph nodes.
- Abdomen – Liver and spleen – Lymph nodes.

Box 12.15: Points to be noted in history

- Swelling – Site – Duration – Rate of growth.
- Similar swellings in other parts of the body.
- Pain
- Fever – Intermittent – Low or high grade.
- Loss of weight – fatigue.

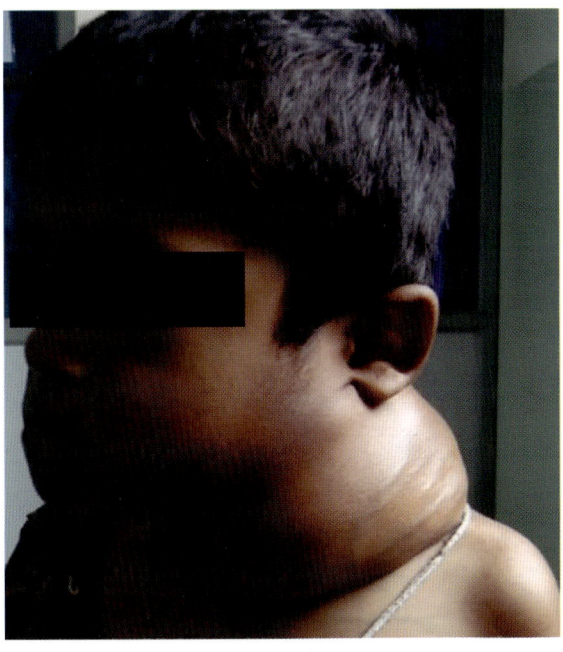

Fig. 12.4: A case of Hodgkin's disease.

Q. 1. What is the clinical diagnosis?

(*a*) Secondary nodes from a squamous cell carcinoma.

(*b*) Hodgkin's lymphoma.

(*c*) NonHodgkin's lymphoma (NHL).

(*d*) Tuberculous lymphadenitis.

The correct answer is (*b*).

As far as **malignancies** in **lymph nodes** are concerned, **secondaries** are much **more common** than a **primary** tumour. But **secondary nodes** from a **squamous cell carcinoma** are a **disease** of an **older age** group. The lymph nodes are **hard**. **Extracapsular spread** occurs early resulting in **fixity** to the adjacent structures.

NHL is seen at a **later age** group. The lymph nodes **vary in size**. Few nodes may be much **larger** in size. The disease may be confined to **one group** of lymph nodes for a **few months**. The consistency is **hard** and **early fixity** is a common feature.

Tuberculous lymphadenitis is a disease of the **young**. But the **rate of growth** is **slow**. **Massive enlargement** over a **short period** of time is **not seen** in tuberculosis. In addition, **matting** and **cold abscess** formation are two features of this disease.

Hodgkin's disease occurs usually in the **second decade** of life. The **cervical** and **axillary** groups of lymph nodes are commonly involved. Associated **fever** and **weight loss** are seen in many patients. The **nodes** are typically **soft, discrete** and **mobile**. The likely diagnosis in this case was a **Hodgkin's lymphoma**.

Q. 2. What were the investigations performed in this patient?

1. **Blood examination: Hb** was 7 gm%. **Eosinophilia** was present. No abnormal cells were seen in the **peripheral blood smear**.

2. **Supraclavicular node biopsy:** A discrete **node** from **level IV** on the **left** side was removed and sent for **histopathological** examination.

3. **CT chest** did not show any **mediastinal mass**. Both the **lungs** were normal.

4. **CT abdomen** was reported as **normal**.

5. **Bone marrow** aspiration **biopsy** was done from the **iliac crest**. The smear did **not show** any **abnormal cells**.

Setting: The clock has moved by one week.

The **biopsy report** was **Hodgkin's lymphoma**. The **pathological type** was **nodular sclerosis**.

Q.3. What was the clinical stage of the disease?

The patient belonged to **stage II B.**

Q.4. How was this patient treated?

The patient received **chemotherapy.** The **ABVD** (Adriamycin, bleomycin, vincristine and dacarbazine) regime was followed. It consisted of **6 cycles** of this **combination chemotherapy** given at an **interval of 28 days**. He made a **good recovery.** The **parents** have been asked to bring **the child** for **regular follow-up**.

Q.5. What is the incidence of Hodgkin's lymphoma?

It is responsible for **1%** of **all cancers**.

Q.6. What are the suspected aetiological factors?

The exact **aetiology** is **not known**. The **following factors** are considered **significant.**

Box 12.18:	Points to be noted regarding aetiology

- Infection with E.B. virus.
- Previous episodes of infectious mononucleosis.
- Increased incidence in HIV patients.
- Family history of Hodgkins lymphoma.

Q.7. What are the common age groups affected by this disease?

It shows a **bimodal** distribution. The **second decade** is the commonest age group. But there is an increased incidence in **persons over 50 years** of age.

Q.8. What are the clinical features of Hodgkin's lymphoma?

Box 12.19:	Points to be noted in the clinical features

- Presence of enlarged group of lymph nodes – Cervical common – Axilla and other groups.
- Duration – Several months
- Associated symptoms – Fever – Night sweats – Itching – Loss of weight and fatigue.
- Lymph nodes – Soft – Described as rubbery – Discrete – Mobile.
- Extracapsular spread – Absent or a late feature.
- Splenomegaly – Less commonly – Hepatomegaly.
- Pain in the nodes after ingestion of alcohol.

Q.9. How are patients with Hodgkin's disease staged clinically?

Patients **without systemic symptoms** are grouped under the term **A** and those with **symptoms as B**

Stage I: Involvement of a **single group** of **nodes** (frequently the neck nodes) or disease confined to a **single extralymphatic site (spleen).**

This is known as **stage I e.**

Stage II: Enlargement of **more than one group** of lymph nodes, but restricted to **one side of the diaphragm (cervical and axillary** nodes enlarged).

Stage III: Enlargement of lymph nodes on **either sides of the diaphragm** or involvement of **single or multiple groups of nodes** associated with **splenomegaly.**

Stage IV: Involvement of the **bone marrow, liver and lung.**

The **final staging** needs to be **redefined** after the **results** of all the **investigations** described below are available. The **treatment protocols** can only be **decided at that stage**.

Box 12.20:	Clinical staging

Asymptomatic – A. With symptoms – B

- **Stage I:** Single group of nodes on one side of diaphragm.
- **Stage IE:** Isolated splenomegaly.
- **Stage II:** Multiple groups on one side of the diaphragm.
- **Stage III:** Single or multiple groups of lymph nodes with splenomegaly.
- **Stage IV:** Involvement of bone marrow, liver and lung.

Q. 10. **What are the investigations needed for these patients?**

1. **Blood examination.** **Anaemia** is a common feature. **Eosinophilia** is frequently observed. The **ESR** levels are **usually raised**. This

is an important **prognostic factor** also. **Uncommonly Reed–Sternberg (R.S.) cells** may be seen.

2. **FNAC** alone is **not adequate**. A **lymph node biopsy** is always performed. The **advantages** of this procedure are as follows.

   (*a*) It **confirms the diagnosis** by the presence of **R.S. cells,** which are derived from **the B cells.** These cells are **large** in size with **abundant finely granular** or **homogenous cytoplasm**. The **pathognomonic** feature is the presence of **two mirror image nuclei (owl eye).**

   (*b*) **Histopathological type** can be determined. This is **significant** in the **prognosis** of the disease.

   (*c*) **Immunohistochemical** studies help in **planning the treatment better.**

   (*d*) Advanced centres are performing **genetic studies** as well. These are useful in the development of **monoclonal antibodies.**

3. **CT chest**. Enlarged **mediastinal lymph nodes** are detected. This has **prognostic value.** In addition **small nodular deposits** in the **lung** parenchyma are also identified. These factors will **alter** the **final staging**.

4. **CT abdomen. Hepato-splenomegaly.** Even if the **liver** is **not enlarged**, the **architectural changes** may indicate **the presence** of the **disease. Nonpalpable lymph node** masses may be picked up by **CT.** Again the final staging is **altered** by these **additional findings**.

5. **Iliac crest bone marrow aspiration biopsy**. It is performed in **all patients except** those in **stage IV**. Presence of **R.S. cells** in the **marrow smear converts** all these patients into **stage IV.**

6. **PETCT** scan has **replaced** all other types of **imaging modalities** in many centres. The involved areas appear as **bright spots** on this scan. It is particularly **useful** in assessing the **response** to the **treatment.** Only **cost** and **availability** are the **limiting factors** for this investigation.

Box 12.21:	Points to be noted regarding investigations

- Blood – Hb, ESR and peripheral blood smear.
- FNAC not done – Limited value – Lymphoma
- Lymph node biopsy – Type of lymphoma. Hodgkin's – Presence of Reed – Sternberg cell.
- Pathological types – Immunohistochemistry – Genetic studies.
- CT chest and abdomen
- PETCT scan – Replacing other scans – Response to treatment.
- Bone marrow biopsy.

Q. 11. What are the pathological types of this disease?

1. **Nodular sclerosis:** This is the **most common type**. Biopsy shows **tumour nodules** with **scattered R.S. cells** with plenty of **reactive lymphocytes** and **eosinophils.** Sections always show **areas of fibrosis**, which is an **essential feature** of this type.

2. **Mixed cellularity:** A type **seen frequently**, it is identified by an **admixture** of **numerous R.S. cells** along with **lymphocytes, histiocytes** and **plasma cells. Fibrosis** is conspicuous by its **absence.**

3. **Lymphocyte predominant.** Sections show plenty of

lymphocytes with **few R.S. cells**. This type has the **most favourable outcome**. But it is an **uncommon** type of the disease.

4. **Lymphocyte depleted:** Microscopy shows a **large number of R.S. cells** that are often **pleomorphic** and very **few lymphocytes**. This type is **rare** and carries a **poor prognosis**, being **anaplastic** in its **behaviour**.

Q. 12. **What are the factors that are responsible for a favourable outcome in this disease?**

(*a*) **Age. Below 45** years.

(*b*) Clinical stage **I and II.**

(*c*) Patients in **group A.**

(*d*) Pathologic type. **Lymphocyte predominant** and **nodular sclerosis**.

(*e*) **Absence** of **extranodal disease**.

(*f*) **ESR below 50.**

(*g*) **CT chest** showing a **mediastinal mass** of less than **one-third** of the **total width** of **the thorax**.

The **remaining patients** belong to an **unfavourable** group.

Box 12.22:	Points denoting the favourable group

- Age – Below 45 years.
- Patients belonging to group A.
- Absence of extra-nodal disease.
- Clinical staging – I and II.
- Pathological type – Nodular sclerosis and lymphocyte predominant.
- CT chest – Nodal mass less than one-third the width of thorax.
- ESR – Below 50.

Q. 13. **What are the treatment protocols for this disease?**

The **treatment** of **Hodgkin's lymphoma** is one of the **success stories** in the management of **cancers** in general. The availability of **newer chemotherapeutic drugs** as well as the **refinements** in the field of **radiotherapy** has made this **possible**.

Stage I and II patients are treated by **chemotherapy.** The time honoured **COPP or MOPP** regimes have been **replaced** by **ABVD** (adriamycin, bleomyin, vincristine and dacarbazine) or **BEACOPP** (bleomycin, etoposide, adriamycin, cyclophosphamide, oncovin, prednisolone and procarbazine) regimes. **Four to six cycles** of treatment at **intervals** of **28 days** is the **usual** strategy. The **response rate** is about **15% more** with the **newer regimes**. **Hodgkin's** lymphoma is a highly **radiosensitive** tumour. Hence **radiotherapy** is added on in patients with **stage III and IV** disease. But there are certain **risks** involved in treating **young patients** with **radiation**. Even in **stage I and II** patients, radiation may be required to treat nodes **persisting** following **chemotherapy.**. A **mediastinal mass** always needs to be treated with **radiotherapy** under **steroid cover**.

Q. 14. What is the role of stem cell transplantation?

Haemopoietic stem cell transplantation is used for patients with a **recurrent disease**. But the results are **better** for those patients who had shown a **response** to the **standard lines of treatment** earlier. These **cells** may be obtained from the **peripheral blood** or from the **bone marrow. The cells** could be collected from the **patient before treatment** or from a **suitable donor**.

Box 12.23:	Points regarding treatment

- Chemotherapy – Newer regimes – (ABVD) Adriamycin, bleomycin, vincristine and dacarbazine
- Bleomycin, etoposide, adriamycin, oncovin, cyclophosphamide, prednisolone and dacarbazine.(BEACOPP)-15% better than COPP or MOPP.
- Stage III& IV – Need chemoradiation.
- Recurrent disease – Haemopoietic stem cell transplantation – Autologous or donor.

A CASE OF NONHODGKIN'S LYMPHOMA

Setting

- Surgical OPD

Chief Complaint

- Swellings in both the groins for the last four months

History of Present Illness

- A **55-year-old man** presented to the OPD with **swellings** in **both groins** of **four months** duration. He had noticed a **small** swelling in the **right groin** about **4 months** ago. It was the **size** of a **marble.** Since then it had been **rapidly increasing** in **size. Two months** later he developed a **similar swelling** in the **left groin,** which also had been **rapidly increasing** in **size.** He did not notice any **swelling** in other parts of the **body.**

- The patient was having **dragging type** of **pain** in both the **groins.** The **pain** was worse on **walking.** It did **not disturb** his **sleep** at night.

- The patient had noticed **swelling** around the **right ankle** for the last **one month**. The swelling became **worse** towards the **evenings**.

- There was no history of **fever**.

- Patient did not complain about **loss of weight**.

- **Past and family histories** were insignificant.

Personal History

- The patient was a **smoker** and used to consume **alcohol** occasionally.

Treatment History

- The patient had **not taken any treatment** for this complaint.

General Physical Examination

- **This** revealed a **well-built** but **poorly nourished** individual. **Pallor** was present. There was no jaundice or clubbing of the fingers.

Local Examination

Inspection: Right Inguinal Region

- A swelling was present in the right inguinal region extending from about 3 cm above the groin crease to 8 cm inferiorly. Horizontally it extended from about 2 cm medial to the anterior superior iliac spine to the midline.

- The **superior and inferior margins** were well **defined.**

- It measured **8 cm by 12 cm** in **size.**

- The **shape** was an **irregular oval.**

- The **surface** was **nodular**.

- The **skin** over the swelling was **stretched** and appeared **reddish** in some places. No **dilated veins** were seen

- The **surrounding area** appeared **normal.**

Palpation: Right Inguinal Region

- The swelling was **warm** and **slightly tender**.

- The swelling appeared to be composed of a **mass of lymph nodes** belonging to the **superficial horizontal** and **vertical inguinal** group as well as the **deep inguinal** group.

- All the **borders** could be **easily made out**.

- The mass was **larger on palpation,** being 10 cm by 14 cm in size.

- The **surface** was **nodular**.

- The **consistency** was **variable.** Most of the areas were **hard.** Few **soft areas** were felt in the **upper part** of the swelling. These areas were **not fluctuant**.

- The **lymph nodes** were **fixed** to **each other.** The **overlying skin** was **fixed** to the swelling in some of the **soft areas**. The swelling was **fixed** to the **deeper structures** with **no mobility**.

Examination of Right Lower Limb

- There was evidence of **lymphoedema** around the **right ankle**. It was **pitting** in nature.

- **No dilated veins** were seen in the limb.

- All the **distal arterial pulsations** were felt **normally**.

- There was **no evidence** of **sensory or motor nerve deficit**.

Examination of Left Inguinal Region

- Most of the **clinical findings** were **similar** to that of the **right side**. The **superficial and deep inguinal lymph nodes** were found to be **enlarged**. The size was **5 cm by 8 cm**. The **consistency** was **uniformly hard**. The **skin** over the swelling was **free.** The swelling was **fixed** to the **deeper structures**.

- **Examination of the left lower limb** did not reveal any **distal pressure effects.**

- **Examination** of the **external genitalia** was normal.

Examination of Abdomen

- **External iliac lymph nodes** were **palpable** on **both sides**. They were about **3 cm to 4 cm** in size and were **fixed. No other group** of **lymph nodes** was palpable in the **abdomen.**

- **Liver and spleen** were **not palpable.**

- **Rectal examination and proctoscopy** did not show any abnormality.

- **No other group of lymph nodes** was found to be **enlarged.**

- Examination of the **respiratory system** was essentially normal.

Box 12.24: Points to be noted in the history
• Swelling – Both inguinal regions – Duration – Rate of growth. • Pain – Aggravating factors. • Distal pressure effects in the limb. • Similar swellings in rest of the body. • Fever – Loss of weight.

Box 12.25:	Points to be noted on inspection of the right inguinal region

- Site and extent - Size and shape - Margins.
- Skin over the swelling.
- Surrounding area.

Box 12.26:	Points to be noted on examination of the left inguinal region

- Mass of nodes – Smaller.
- Consistency – Hard.
- Skin – Free.
- Fixed to deeper structures.
- No distal pressure effects.

Box 12.27:	Points to be noted in the remaining part of the clinical examination

- External iliac nodes – Palpable and fixed.
- External genitalia – Normal.
- Spleen and liver not palpable.
- No other group of nodes enlarged.
- Respiratory system – Normal.
- P.R. and proctoscopy – Normal.

Q. 1. What was the clinical diagnosis?

(a) Chronic nonspecific lymphadenitis.

(b) Secondary deposits in inguinal nodes.

(e) Hodgkin's lymphoma.

(d) NonHodgkin's lymphoma.

The correct diagnosis is (*d*)**.**

Most **Indians** have **bilateral enlarged inguinal nodes** due to **chronic nonspecific infection.** This is caused by **ascending infection from the feet owing to their habit of walking barefoot.** But the nodes are usually **small** in **size, nontender, firm and mobile**. **Massively enlarged** nodes that are **fixed** along with the presence of **fixed external iliac** nodes are **not seen** in this condition.

Secondaries in lymph nodes, as is well known, are **more** common than **primary malignant tumours**. But the **primary** is almost always **detected** in **these cases**. It could be a **melanoma** in the limb. A site for a **primary** that is easily missed is the **anal canal**. Examination in this case did **not show** any **malignant tumour** in the **drainage area**. An **occult primary** at this **site** is **most uncommon.**

Hodgkin's disease can occur at **this age** (**bimodal distribution**). The **inguinal group** is **not** a **frequent site**. The **nodes** will be **soft, discrete and mobile**. An enlarged **spleen** is more **often** seen. **Systemic symptoms** are also more **common**. Lymph node **biopsy** will be confirmatory.

The **clinical picture is suggestive of NHL**. The nodes can achieve a **massive size** in this **condition**. The nodes are **hard. Necrotic** areas will be **soft. Extracapsular** spread occurs **early** leading to **adherence** to **each other** as well as to **deeper structures**. Unlike a **Hodgkin's** lymphoma, which has a **predilection** for **cervical** and axillary groups, **NHL** can involve **any group of lymph nodes**.

Q. 2. **What were the investigations done in this patient?**

Blood examination: Hb was 8.5 gm%. The **ESR** was 55 mm. The **peripheral blood smear did not** show any **abnormal cells**.

Lymph node biopsy: A **node** that was **discrete** in the left inguinal group was chosen for **biopsy.**

CT abdomen: Liver and spleen were not enlarged. **Bilateral enlarged external iliac** nodes were noted. No **other group** of nodes was detected.

CT chest was normal.

Bone marrow biopsy did not reveal any abnormal cells.

Setting: A week later. The **biopsy** report was a **large B cell lymphoma** type of **NHL.**

Q. 3. **What was the stage of the disease?**

The final staging was **stage II A.**

Q. 4. **What was the treatment protocol advised for this patient?**

The patient was put on **COPP** **(cyclophosphamide, oncovin, prednisolone and procarbazine)** regime. The **first two** drugs were given **intravenously** and the **latter two** by the **oral route.** He had a total of **six cycles** at intervals of 28 days. There was only a **partial response**. The **size** of **both the inguinal masses** had **come down**. The **oedema** at the **ankle** had become **worse.** A **repeat CT** showed partial **obstruction** of the **right external iliac vein**.

The patient was given a course of **EBRT.**

There were **persisting nodes** at the **end of EBRT**. He was advised a **repeat course** of **chemotherapy** along with **Rituximab**. Since he could **not afford** the treatment, he was **discharged** from the hospital.

Q. 5. **What could have been the outcome of this patient?**

The **outcome** would be **poor.** The **lifespan** would have been only **some months**. **Death** could have been caused by **erosion** of the **femoral vessels** by the **tumour.** The other **factor** responsible for **death** could be severe **intercurrent infection** caused by **reduced immunity** levels.

Q. 6. **What are the general characteristics of NHL?**

Nonhodgkin's lymphomas present a more **complex group** of diseases as **compared with Hodgkin's** lymphoma. It is best described as a **heterogeneous group** of **lymphocytic disorders** with different morphological appearances, clinical presentations and a variable response to therapy. NHL represents about 4% of all malignant tumours. It is the most common haemopoietic malignancy in adults. There is some evidence to show the increasing frequency of the disease. Recent advances in immunohistochemistry and genetic studies have been helpful in the better understanding of the disease. Currently, the different types of NHL are thought to represent neoplastic cells arrested at various stages of differentiation of the B cell or T cell lymphocyte.

Q. 7. What are the important aetiological factors?

In addition to the factors mentioned under Hodgkin's lymphoma, the following are significant.

(*a*) Patients who have undergone transplantation and are on immunosuppressive therapy have a higher incidence.

(*b*) Certain pesticides have also been incriminated in the aetiology.

Q. 8. What are the differences in the clinical presentation of NHL as compared with Hodgkin's lymphoma?

The disease may be restricted to one group of nodes or only the spleen. Within a group some lymph nodes may be massively enlarged. The consistency is hard. Necrosis causes softening of the gland. Extracapsular spread occurs early with fixity to the skin and deeper structures. The clinical presentation of extranodal tumours depends on the site of the tumour. The biological behaviour is much more diverse. Hence the outlook also differs to a large extent.

Q. 9. What is the importance of examination of the external genitalia in this patient?

Massive inguinal node enlargement can cause lymphoedema of the scrotum and the penis.

Q. 10. Why is a per rectal (P.R.) examination important in the presence of enlarged inguinal nodes in this patient?

The lymphatic drainage of the anal canal is to the deep inguinal nodes. A primary malignancy in the anal canal can be missed if a P.R is not done.

Q. 11. How are patients with NHL staged clinically?

The staging is the **same** as for **Hodgkin's** disease. But the **incidence** of involvement of a **single group** is **higher**. **Extranodal disease** occurs more **frequently** like an **isolated splenic** involvement. **Majority** of patients belong to **group A,** having **no systemic symptoms**.

Q. 12. What are the pathological types of NHL?

A **large number** of **histopathological** types have been **described**. It is also more **complicated** as **compared with Hodgkin's lymphoma**. The **propensity** of the tumour to arise from **extranodal sites** more often makes **understanding** these types **more difficult**. The **basic classification** is as follows.

B cell tumours:

1. **Diffuse large B cell lymphoma:** This is the most common variety **(30%)**. The tumour is composed of **large immature lymphocytes**. These are **rapidly growing aggressive tumours**, involving the **abdominal** or **mediastinal group** of nodes frequently.

2. **Follicular lymphoma:** The term is used because **microscopically** the **cells** tend to **grow in a circular (follicular) pattern** in the lymph **nodes**. They are in general **slow growing** tumours. But over a period of **time**, they may **morph** into the more **aggressive large cell lymphoma.**

3. **Small cell lymphocytic lymphoma** is considered to be a **variant** of **chronic lymphocytic leukaemia.**

4. **MALT Lymphoma:** These are **extranodal** in origin. **MALT (mucosa-associated lymphoid tissue)** tumours are seen in **many parts** of the body. But the **stomach** is the most **common site** and is probably caused by **infection** with *H. Pylori.*

5. **Burkitt's Lymphoma:** This is an **uncommon type**, and was first described by **Burkitt** in **children** and **young adults in Africa**, involving the **jaw and facial bones**. Infection with **Epstein Barr virus** is said to be the **aetiological** factor. But the tumour may also manifest as a **large abdominal mass**. **Spread** to the **brain** and the **CSF** are the **special characteristics** of this type of tumour.

T cell tumours are **rare.** Many types have been described, but the following **two** are important.

1. **Precursor T cell lymphoblastic lymphoma:** The **commonest site** for this type is the **thymus** gland. So it produces a clinical picture of a **mediastinal mass** with **compression** of the **superior vena cava** and **trachea**. It affects **young men** most frequently.

2. **Peripheral T cell lymphoma:** They arise from more **mature** forms of **T cells**. They can be **nodal** or **extranodal** in their presentations. The **extranodal** sites are **skin, air passages** and **intestines**.

Box 12.28:	Points to be noted in pathological types of B cell and T cell NHL

- Diffuse B cell lymphoma. 30% – Large immature lymphocytes. – Abdominal and mediastinal nodes. Aggressive tumour.
- Follicular lymphoma – Cells arranged in a follicular pattern.
- Slow growing tumour – Later aggressive.
- Small cell lymphoma – Variant of chronic lymphocytic leukaemia.
- MALT (mucosa-assisted lymphoid tissue) lymphoma – Extranodal – Stomach – Common site – H. Pylori.
- Burkitt's lymphoma – Africa – Extranodal – Children and young adults – Jaw and facial bones.
- Infection with E.B.virus – Implicated in aetiology.
  - Spread via CSF to brain.
  - T Precursor cell – Thymus – SVC syndrome.
  - Mature T cells - Skin, intestine.

Q. 13. How are NHL classified according to their biological behaviour?

(*a*) **Indolent type:** These are **slow growing** tumours with a **better prognosis**.

Follicular, small cell lymphocytic and MALT lymphoma belong to this group.

(*b*) **Aggressive Type:** Large B cell, **Burkitt's and T cell precursor lymphoblastic lymphomas**.

These are **rapidly growing** tumours with a **poor prognosis.**

Box 12.29:	Points to be noted regarding T cell tumours

- Rare tumours.
- Precursor T cell lymphoblastic lymphoma – Thymus.
- Mediastinal mass – Compression of adjacent structures – Young adults.
- Peripheral T cell tumours – More mature T cells.
- Nodal or extranodal – Skin, air passages and intestine.

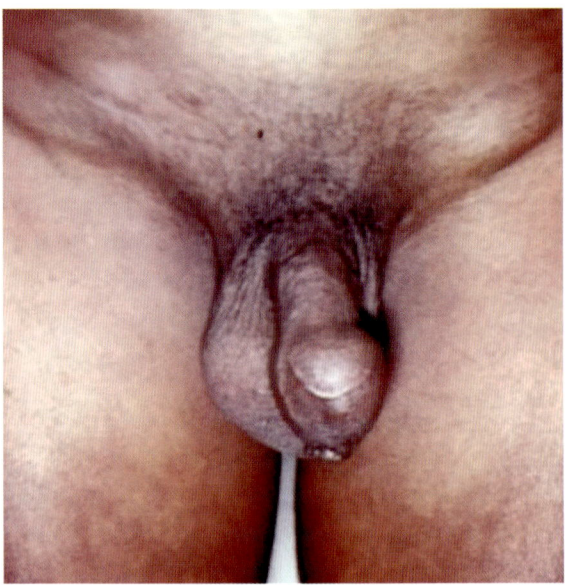

Fig. 12.5: NHL involving bilateral inguinal lymph nodes.

Q. 14. What are investigations to be done in a case of NHL?

These are the **same** as for **Hodgkin's** lymphoma. But a **peripheral blood smear** is more important to rule out **leukaemia.**

Imaging modalities like **US, CT and MRI** play a **major** role since **many** of the tumours are **extranodal.**

PET CT is also employed more **frequently** to assess the response to treatment.

Lymph node biopsy is as **crucial** as in the case of **Hodgkin's** disease.

Extranodal or **deep seated masses** are diagnosed by a **CT-guided biopsy**.

Box 12.30:	Points to be noted regarding the investigations

- Peripheral blood smear.
- Lymph node biopsy.
- Extranodal sites – CT-guided biopsy.
- US,CT, MRI and PET CT.

Q. 15. What are the principles of treatment for NHL?

Chemotherapy is the **primary line** of treatment. **COPP (Cyclophosphamide, oncovin, prednisolone** and **procarbazine**) is the favoured regime. The first two drugs are administered intravenously and the latter two orally. **Mustine hydrochloride** can be **substituted** for cyclophosphamide (MOPP). The usual pattern is to give **four cycles** of this treatment at an interval of **28 days**. Though response to **initial chemotherapy** is **satisfactory, recurrences** are **common.** These tumours are **not** as **radiosensitive** as **Hodgkin's** lymphoma. Hence **radiotherapy** is more often used for **advanced** or **recurrent** disease. **Chemoradiation** can be given **concurrently** or **radiation may follow chemotherapy.**

Rituximab, a **monoclonal antibody,** has been found to be **useful** in the management of **NHL.** Its action is against a **cell surface antigen** secreted by **B cells, CD20.** The treatment protocols involving rituximab are as follows. It is used **most frequently** for **large B cell** tumours **recurring** after **chemotherapy**. It has also been **combined with conventional therapy,** especially for **aggressive tumours**. The drug has been tried as a **sole agent** for patients with the **follicular type** of **NHL.** The advent of **rituximab** has certainly **increased the disease-free interval** at least in a **group of B cell** type of NHL. The number of patients living at the end of **five years** without the disease is only about **60%.**

Q. 16. What is the prognosis?

In general patients with **NHL** do **not do as well** as patients with **Hodgkin's**. lymphoma As mentioned earlier, **recurrences** are more **common** especially in the **aggressive** group.

The causes of **death** include the following.

(*a*) **Respiratory distress** due to a large **mediastinal mass.**

(*b*) **Intercurrent infection** resulting from **immunodeficiency.**

(*c*) **Acute renal failure** due to **hyperuricemia** due to massive **tumour necrosis.**

Q. 17. What does the term unknown or occult primary mean?

It refers to the **presence** of **secondaries** in patients where a **primary tumour cannot be detected** on **clinical examination**. Most often the **secondaries** are seen in **lymph nodes**. The **neck** is the **commonest site**. Lymph nodes involved belong to **level II or III**, with a possible primary in the **head and neck. Level III and Level IV group** is **not** usually **discussed** in this context.

Q. 18. How often are these cases seen in clinical practice?

The reported incidence was as high as **9%** of **head and neck**

cancers. With the advent of various **modern investigations** it has come down to about **3%.**

Q. 19. What is the common mode of presentation?

1. **Elderly or middle-aged males** form the most common group.

2. Most of them are **smokers** or **tobacco chewers.**

3. The presenting complaint is a **swelling** in the **upper part** of the **neck.**

4. The **duration** varies from a **few weeks to months**. But the **rate** of growth is quite **rapid.**

5. **Pain** is a **late** symptom.

6. It is the **total absence** of **any symptom** referable to a **primary tumour** that makes this **group of patients unique** in their character.

Box 12.31: Points regarding history
• Elderly males – Smokers, tobacco chewers
• Swelling in the upper or middle level of the neck.
• Duration – Few months.
• Rate of growth – Rapid.
• Pain is a late symptom.
• No symptom of the primary tumour.

Q. 20. What are the inspection findings?

(*a*) A **swelling** will be visible in the **upper part of the neck** in relation to the **sternomastoid** muscle. Occasionally the swellings may **be bilateral**.

(*b*) **The size** may be **variable**. Many are more than **6 cm in size**.

(*c*) The **upper and lower margins** are usually well **defined**.

(*d*) The **shape** is **usually irregular**.

(*e*) The **surface** may be **smooth or nodular**.

(*f*) The **skin** over the swelling often appears to be **stretched.**

Q. 21. What are the palpatory findings?

(*a*) **Warmth** and **tenderness** are usually absent.

(*b*) The **consistency** is invariably **hard**.

(*c*) The swelling may be **arising** from a **single** node of level **II or III** or **multiple nodes** that are often **adherent to each other** forming a **single**

mass. **Massive enlargement** of these two groups may be associated with **additional palpable nodes** belonging to other levels.

(*d*) The mass may have **restricted mobility,** or more frequently, be **completely fixed** to the deeper structures.

(*e*) It is **deep to the sternomastoid** and almost always **adherent** to the muscle.

(*f*) **Fixity** to the overlying **skin** occurs only in **the late stage** of the disease.

(*g*) The thyroid gland is palpated for enlargement for evidence of malignancy.

(*h*) A laryngeal click is elicited by moving the larynx in a horizontal direction. Absence of the click suggests an extrinsic carcinoma of the larynx.

Q. 22. What is the next step of clinical examination?

Examination of the **oral cavity** is performed to detect an **asymptomatic malignancy.** A methodical **inspection** and **palpation** of this region may reveal the presence of a primary. Two anatomical sites need a special mention. They are the **base** of the **tongue** and the **tonsil,** which may either **not** be **visible** or appear **normal** on **inspection.** But **induration** may be felt on **palpation** of these two areas, indicating **malignancy.** But as mentioned earlier, in **most cases, no positive findings** are present.

Q. 23. What are the classical sites of occult primary malignant tumours?

(*a*) **Nasopharynx.**

(*b*) **Fossa of Rosenmuller.**

(*c*) **Vallecular fossa.**

(*d*) **Posterior one-third of the tongue.**

(*e*) **Subglottic area.**

These **tumours** can only be **detected** by **investigations.**

Box 12.34: Classical occult primary sites

- Nasopharynx.
- Fossa of Rosenmuller.
- Vallecular fossa.
- Posterior third of the tongue.
- Subglottic area.

Q. 24. How is the diagnosis of malignancy confirmed?

FNAC shows a **squamous cell carcinoma.** The **only other condition** that it has to be distinguished from is an **NHL.** But as has been repeatedly stressed, **secondaries** are much **more common** than primary malignancy in **lymph nodes.**

Core needle biopsy (CNB) is performed only if **FNAC was nonconclusive.**

Q. 25. What are the investigations done to detect a primary tumour?

1. **Panendoscopy: Endoscopic examination** of the entire **suspicious area** is the next step. In addition to the **naso, oro** and **hypopharynx,** the **cervical oesophagus** (**post cricoid** region is a notorious area), the **larynx** and the **subglottic** regions are examined for a **primary** tumour. In **most cases,** the search is **futile.** Even when the appearance is **normal, biopsies** are taken from all these areas (**blind biopsy**). A **tonsillectomy** has been advised as a **diagnostic procedure,** to detect a primary tumour. But the **success rate** is very low.

2. **X-ray chest. Secondaries** are **rare.** But **doubtful** lesions on X-ray need a **CT** chest to confirm the same.

3. **CT scan of the head and neck**. The advent of **CT** raised hopes of identifying a primary in **more number of patients** belonging to this group. Occasionally, a **primary** in the **paranasal sinuses** may be detected. If any **abnormality** is found in the catchment area, a **repeat endoscopy** and **biopsy** is performed. But in **most instances** the **CT pictures** are **normal**.

   CT scan also shows the **extent of infiltration** of the **important** adjacent **structures** by the **lymph nodes** in the **neck**. **Resectability** is determined by this test. **Involvement** of the **carotid artery** indicates **inoperability.**

4. **PET CT** scan. With the advent of this scan, the **incidence** of **occult primary** in head and neck cancers has **come down** from about **10%** to **3%**. When present, **both the primary** and the **nodes** are **identified** by this scan. The **disadvantage** of this scan is the **20% false positive** rate.

Box 12.35:	Points to be noted regarding investigations

- Panendoscopy – Essentially normal – Blind biopsy.
- X-ray chest – CT if needed.
- CT head and neck – Detect primary – Repeat scopy and biopsy.
- CT of lymph nodes – Resectability – Invasion of adjacent structures.
- Carotid artery involvement – Inoperability.
- PET CT scan – Identifies primary most frequently – False +ve rates high.

Q. 26. What are the principles of treatment?

Treatment of these patients **poses** both **ethical** and **technical problems**. The **basic principle** in the management of any cancer is **control of the primary**. Hence the **rationale of treating** the **secondary nodes before treating the primary** is rather **difficult** to **explain**. The following are the **guidelines** on which the **treatment strategies** are **planned** at the present time.

Squamous cell cancers of the **head and neck** are grouped under the term **locoregional cancers. Distant metastases** are **uncommon,** and when they do **develop**, the duration is **after several years**. Therefore adequate locoregional treatment results in a **long disease-free interval**. Thus the **management** of the **nodes** is **beneficial** to the patient.

Squamous cell cancers are known to **spread beyond** the capsule **early** in the course of the disease. Such an **extracapsular spread** of these nodes **involves important adjacent structures**. Level **II and III** nodes are in **close proximity** to the **great vessels** in the neck. **Erosion** of these vessels results in **fatal massive bleed. Proper treatment** of the lymph nodes can **prevent** this **life-threatening complication**.

In **some cases**, the **primary** tumour becomes **manifest clinically** after a **period of time**. Depending upon the **site** and **extent** of the **tumour**, the **treatment** can be **planned** at that stage, thus **improving the outcome**.

Radiotherapy forms an **integral part** of the **treatment** for this group. The **field of radiation includes** most of the **possible primary sites** of malignancy. Hence a **small unrecognised primary** tumour may be **controlled** by this **treatment**

A few patients go through a **normal lifespan, without** the appearance of a **primary tumour**, following **adequate treatment** of the **secondary nodes**. In some of these cases, even a **postmortem examination** does not **reveal any primary**.

But all these **strategies** must be **tempered** by the fact that the very **appearance of the secondaries before the primary becomes manifest** indicates a **biologically aggressive tumour.**

Box 12.36:	Treatment strategies

- Squamous cell cancers are locoregional.
- Distant metastases – Uncommon – After several years.
- Erosion of great vessels – Exsanguinating bleed.
- Radiation – Controls possible primary.
- Primary detected later – Treated by radiation.
- A few patients – Normal lifespan.
- Appearance of secondary before primary – Aggressive tumour.

Q. 27. How are these patients treated?

Cervical block dissection is the operation of choice for **patients** presenting with **resectabe (mobile) nodes less** than **6 cm in size**. Depending upon the **stage** of the disease, certain **operative modifications** can be employed. This would mean **conservation** of the **internal jugular vein, spinal accessory nerve** and the **sternomastoid**. But in **most** of **our patients** these **modifications** are **not possible** since the **muscle** is invariably **fixed to the nodes**. As mentioned above, a **preoperative CT** is a **useful guide** in planning the **operation**. Following surgery, a course of

EBRT is given to all the patients. The **entire susceptible sites** of the **primary tumour** as well as the **operated area** are included in the **field of radiation**.

Patients presenting with **nodes larger than 6 cm,** or **fixed nodes** and nodes found to be **unresectable** on **CT scan**, are treated by an initial course of **chemoradiation (neoadjuvant)**. **Two to three cycles** of **Cisplatin and Bleomycin** are given along with **EBRT.** If the nodes **regress in size**, and a repeat **CT shows resectability**, these patients undergo a **radical neck lymphadenectomy. Following surgery** they are also given **radiotherapy** as in the previous group.

Patients who **do not respond** to **chemoradiation** are treated by **palliative EBRT.** In this group, the **prognosis is poor**.

Successfully treated patients need **yearly surveillance**. A **complete physical examination** followed by **panendoscopy** is the basic strategy. **CT and PET CT** are advised only in **selected cases**.

Box 12.37:	Points regarding treatment

- Mobile nodes proved resectable by CT if needed, undergo a radical lymphadenectomy.
- Since in most cases, the sternomastoid is adherent, a classical block dissection is performed.
- In a few selected cases, modifications can be used to conserve the internal jugular vein, the spinal accessory nerve and the sternomastoid muscle.
- Postoperative EBRT. The area of radiation includes all possible
- primary sites and the operated area.
- Nodes more than 6 cm. or fixed nodes – Preoperative chemoradiation.
- Cisplatin, bleomycin and EBRT – Concurrent treatment. Down staging – Radical surgery.
- Inoperable cases – Palliative chemoradiation.
- Yearly surveillance – Panendoscopy – CT and PET CT if needed.

A CASE OF VARICOSE VEINS

Setting

- Surgical OPD.

Chief Complaint

- **Chronic ulcer** in the right leg for **2 years.**
- **Dilated and prominent veins** in the **right lower limb** of **10 years duration**

Occupation

- The patient was working as a **barber** for the last **20 years**.

History of Present Illness

- A 45 year old man presented to the surgical OPD with the chief complaint of a **nonhealing ulcer** in the lower part of the right leg..

- The patient had developed a **small ulcer** on the inner aspect of the right ankle about 2 years ago. He had **itching** over that area for **one year** before he developed the ulcer. At that stage he had noticed an **eczematous** change with a **watery discharge**. The overlying skin had broken down to form an **ulcer.** The size of the ulcer had **gradually increased** in size over the last two years.

- The ulcer was **not painful** There was no history of **foul smelling discharge** or episodes of **bleeding** from the ulcer.

- The patient had noticed **prominent and dilated veins** on the inner aspect of the right lower limb for the past **10 years**. They had **enlarged to a great extent** during this period.

- He had dragging **pain** extending down the leg especially towards evenings. The pain was **relieved at night**. There were no episodes of **severe pain**.

- He had noticed **darkening of the skin** of the **lower part of the right leg** over the last 3 years.

- There was no history of **swelling** of the limb.

- He had no **abdominal complaints**.

- He was **able to work** during this period.

Past History

- He did not suffer from any **major illness** in the past.

Family History

- **No other member of the family had similar** complaints**.**

Personal History

- He was a smoker for the last 30 years. He did not chew paan or consume alcohol.

Treatment History

- He had been under the treatment of a local doctor for several years.

The doctor used to dress the ulcer and give him some capsules intermittently without any relief. Later the patient used to dress the ulcer himself after application of Betadine ointment.

- General physical examination.
- The patient appeared healthy and all the clinical parameters were within normal limits.

Local Examination

- The gait was normal.
- The patient was made to **stand** and expose both **lower limbs completely**.
- The right lower limb showed **grossly dilated** and **tortuous veins** on the **medial aspect of the leg and thigh** indicating that the **long saphenous vein** was affected.
- The **short saphenous vein territory** did not reveal any **dilated veins**.
- No **prominent veins** were visible on the **posterior aspect of the thigh.**
- The **left lower limb** did not show **any varicosity.**
- The following **tests** were performed in the **right lower limb.**
- The Trendelenburg test was positive indicating **saphenofemoral incompetency**.
- The **three bandage test** showed that the **perforators below the knee** and **middle** of the **leg** were **incompetent**

- Fegan's **test. Defects** in the **deep fascia** were felt **below the knee** and **middle of the leg**
- Scwartz's **test** showed that the **valves** along the **long saphenous vein** were **incompetent.**
- **Morrissey's test.** When the patient was made to **cough,** an **impulse** in the **nature** of a **fluid thrill** was felt at the **saphenous opening.**
- **Perthe's test.** The patient did not **complain** of **pain** when he was asked to **walk briskly** for **five minutes** after the vein was **emptied** and a bandage **applied at the saphenofemoral junction.**

Examination of the Ulcer

- **A single ulcer** was present over the **right medial malleolus.** It was **oval in shape** and measured **5cm by 3 cm in size.**
- The **margin** was regular. The floor had **pale granulation tissue and slough** with minimal discharge. There was **no bleeding** from the floor of the ulcer.
- The edges were **sloping** and there was **no induration**.
- The **base** was formed by the **medial surface** of the **tibia** and the ulcer was **immobile.**
- Movements of the ankle joint were restricted.
- Enlarged multiple **lymph nodes** were palpated in the **right inguinal**

region. They were **soft, nontender and small** in size.

- Pigmentation. The **lower half** of the right leg showed **hyperpigmentation** on the **anteromedial surface**

- **Lipodermatosclerosis.** The area surrounding the ulcer was **hard to palpate. The skin and subcutaneous tissue** were **thickened** and **adherent** to the **tibia.**

- There was no thickening of the tibia.

- On **measurement** of the **girth of the limb** no **swelling** was detected

- All the **pulsations** were felt **normally.**

- There was no **lymphoedema.**

- No **motor or sensory deficit** was detected

Examination of the Abdomen

- **No mass** was identified in the **lower abdomen.**

- **Examination of other systems** was normal.

Q. 1.   What was the clinical diagnosis?

Varicosity of the **long saphenous vein** with an **ulcer** was the obvious diagnosis. The clinical picture was very typical of this condition.

Q. 2.   What were the investigations done in this patient?

Pus from the floor of the ulcer was sent for **culture and sensitivity.** There was no bacterial growth.

Duplex US study of the right lower limb was done. The arterial system was normal.

The **deep veins** and the related **valves** were normal.

The **saphenofemoral junction** was **incompetent. Incompetent perforators** were found **below the knee, middle of the leg** and around the **ankle.** These sites were marked to help the surgeon during the operation.

Q. 3.   What was the indication for treating this patient?

He had **symptomatic varicosity** along with **complications** including an ulcer.

Q. 4.   How was this patient treated?

The patient was **admitted** to the hospital He was told to abstain from smoking completely. He was made to **lie in bed** for practically **24 hours of** the day. The foot end of the **bed** was **raised** to reduce venous stasis. The **ulcer** was dressed **daily.** A **pressure bandage** was applied from the base of the toes to the groin

Setting: 10 days later.

Q. 5. What was the operative procedure?

The patient underwent a **flush ligation** of the **long saphenous** vein at the saphenofemoral junction. The long saphenous vein was then **disconnected** (**Trendelenburg operation**). Tiny incisions were made at the site of the **incompetent perforators.** The skin and the deep fascia were incised exposing these veins. These were **ligated and divided**. A couple of **large tributaries** joining the long saphenous vein were **avulsed** through the same incisions. After skin closure, a **pressure bandage** was applied over the limb. The limb was kept in an **elevated** position. After a week the sutures were removed. The incision at the ankle was infected and hence took about 10 days to heal. The **ulcer** was then covered with a **split skin graft.**

Q. 6. What was the advice given to the patient at the time of discharge?

He was to **abstain** from **smoking** permanently. He was advised to wear an **elastic stockinet** for six months and to keep his right lower limb **elevated** at night.

At his return to the OPD six months later he was **asymptomatic** but was worried about the **hyperpigmentation** of the lower part of the leg. It was explained to him that this may **improve to some extent** over a period of time.

Q. 7. Define varicose veins.

When the veins appear **dilated tortuous and elongated** they are known as **varicose veins**. All prominent or dilated veins do not fit into this category.

Q. 8. Which are the other sites where varicose veins are present?

Dilated veins at the gastrooesophageal junction. These are known as varices. If the **pampiniform plexus** of veins in the **spermatic cord** were to be involved these are known as **varicoceles.**

Q. 9. What is the economic importance of this disease?

Varicose vein is a **very common** disease. Once **complications** develop, the **morbidity increases** to a large extent. This results in long term **absenteeism** from work. If a proper audit were to be undertaken it would show a loss of several **million of manhours.**

Q. 10. Name the occupations commonly associated with this condition.

It is more common in those occupations wherein a person has to be **on his feet** for a **long time. Barbers** are probably at the top of the list followed by **traffic** constables, **bus conductors** etc. But there are patients who do not fall in this group. A **congenital weakness** of the **vein wall and valves** may be the causative factor. The incidence in **women** has **come down** following a dramatic fall in **multiparity.**

Q. 11. **How is the history taken in these cases?**

Chief complaint: Presence of **dilated tortuous veins** in the lower limb of **several years** duration is the main complaint. At this stage the patients are **asymptomatic** and rarely seek medical advice.

Pain: This is a **late symptom**. It may be of **dragging type** and is worse towards evenings It is due to the **stretching** of the **medial wall** of the veins.

The remaining symptoms are due to **complications**.

Acute complications are thrombophle-bitis and bleeding

Thrombophlebitis manifests by the presence of **severe pain** radiating down the limb with fever. The vein is **tender, firm and noncompressible** A **red streak** may be seen along the path of the vein.

Bleeding is a **dramatic complication**. This is never massive but brings the patient to the hospital. It occurs when the **overlying skin is stretched** and becomes very **thin** and gives way. **Minor trauma** may precipitate this complication. The fact that the **central veins** are **valveless** and the **valves** along the superficial veins are **incompetent makes for a single column of blood.** Hence the **bleeding** is practically from the **right atrium**. Once the patient is made to lie down **supine** and the limb is **elevated** above the **level of the heart**, the bleeding **stops**. A **firm pressure bandage** and keeping the **limb elevated** for forty eight hours is the complete treatment.

Chronic complications include **eczema, ulceration, pigmentation** and **lipodermatosclerosis** these are described later.

Box 12.38: Points regarding history
• Dilated veins – several years.
• Pain- late symptom
• Acute complications- thrombophlebitis and bleeding
• Chronic complications –eczema, ulcer, pigmentation and lipodermatosclerosis

Past history: A previous history of **major surgery** is very important since it can lead to **DVT**. The varicosities then become **secondary** in nature.

Family history: There is an **increased incidence** in other members of the family especially when the cause could be a **congenital weakness** in the **vein wall**.

Pregnancy is often associated with varicosity. The **pressure of the gravid uterus** on the iliac veins is one factor. The **high level of progesterone** is likely to **relax** the muscles in the **medial wall** of the vein aggravating the condition.

Q. 12. **How does the method of local examination differ from the traditional in these cases?**

Usually clinical examination of a case proceeds along well established lines like **inspection, palpation** etc. But in these cases it may lead to some **confusion.** Hence a **step wise examination** has been found to be more reliable. The following table mentions the important steps in a case of varicose veins.

Box 12.39:	Points regarding the steps of local examination
1. Side and system.	
2. Various clinical tests.	
3. Complications.	
4. Evidence of DVT.	
5. Examination of regional lymph nodes.	
6. Examination of the abdomen.	

Q. 13. **What are the clinical findings in step 1?**

The patient must be made to **stand** with both the **lower limbs completely exposed** (easier in men). The examination must be conducted in **good light** (especially popliteal fossa).

(*a*) **Side:** The varicosity may be either **unilateral or bilateral**. In bilateral cases **one side** may show more **advanced disease.**

(*b*) **System involved:** The varicosity of the **long saphenous system** is easily identified Presence of dilated veins on the **medial aspect** of the **limb** makes recognition easy. On the contrary, the **short saphenous system** needs a more **careful examination**. The **politeal fossa** and the posterior aspect of the **leg** may show dilated tortuous veins.

(*c*) A small number of patients have an **ulcer** over the **lateral malleolus** associated with **long saphenous** varicosity. This anomaly can be explained by the presence of an **incompetent communicator** vein connecting the two systems. This vein starts from the **middle** of the **posterior aspect** of **the leg** to run upwards and medially to join the **long saphenous vein above** the **knee**.

(*d*) The **posterior surface of the thigh** may show **dilated veins**.

It is an uncommon sign, being an **indirect evidence** of **DVT.** When **the deep veins** are **blocked**, these veins offer an **alternative route** .

Box 12.40:	Points to be noted regarding the step 1 of local examination

- Side. Right and or left.
- System. Long or short saphenous or both.
- Anomalous position of the varicose ulcer.
- Dilated veins on the posterior surface of the thigh.

Q. 14. **What are the tests performed in step 2 of the local examination?**

(*a*) **Trendelenburg test:** The purpose of the test is to demonstrate **saphenofemoral incompetency**. The patient is made to lie down **supine.** The limb is **elevated** and the **long saphenous vein is emptied** by milking movements from below upwards. The **saphenofemoral junction** is now identified. It is located **4 cm below and medial** to the **pubic tubercle**. An easier method is to feel the pulsations of the **femoral artery** at the **midinguinal point**. The junction lies **medial** to this point. The **thumb** is placed at this point to **occlude the junction**. Maintaining the pressure, the patient is made to **stand**.

When the pressure of the thumb is **released** if there is a **rapid flow of blood** from the **groin downwards** it indicates an **incompetent saphenofemoral junction**. A **venous bandage** applied at the groin instead of the thumb is more useful especially in **obese patients**.

In patients with **short saphenous varicosity**, the test is performed at the the shortsaphenofemoral junction in the **popliteal fossa**.

Trendelenburg test 2. This is used to detect **incompetent perforators**. Maintaining the pressure, the patient is made to **stand**. If there is **rapid** filling of blood from **below upwards,** it suggests the presence of **incompetent perforators**.

The **explanation** for a positive test no 1 is as follows. When a person is in a **standing position**, the pressure in the **deep veins** is **highe**r than the **superficial veins**. In addition the flow is **against gravity**. The unidirectional flow from **below upwards** is helped by several factors including **valves** in the veins. But the **central veins** are

valveless. The first valve is in the **femoral vein** close to the **saphenofemoral junction.** Thus in the **erect** position, the blood in the **deep venous system** is in the form of a **single fluid column** extending from the **right atrium** to the femoral vein. When a person is in a **standing position** for a **long time**, there is **stasis** of blood resulting in **dilatation of the femoral vein.** It also tends to **increase the size** of the **opening** at the **saphenofemoral junction** rendering the **valve incompetent.** Blood is able to run down from the **femoral** to the **long saphenous vein** resulting in varicosity.

(*b*) **Three bandage test:** This test detects the presence of **incompetent perforators.** Perforator veins are those that **connect** the **superficial** to the **deep** venous system. Since these are the **only veins** to **perforate** the **deep fascia,** these are known as **perforators.** In the anatomical sense, even the **terminal parts** of the **long and short saphenous veins** could be considered as **perforators.** **Communicators** are veins that run in the **subcutaneous** plane **connecting** the **two**

saphenous systems. Several have been described but the most important one has been described earlier.

The **flow of blood** in these veins is unidirectional from the **superficial** to the **deep system** against the **pressure gradient**. Two factors are responsible for this phenomenon. The **stragically placed valves** help to some extent. The action of the **calf pump (peripheral heart)** is more **significant.** The **venous return** in the leg is collected in a **plexus of veins** in the **soleus muscle. Contraction** of the **soleus** muscle **forces** the blood into the **deep veins. Reflux** is **prevented** by the presence of **valves** in the veins. **Relaxation** of the muscle induces a **negative pressure** in the **venous plexus**, drawing blood from the **superficial system** via the **perforators.** Thus during **walking** there is a **rhythmic contraction** and **relaxation** of the **soleus** muscle. Thus its action is **compared** to that of the **heart.** But if the person were to **stand** for a **long time**, the **soleus** is in a state of **tonic contraction.** Thus the blood **accumulates** in the **perforators** causing dilatation. The **valves** become **incompetent.** Further when the person starts **walking,** the **contractions** of the **soleus** now force the blood in a **reverse direction** via the incompetent **perforators.** This leads to **varicosity of the superficial veins**. Thus **a vicious cycle** is established **aggravating** the condition.

The **aim** of the three bandage test is **to locate the sites** of these **perforators.** With the patient supine, the **long saphenous** vein is **emptied. Bandages** are applied at the following sites to **occlude the perforators**. The sites are at the **groin, above the knee, below the knee** and at the **ankle.** The patient is now made to **stand.** With all the bandages in place, if a **bunch of dilated** veins appear at any site in the limb, it suggests the presence of **incompetent perforators** at this site. The bandages are then **released** from **below upwards.** If **dilated veins appear** at these **sites after release of the bandage,** they indicate the presence of **incompetent perforators.** When the bandage at the groin is released, the Trendelenburg test is being repeated.

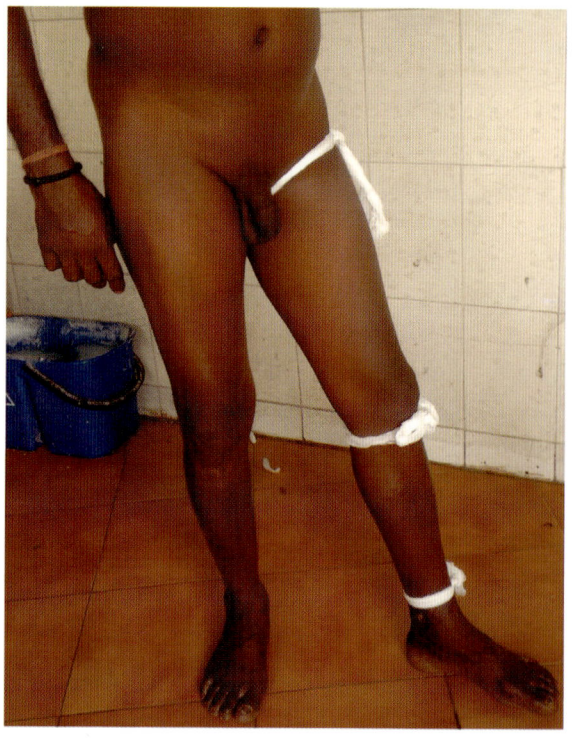

Fig. 12.6: Three bandage test.

(*c*) **Fegans test:** The rationale behind this test is the same. When a **perforator pierces** the deep fascia it creates a defect in the fascia. But it is **too small** to be detected clinically**. Incompetent perforators** are much larger in size and hence the **defects** also are **much bigger**. These can be **palpated** during clinical examination.

With the patient **standing,** the sites of the most **prominent veins** are **marked**. With the patient **supine** the veins are **emptied**. A finger is run along the **course** of the **long saphenous** vein. If the **finger dips in** suddenly, it indicates a **large defect** in the **fascia** confirming the presence of an **incompetent perforator**. The common sites are **below the knee**, at the **middle of the leg** and **around the ankle**.

But this test has certain **limitations. Lipodermatosis** binds the skin to the fascia and hence in the **lower part of the leg** this test **cannot be** performed. Again in the **thigh segment, the deep fascia** is separated from the skin by a **thick layer of fat**. Hence **detection of defects** is not possible.

(*d*) **Schwartz's test: Incompetency** of **the valves** along the **long saphenous** vein is demonstrated by Schwartz's test. Patient is made to **stand** and a **tap is** given by the finger at the **ankle** over the vein. A finger kept over the **most prominent part** of the vein in the **thigh** feels the **impulse**. Since the **valves are incompetent** the blood within is reduced to a **single fluid column** allowing the **impulse** to travel from the **ankle to the thigh**.

(*e*) **Morrissey's test:** The patient is asked to **stand and**

cough. An **impulse** in the nature of a **fluid thrill** felt at the **saphenous opening** indicates **saphenofemoral incompetency.**

(*f*) **Perthe's test:** The test is performed to **demonstrate** the **patency** of the **deep venous system**. With the patient supine, the limb is **elevated** and the **long saphenous** vein is **emptied**. A **venous bandage** is applied at the **groin** to **block** the **saphenofemoral junction**. The patient is asked to **walk briskly** for about **5 minutes**. Appearance of **severe cramp like pain** in the calf muscles along with all the superficial veins becoming **engorged,** is taken as a **positive test**. Since the **superficial vein** is **blocked by a bandage** and if the deep veins are **thrombosed,** the **blood accumulates** in the limb releasing **P factor** causing severe **pain.**

Unfortunately this test has **limitations**. It has a **high percentage** of **false negatives**. A **thrombosed vein** often undergoes **recanalisation**. Recanalised veins act **as conduits** for the flow of blood. But they are **devoid** of the **muscles** in the

medial coat as well as **valves.** Hence functionally these are **poor substitutes** for a **normal deep vein** despite a Perthe's **test being negative.**

(*g*) **Rarely** varicose veins may be **secondary** to a **congenital arteriovenous malformation.** Association of **local gigantism** and other features will help to diagnose this condition.

Box 12.41: Points regarding various tests

- Trendenlenburg test 1 and 2.
- Three bandage test.
- Fegan's test.
- Morrissey's test.
- Perthe's test.
- Congenital arteriovenous malformation

Q. 15. Step 3: What are the complications and what is the pathophysiological basis for these complications?

All the **complications** are the result of persistent **VENOUS HYPERTENSION. Reflux** of blood due to **changes** described earlier lead to **these complications.** The venous pressure is **highest** at the level of the **ankle.**

(*a*) **Pigmentation:** Due to an increase in pressure, small **venules** and **capillaries rupture** leading to **extravasation** of blood in the **subcutaneous tissue.** The **haemosiderin pigment**

released from the **RBCs** leads to **pigmentation.** It is seen in the **lower part of the leg** and around the **ankle.** In most instances this complication is **irreversible.**

(*b*) **Varicose eczema:** The same pigment is responsible for inducing a **chemical dermatitis. Itching** is the chief complaint. The skin at the **ankle** shows evidence of **eczema** with a **watery discharge.** Within a short time it is converted into a **bacterial dermatitis. Scratching** by the patient hastens this process. The skin is **reddish** with **blisters** that **break down frequently.**

(*c*) **Varicose ulcer:** Most of **our patients** seek treatment only **at this stage. Ulceration** is a sequel to **eczema.** Once **infection** supervenes, the **skin breaks down** resulting in ulceration. The **medial and the lateral malleoli** are the most common sites. **Long saphenous** varicosity leads to an ulcer over the **medial malleolus** and **vice versa. An exception** has already been described.

The **ulcer** is **single, oval in shape** with the floor comprising of **pale granulation tissue.** The edges are **sloping** and the base is formed by the underlying **bone. Chronic inflammation** leads to **abundant fibrosis** and hence there may some degree of **hardness** at the base.

(*d*) **Lipodermatosclerosis:** This complication causes **severe morbidity**. It is seen along with an **ulcer** in most patients. The **skin** over the **lower part of the leg** and around the ankle is **markedly thickened**. The **subcutaneous fat** is replaced by **dense fibrous tissue** that binds the **skin** to the **deeper structures**. With pigmentation added, the area comes to resemble **toughend dark leather.**

The **aetiopathology** of this condition is rather **complex. Venous hypertension** causes **increased capillary permeability**. This allows the **WBCs** to move into the **perivenous tissues**. These **liberate cytokines** inducing an **inflammatory reaction** resulting in **fibrosis.** Since the reaction occurs all **round** a **vessel,** it is known as a **fibrous cuff,** narrowing the **lumen further**. This leads to increased venous pressure, setting in a **vicious cycle**. This fibrosis ultimately leads **to lipodermatosclerosis**.

An additional factor is the **change in the valves**. **Maximum** venous pressure is present at the **base** of the **leaflets** that form the **valve.** Hence the **fibrosis** at these sites will be much **more.** Thus the valves **become deformed** and **the leak** across these valves will become **worse.**

The **following complications** are not seen **frequently** at the present time.

(*e*) **Periosteitits of the tibia or less commonly the fibula**. In **long standing** ulcers, the **inflammation extends** to involve the **periosteum**. This leads to **deposition of new bone** under the periosteum due to the action of **the osteoblasts**. **Comparision** with the width of the **bone** on the **opposite side** helps to detect this complication. **Xray** is confirmatory. It does not need any specific treatment.

(*f*) **Calcification:** The portion of the **long saphenous vein** below the **knee** may get **calcified** following **thrombosis.** The vein feels hard on the surface of the tibia. It is easily recognized **on Xray**. Again it is an inconsequential complication.

(*g*) **Talipes equinus deformity** of the foot. It is associated with **ulcers** of **several years** duration. To **reduce the discomfort** while walking, the patient changes his **gait**. The **heel is raised off** the ground. The resulting **contracture** of the **Tendo Achilles** produces an **equinus deformity**.

(*h*) **Marjolin's ulcer:** It is a **squamous cell carcinoma**. It occurs in patients who had **irregular and intermittent treatment** for their varicose ulcers. The ulcers **heal** to **break down** repeatedly at intervals of **weeks or months**. Over a **period of time** the squamous epithelium undergoes a **malignant transformation**.

There is **considerable delay** in the diagnosis since the patient had **several episodes** of the ulcer healing and recurring again. Only when the ulcer assumes a **large size** or starts **bleeding**, treatment is sought for.

Box 12.42:	Points regarding complications

- Pigmentation.
- Varicose eczema.
- Varicose ulcer.
- Lipodermatosclerosis.
- Periosteitis.
- Calcification.
- Equinus deformity of the foot.
- Marjolin's ulcer.

Q. 16. What constitutes step 4 of the local examination?

Examination for deep vein thrombosis (DVT) Presence of **DVT** makes varicose veins **secondary** in nature. **Acute DVT** presents with **dramatic symptoms** and **signs. Various tests** have also been described to identify this condition. On the other hand, **chronic DVT** is a **silent disease**. A **high degree of suspicion** is absolutely essential. It may be a **sequel** of previous **major trauma or surgery. None** of the **tests** described for the acute stage are **useful.** An **increase in the girth** of the limb especially the **thigh segment** may be the only clue (**champagne bottle appearance**). Measurement of the **girth** both at the thigh and leg is necessary. **Often Duplex US studies** are needed to confirm the diagnosis.

Box 12.43:	Points to be noted regarding step 4

- Presence of DVT- secondary varicosity.
- Acute stage – easy diagnosis- symptoms signs and tests.
- Chronic- high degree of suspicion- girth of the limb- Champagne bottle shape.
- Duplex US study.

Q. 17. Describe step 5 of the local examination.

Palpation of the regional lymph nodes.

In the presence of **sepsis,** the **lymph nodes** either in the **inguinal or popliteal** region are enlarged. These are **firm, nontender and mobile**.

Q. 18. **What are the areas to be examined in step 6 of the local examination?**

Palpation of the abdomen: Large lower abdominal masses may press on **the veins** to produce secondary varicosity. **Malignant external iliac nodes** are a good example. The **thigh segment** may show **more dilated veins** compared to the rest of the limb. A **gravid uterus** has already been referred to.

Box 12.44:	Points to be noted in steps 5 and 6

- Enlarged lymph nodes- firm, nontender and mobile.
- Abdominal masses- Ext.iliac nodes.
- Gravid uterus.

Q. 19. **Why are investigations needed when obvious clinical signs are present to prove the diagnosis?**

1. The **clinical tests** are **subjective** in nature. The **quality of examination** decides the results. The results of these tests are **not** always **totally reproducible**. The **Trendelenburg test** is **difficult** to perform in an **obese female**. The **thumb** may get **displaced** during **change of posture.**

2. **All the incompetent perforators** may not be **detected** by clinical examination, increasing the rate of recurrence.

3. The status of the **deep veins** cannot be determined by **clinical tests alone**. The **Perthe's test** is associated with a high percentage of **false negatives**.

4. Most importantly, **no clinical tests** are available to **demonstrate incompetency** of the **valves** in the **deep venous system**. These can result in secondary varicosity.

Box 12.45:	Points regarding the need for investigations

- Clinical tests are subjective- results variable.
- All incompetent perforators not detected.
- Status of the deep veins.
- No tests to demonstrate incompetent valves in the deep veins.

Q. 20. **What are the investigations done in these patients?**

1. **Duplex US studies:** The use of the **grey scale US** with a **Colour Doppler** has made understanding of the **disease** much better. Hence the **treatment** has become **more rational**.

It **confirms** the results of the various **clinical tests** performed earlier. The results are **objective** and can be **recorded. Additional incompetent perforators** are detected by this study. The state of the **deep veins** is **defined clearly.** This is most important when **treatment strategies** have to be planned. **Incompetency of** the **valves** in the **deep venous system** can only be **identified** with the help of investigations. **Reflux** of blood during a **Valsalva manoeuvre** demonstrates **deep vein valvular incompetency.** The test identifies the varicosity as of the **secondary** type.

Advantages: It is **available** in most parts of the country. It is **cost effective.** It is **also noninvasive.** No **radiation** is involved and is therefore **safe** in **pregnant women.**

Disadvantage: The only disadvantage is that the study is **operator dependent.** But in this era of **specialization** we have **dedicated ultrasonoligists** who study vascular diseases only.

2. **Venography (phlebography):** In this study, a **radio opaque contrast** containing **iodine** is **injected** into the vein to define the **venous abnormalities** in the limb. In an **ascending venogram,** the contrast is injected at the **ankle** and a series of Xrays are taken. In a **descending venogram,** the contrast is injected into the **femoral vein** at the **groin** and Xrays are taken during a **Valsavla manoeuvre. Reflux** of blood along the **femoral and popliteal veins** indicate **deep vein valvular incompetency.** After the **advent of US,** venograms are **rarely performed.**

Disadvantages:

(*a*) It is an **invasive investigation.** Local complications like **haematoma** or **extravasation** of the contrast add to the morbidity.

(*b*) **Hypersensitivity** to iodine can lead to life threatening **anaphylactic reactions.**

(*c*) **Interpretation of the Xrays** is **difficult** since three dimensional structures are reduced to two dimensional pictures. **Overlapping** of the veins makes reading of these Xrays **more complex.**

3. **Plain Xray** may show **increased density** of the **tibia** in the presence of **periosteitis. Calcified vein** may also be seen.

4. **Culture and sensitivity** of the **pus** present in the floor of an **ulcer** are needed since the patient would have received plenty of **antimicrobials earlier**.

5. If a **malignant change** is suspected of the **varicose ulcer**, multiple **edge biopsies** are done.

Box 12.46: Points regarding investigations

- Duplex US study.
- Venography.
- Plain Xray of the leg.
- Pus culture and sensitivity
- Edge biopsy if malignancy is suspected.

Q. 21. What is the CEAP classification?

Futher classified as

C 0 No visible or palpable varicose veins.

C 1 Telagiectic or reticular veins.

C 2 Varicose veins.

C 3 Oedema.

C 4 Healed varicose ulcer.

C 5 Active varicose ulcer.

E. Aetiological.

Ec. Congenital

Ep. Primary.

Es. Secondary- Post thrombotic.

A Anatomical

S. Superficial veins.

P. Perforators veins.

D. Deep veins.

P. Pathophysiological.

Pr. Reflux.

Po. Obstruction.

Pr,o. Reflux with obstruction.

Pn. No venous pathophysiology.

Q. 22. How are varicose veins classified according to the aetio;ogy?

1. **Primary or idiopathic:** These patients have no **demonstrable aetiology**. **Certain occupations** like that of **barbers** have a **higher risk** of developing the disease. It may also be the result of **congenital weakness** of the vein wall or a deficiency in the valves.

2. **Secondary:** These are secondary to a primary disease. **DVT** leading to a **post thrombotic state** is the commonest cause. **Abdominal masses** including a **gravid uterus** can also produce secondary varicosity.

3. **Rarely secondary** varicosity may be a manifestation of **congenital arteriovenous malformation**.

Q. 23. Is the presence of varicose vein an indication for treatment?

In the **presence** of **complications treatment** is always **needed**.

Most of **our patients** fall into this category. The **rate** at which **complications** develop is **variable.** Some of the patients have **grossly dilated veins** with most of the **clinical tests** being **positive but do not have** any **complications** for many **years.** On the other hand, **few patients** with a **single incompetent perforator** at the ankle develop **pigmentation** and **ulceration** within a **short period** of time.

The treatment of **asymptomatic primary** varicose veins is based on **personal preferences.** The main indication for treatment is **cosmetic disfigurement**. In the **West,** where **body image** is of great concern, the **number** of patients may be much **more.** In our country, some belonging to the **higher strata of society** may demand treatment at this stage.

Q. 24. **What are the surgical procedures employed for the treatment of primary varicose veins?**

1. **Trendelenburg's operation:** It is indicated in patients with **saphenofemoral incompetency.** It consists of **flush ligation** and **division** of the **long saphenous** vein as close to the **saphenofemoral junction** as possible. Flush ligation is required to **prevent** the development of a **saphenavarix** at a later date. But this classical operation is **associated** with **recurrences.** Hence attempts are being made to **modify** the procedure to **reduce** the **recurrences.**

Operative details: An oblique incision is made at **the groin crease** dividing the skin and the subcutaneous tissue. The **long saphenous** vein is now identified. If large **lymph nodes** are found at this site they may need to be **separated** for proper visualization. The **three named tributaries** that join the long saphenous vein are **ligated and divided**. They are the **superficial epigastric**, the **superficial circumflex** and the **external pudendal** veins. **Unnamed tributaries** if present are also treated in the same way. These steps are needed to **reduce** the **risk** of recurrence. The **cribriform fascia** is incised and the **saphenofemoral junction** is clearly **defined.** The **long saphenous vein** is ligated **flush (juxtrafemoral)** with the **femoral vein** and divided between **ligatures.** Closure of the incision in layers completes the operation.

If the **short saphenous** venous system is affected, a similar operation is conducted at the **popliteal fossa** with flush ligation of the **short saphenous** vein. The operation is **more difficult** for the following reasons.

(*a*) The **popliteal fossa** is a **narrow space** bound by tendons.

(*b*) The **saphenopopliteal junction** is **deeply** placed.

(*c*) The **neurovascular structures** are in very **close proximity** of the venous junction.

Hence the **recurrence** rate **is higher** with this operation.

2. **Subfascial ligation** of the perforator veins. This procedure is usually **combined** with a **Trendelenburg's operation**. The reason for **a subfascial** ligation is that in the **subcutaneous plane** it is not possible to **distinguish** between a **communicator vein** and a **perforator.** As mentioned earlier, these are the **only veins that perforate** the **deep fascia.**

In the past before US became available, the operation needed a **long incision** extending from **below the knee** upto the **ankle** dividing the skin and deep fascia to **expose** the **perforators..** This procedure is **not suitable** when the indication is basically **cosmesis.** It is therefore **no longer performed**

US guided perforator ligation: It is now the most popular procedure. **Tiny incisions** are made over **sites** marked by the **ultrasonologist** earlier. The **skin** and the **deep fascia** are incised exposing the **large perforators.** These are ligated and divided subfascially. A subcutaneous ligation may either lead to a **recurrence** or **an unsightly bulge** at these sites.

Minimal access surgery: This is the **ideal operation** if **cosmesis** is the **primary indication.** Through a **small incision** at the medial aspect of the popliteal fossa, an **endoscope** is introduced into the **subfascial plane,** A **space** is created between the **fascia and the muscles.** The **perforators** are easily **visualized, clipped and divided.** The procedure is known as subfascial endoscopic perforator surgery **(SEPS).**

3. **Vein stripping procedure:** It was commonly **combined** with a **Trendelenburg procedure** in the past. The principle was to strip the vein with the help of **Myer's vein stripper**. After completing the Trendelenburg procedure, an **incision** was made at the **ankle** to expose the vein. The **narrow smooth end** of the instrument was then introduced into the lumen and **pushed upwards** along the vein until it emerged at the **groin** through the vein. **Additional incisions** may be needed at the knee in cases of **extreme tortuosity**. Once the instrument reached the **groin,** a **dome shaped head** was attached to the vein. The **stripper** was **firmly anchored** to the **vein** at **both ends**. **Steady traction** was applied to the stripper at the **lower end** to strip the vein from **above downwards**. Firm pressure bandage was applied during this stage to **prevent bleeding** from the **tributaries** which were being **sheared off** due to the traction.

The **short saphenous** vein should **never** be **stripped** because of its **close proximity** to the **sural nerve**, makes **sural neuralgia** a **certainity.**

4. **Avulsion** of the **cosmetically** disfiguring **tortuous tributaries**. Through tiny incisions these tributaries are avulsed.

Box 12.47:	Points regarding surgical procedures

- Trendelenburg operation.
- Subfascial ligation of incompetent perforators.
- Vein stripping.
- Avulsion of tributaries.

Q. 25. **What are the nonsurgical methods of treatment?**

Occlusive sclerotherapy. Sclerosing agents are used to induce **endothelial damage** resulting in **thrombosis**. As the thrombus gets **organized** into **fibrous tissue,** the **lumen** of the vein is **obliterated.** These were used for either **recurrent** or **residual veins after surgery in the past**. Traditionally sclerotherapy was used to treat **localized bunch** of varicosities also. Sodium tetradecyl sulphate (**STD**) was the agent used.

Technique of sclerotherapy. With the help of a **tourniquet** the **veins** are made **prominent**. Once the vein is **entered,** the tourniquet is **released** and the vein is **emptied.** The drug is now **injected** into the vein and a **firm pressure bandage** is applied over the limb to **maintain contact** of the drug with the endothelium. The patient is advised **rest** for about **forty eight hours**. The danger is that of the drug reaching the **deep veins** resulting in **DVT** or even worse, a fatal **pulmonary embolism.**

Q. 26. What are the modern methods of endovascular sclerotherapy?

Over th years it became **evident** that the **Trendelenburg operation** had a significant rate of **recurren**ce. Recurrences could be due to **faulty surgery**. But even with a **flush ligation**, **recurrences** have been reported. **Neovascularisation** could be one of the reasons. Hence a large number of **less invasive procedures** have now been described as **the primary line** of treatment.

Foam sclerotherapy: A **long catheter** is introduced into the **long saphenous** vein at the **groin** and is manipulated till the **ankle,** usually under **US** guidance. The **sclerosing agent** is converted into a **foam** by mixing it with **air.** This helps the drug to reach a **larger surface area** of the vein. As the catheter is being **withdrawn** the drug is **injected.** The **entire vein** is thus **sclerosed**. But the **complications** mentioned earlier can also **occur** by this method.

Endovascular laser or use of **radio frequency probes** work on **the same principle as sclerotherapy.**

Box 12.48:	Points regarding nonsurgical methods of treatment
	• Occlusive sclerotherapy- residual or recurrent varicosities.
	• STD-Endothelial damage- thrombosis- fibrosis- occlusion.
	• Foam sclerotherapy- large surface area- primary line of treatment.
	• Endovascular laser or use of radio frequency probes.

Q. 27. How are secondary varicose veins treated?

The treatment is essentially **conservative**. Application of a **firm pressure bandage** keeps the **veins empty** and relieves **the symptoms**. The bandage is to be kept in place as long as the patient is in the **standing** position. The limb may be kept in an **elevated** position at night. But the amount of **pressure may vary** if the patient is made to apply the bandage. This disadvantage is nullified by the application of a **graduated pressure compression stockinet**, available in the market. The **maximum** pressure is at the **ankle** and is **reduced** gradually till the **groin**.

■■■

Hernias

13

A CASE OF INGUINAL HERNIA

Setting

- Surgical OPD

Chief Complaint

- **Swelling** in the **left inguinoscrotal region** of **4 years duration**.

Occupation

- **Manual labour** involving lifting of **heavy weights**.

History of Present Illness

- A **48**-year-old man presented to the OPD with a complaint of a **swelling** in the **left inguinoscrotal region** of **4 years duration**. The patient noticed a **small swelling** in the **left groin 4 years** ago. It used to **appear** on **straining and coughing** and used to **disappear completely. Six months later**, the **swelling** used to **appear** in the **standing position** and became **smaller on lying down**.

It started **descending** down to the **scrotum** about a **year ago**. The patient noticed that the **swelling** became **bigger** on **straining.** At that **stage** the patient was **able** to **reduce** the **swelling**. The **reduction** was **easy** and **not painful**. For the last **three months**, the patient is **unable** to **reduce** it **completely.**

- The patient complained of **dragging pain** more towards the **evening**. The pain was **relieved** at **night.**
- He did **not** have **chronic cough** or **breathlessness.**
- He did **not** complain of **urinary problems**.
- There was **no** history of **constipation.**
- **Past and family histories** were not significant.

Personal History

- The patient was a **beedi smoker** for the last **30 years**. He was also **consuming alcohol** daily.

Treatment History

- He had **not** taken any **treatment** for this condition.
- **General physical examination** did not reveal any abnormality.

Local Examination

Inspection

- **Patient in standing position.** There was a **left-sided inguinoscrotal swelling**. It **extended** from **above** the **groin crease** to the **bottom** of the **scrotum**. The **margins** were **well defined**.
- The **size** was **15 cm by 10 cm**. The **shape** was an **oblique oval**.
- The **surface** was **smooth.**
- There was an **expansile impulse** on **coughing.** There was **no swelling** in the **right inguinal region** on **coughing**
- The **skin** over the **scrotal part** of the **swelling** was **stretched. Rugosities** were **absent.**
- **Visible peristalsis** was not seen in the **scrotal part** of the swelling.
- **Inspection** with the patient in **supine position**. There were **no changes** in the **physical findings.**

Palpation

- Patient in supine position.
- The **site** and **extent** were confirmed. The swelling was felt to be **extending** from **above** the **inguinal ligament** to the **bottom** of the **scrotum.**
- The **swelling** was neither **warm** nor **tender.**
- There was a **palpable expansile impulse** on **coughing.**
- The **size and shape** were confirmed. The **borders** were **distinct.**
- The **surface** on palpation was **lobular.**
- The **consistency** was **soft.**
- The **swelling** was **reduced** with **some** amount of **difficulty.** The **patient** did not **experience** any **discomfort** during **reduction**.
- **Deep ring occlusion test**. The **swelling did not appear** when the patient was asked to **cough** with the **deep ring occluded** by the **thumb**.
- **Zieman's test.** The **impulse** was felt by the **index finger**.
- The **external ring invagination test**. The **external ring** was **grossly enlarged** admitting more than **two fingers.**
- Following **reduction** of the **swelling,** the **testis** was **palpable**. It was **normal.**
- There was **no palpable expansile impulse** on coughing on the **right side**.
- The **right testis** was **normal.**
- The **bulbous urethra** felt **soft** on Perenium.

Percussion

- The swelling was **resonant.**

Auscultation

- **No bowel sounds** were heard over the swelling.
- The **tone** of the **abdominal muscles** was **good.**
- Examination of the **respiratory system** did not reveal any abnormality.
- **Other systems** were clinically normal.

Q. 1. **What was the clinical diagnosis in this patient?**

Left-sided complete indirect inguinal hernia with **bowel** as the content.

Hernia was **identified** because of the presence of **expansile impulse** on **coughing** and **reducibility**.

Inguinal hernia was diagnosed because the **swelling** was **above** the **inguinal ligament** and it was **descending down** into the **scrotum.**

It was of the **indirect type** as demonstrated by the **deep ring occlusion test**. It was a **complete hernia** because it **descended down** to the **bottom** of the **scrotum.**

Bowel was probably the **content** since it was **resonant** on **percussion.**

Q. 2. **What were the investigations performed in this patient?**

No investigations were needed to **confirm the diagnosis.**

Chest X-ray was normal.

Q. 3. **What was the treatment adopted for this patient?**

He was advised to **undergo** a **hernioplasty.** The patient was discharged and asked to **return** after **3 weeks** for the **operation. In the meantime** he was **advised to stop smoking** completely as he was known to be a heavy smoker. *Setting.* 3 weeks later.

The patient was **readmitted** for the **operation.** He underwent a **hernioplasty**. The **contents** of the hernia sac included both **greater omentum** and **small intestine**. A **prolene mesh** was used to **strengthen** the **posterior wall** of the **inguinal canal.**

The **patient** had a **smooth postoperative** period. He was **advised** to **abstain** from **heavy manual work** for **six weeks**.

He returned to the OPD **6 weeks later**. The **incision** had **healed well.** He was told to **go back to work**. He was also **advised** to **abstain** from **smoking.**

Q. 4. **Define a hernia.**

Hernia is **defined** as an **abnormal protrusion of contents** of a **cavity** through a **defect** in the **wall** of that **cavity.**

Q. 5. Describe the anatomy of the inguinal canal.

A thorough knowledge of the **anatomy of the inguinal canal** is essential to **understand** this common **surgical disease.** The **canal** is basically a **defect** in the **anterior abdominal wall,** for the **passage** of the **spermatic cord** in the male and the **round ligament** in the female. The anterior wall is formed by the **aponeurosis** of the **external oblique** muscle and a **part** of the **conjoint tendon laterally.** The **posterior wall consists** of the **fascia transversalis** in its **entire extent,** and **strengthened** by the **conjoint tendon** on the **medial aspect.** The **arched fibres** of the **conjoint tendon** form the **roof,** and the **floor** comprises of the **grooved surface** of the **inguinal ligament.** The **key structure,** to understand the **anatomy clearly,** is the **conjoint tendon.** It forms a **part of the anterior wall** and then **curves** over the **cord** to be a part of the **posterior wall medially.** The internal ring is a **window** in the **transversalis fascia,** for the **passage** of the **spermatic cord,** and is said to be **surrounded** by a few **fibres** of the **internal oblique muscle,** forming a doubtful **sphincter.** The **external ring** is a **triangular defect** in the **external oblique**

for the exit of the spermatic cord. This **opening** is **adequate** for the **passage** of the **cord** and **admits** the **tip of the little finger** only if this **structure** were to be **absent.** The **nerves** in relation to the **canal** are the **genital branch** of the **genitofemoral,** the **ilioinguinal** and the **iliohypogastric nerves.**

An **inguinal shutter mechanism** has been described, that **reduces** the **risk** of the **occurrence** of a **hernia.** When the **intra-abdominal pressure increases,** the **following factors** cause a **narrowing** of the **defect.** The **sphincteric action** of the **internal oblique compresses** the **internal ring.** Again the **contractions** of the **conjoint tendon** bring the **roof down.** The **external oblique pulls** up the **floor** and also **reduces** the **size** of the **external ring. Professions** that involve **lifting of heavy weights** regularly **enhance** the **risk** of development of a **hernia.** An **indirect inguinal hernia** is said to **occur** in the presence of a **persistent patent processus vaginalis** and a **direct** one, the result of a **weak fascia transversalis.**

Q. 6. What are the points to be considered in taking history in a case of inguinal hernia?

Age and gender. Inguinal hernia is seen in **young infants** as well as

adults and **elderly patients**. The disease is seen **more frequently** in **males**. But it is important to **note** that in **females,** an **inguinal hernia** is **more common** than a **femoral hernia.**

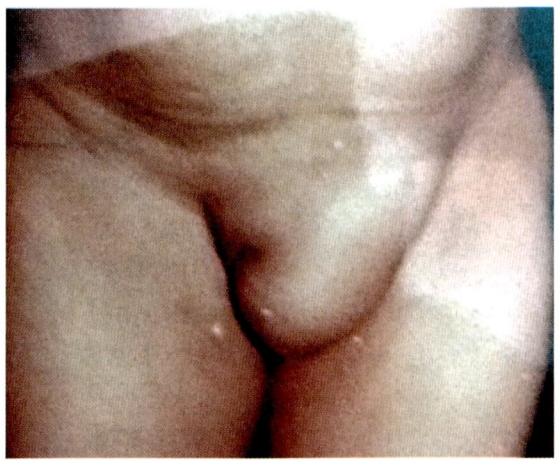

Fig. 13.1: Complete inguinal hernia in a female.

Swelling: The most **common complaint** is a **swelling** in the **groin.** Initially, the **size** is quite **small.** Over a **period of time** it **enlarges,** and the **patient** may notice that it **descends down** to the **scrotum.** The **swelling** becomes **more prominent** when the **patient stands up** or **during straining and coughing**, due to **increase** in **intra-abdominal pressure**. In the **early stages,** the **swelling disappears completely** on **lying down.** But later, especially when the **size is larger** or it is **inguinoscrotal,** the **swelling** may get **reduced partially** or **not at all.** Under

these **circumstances**, the **patient** almost always **tries** to **reduce** the **swelling** himself. Then the **following questions** need to be asked.

(*a*) Is the **reduction easy or difficult?**

(*b*) Is **reduction painful?**

(*c*) Is the **reduction partial or complete**?

This **information** is important to **assess** the **risk** of the **complications**.

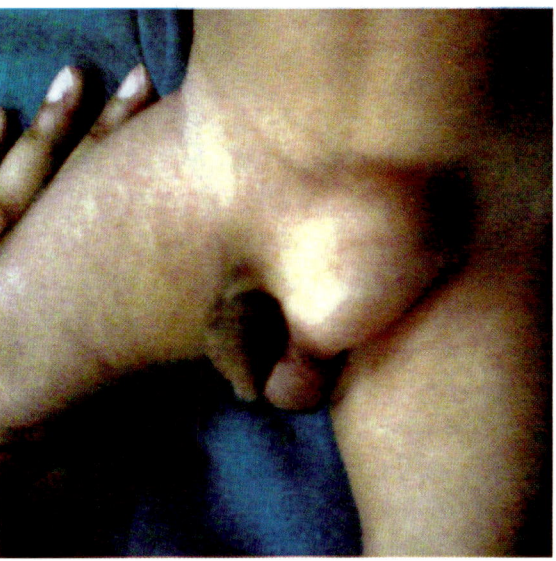

Fig. 13.2: Inguinal hernia in an infant.

PAIN Surprisingly, a small **hernia** may be **painful** because of the **narrow internal ring,** but majority of the **large hernias** are **painless**. Pain, when **present**, is of the **dull** or **dragging** type, due to **traction** on the **nerves** in the **mesentery** or an **adherent omentum.** In a **small group of patients**, particularly if they are **obese**, **pain** may be the **presenting symptom**, and if the **swelling** is **not obvious**, an **ultrasonography** is performed to clinch the **diagnosis.**

The **second group** of **symptoms** cause a **persistent increase** in the **intra-abdominal pressure.** These are usually referred to as **precipitating factors.** They may **precipitate** a **hernia** in the presence of **anatomical factors** mentioned above such as **persistent processus vaginalis** or **weak fascia transversalis.**

The precipitating factors include the following.

(*a*) **Respiratory symptoms** such as **chronic cough**, **breathlessness** etc. If the **patient** has any of **these symptoms**, all **further details** related to the **system** needs to be **asked for.**

(*b*) **Urinary symptoms** such as **difficulty** in **passing urine** etc. In **older males**, it is **mandatory** to elicit detailed **information** regarding **benign hypertrophy** of the **prostate.**

(*c*) **Chronic constipation.** If the answer is **positive**, **information** regarding **bleeding per rectum** and **tenesmus** are **inquired** into.

Personal history. History of **smoking** is **vital** because it causes **chronic bronchitis.** Persons who are **chronic smokers**, may have **severe cough** in the **postoperative period.** It is wiser to get such **patients** to **abstain** from this **habit** for about **six weeks** before performing **elective surgery.**

Local examination.

Inspection

Inspection always **starts** with the **patient** in a **standing position** and being made to **cough,** because the **risk** of **missing** a **small hernia** in an **obese patient** when he is **supine** is **real.** The **side** and **position** of the swelling, whether **inguinal** or **inguinoscrotal** are noted. Many **elderly males** have **bilateral swellings.** Hence **both groins** need to be **inspected** carefully. In a case of **inguinal hernia,** part of the **swelling** is seen to be **above** the **groin crease.**

Size and shape: The **shape** is classically described as **pear shaped.** The **size** varies, with a **giant hernia** descending **down** almost to the level of **middle** of the **thigh.**

Borders of the **swelling** are usually **well defined**

EXPANSILE impulse on **coughing** is the most **important inspection sign.** Interestingly, this is one of the **very few signs** where **inspection scores over palpation.**

Visible peristalsis: This sign is **likely** to be **positive** only in **some cases** of **inguinoscrotal hernia.** The **peristaltic movement** of the **bowel** present in the **hernia sac** is seen in the **scrotal part** of the **swelling** since all the **overlying layers are stretched** out and **thin.**

Inspection with the **patient** in the **supine position.** There are **three possibilities.**

(*a*) The **swelling disappears completely.**

(*b*) The **size** becomes smaller. Details regarding the **size, extent** and **shape** are to be **noted** at this **stage** again.

(*c*) The **size** of the **swelling** remains the **same.**

Palpation: In the group (*a*) mentioned above, **part of the palpation** is done with the **patient standing**, making the **examination** rather **difficult.** In all **other cases** palpation is done with the **patient** in the **supine position.**

Warmth and tenderness. Most of these swellings are neither tender nor warm.

Extent of the **hernia** is made out more **accurately** by palpation. If the hernia is **confined** to the **inguinal canal**, most often of the **indirect type**, it is known as a **bubonocele.** In the **remaining cases**, the **lower limit** may be at the **root**, the **middle** or the **bottom** of the **scrotum.**

Consistency is **soft:** A **granular feeling** gives the impression of the contents being **omentum.** An **elastic** feel suggests the presence of **bowel.**

Percussion: Resonance indicates bowel, and in general, a **dull note** signifies **omentum.** But the test is of **limited** value.

Auscultation: If **bowel sounds** are heard, it suggests **bowel** as the content.

Reduction: An **effort** is now made to **reduce** the **contents** back into the **abdominal cavity.** Commonly, the **inguinoscrotal variety** is more **difficult** to reduce. A **bimanual method** is employed for this **purpose.** With the patient **supine,** the **knee** and the **hip joints** are **flexed.** In addition, the **hip** is **internally rotated.** In this **position,** the **muscles** are **relaxed** and the **canal** is most **capacious.** The **right hand** is now **placed** at the **lower limit** of the **swelling** to apply **gentle pressure** to **push** the **swelling** in an **upward direction**, and the

left hand being **placed** at the **level** of the **external ring guides** the **contents** into the **peritoneal cavity** by application of pressure in an **anteroposterior direction**. At any stage of this **reduction**, if the **patient** complains of **pain**, the **test** should be **stopped**. The **results** of this test may be as follows.

(*a*) The **reduction** is **easy** and **complete**.

(*b*) The **reduction** is more **difficult** and takes a **longer time**.

(*c*) The **reduction** is **incomplete** and **contents** are still **felt** in the **proximal** part of the **hernial sac**. **Failure** to **reduce** the **contents completely** may be due to an **adherent omentum** or a **large segment** of the **small intestine** occupying the sac, preventing the return via a **small internal ring**.

Q. 7. Describe the deep ring occlusion test.

The test can be **performed** only if the **contents** can be **completely reduced**. The **deep** or the **internal ring** is situated **4 cm above** and **lateral** to the **pubic tubercle**. Clinically, the **pulsation** of the **femoral artery** at the **midinguinal point**

offers an easy **landmark** to perform this **test**. The **thumb** (corresponding to the **size** of the **normal ring**) is placed **1.25 cm above** this **point** and the **patient** is asked to **cough**. If the **swelling appears**, the hernia is of the **direct type** and **vice versa**. The **neck** of the **direct hernia sac** is formed by the **Hasselbach's triangle**. The **boundaries** are the **lateral border** of the **rectus** abdominis **medially** and the **inferior epigastric artery** on the **lateral** side; the **inferior margin** is formed by the **inguinal ligament**. It is necessary to perform this **test** because all **complications** are more **frequently seen** in an **indirect hernia,** owing to the **narrow** size of the **internal ring** as well as the **oblique nature** of the **inguinal canal**. The **limitation** of this test is that in a **large indirect hernia**, particularly **inguinoscrotal** in nature, the **internal ring** is very much **enlarged**. Under **these circumstances**, the **swelling** does **appear despite occluding** the **internal ring** with the **thumb**, and an **indirect hernia** may be mistaken for a **direc**t one. But with the almost **universal use** of a **prolene mesh** in the **repair** of this condition, this **limitation** is **not significant**.

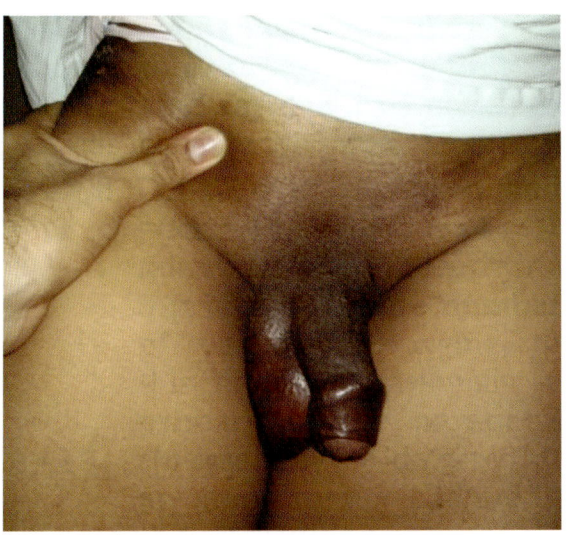

Fig. 13.3: Deep ring occlusion test.

Q. 8. How is the external ring invagination test performed?

External ring invagination test: The **purpose** of this **test** is to **determine** the **size** of the **external ring**. The **normal ring admits** the **tip** of the **little finger**. But this **space** is **occupied** by the spermatic **cord** in the **male**. Hence any **effort** to **do** the **test**, when the **ring** is **not enlarged**, results in **severe discomfort** to the **patient**, since the **testicular nerves** are being **compressed** during this **procedure**. The **method** of **performing** the **test** is as follows. The **little finger** is **invaginated** along the **scrotum** into the **external ring**. The oblique **pubic crest** is the **guide** to the proper **anatomical plane**. Once the **bony crest** is **felt**, the **finger** is moved **anteriorly** and the **edges** of the **ring** can easily

be **made out**. An **enlarged ring** assumes a **semicircular shape**. If there is any **doubt** about the **ring** at this stage, the **patient** is asked to **contract** his **abdominal muscles**, making the **edge** more **prominent**. If the **finger slips in** easily, with **no discomfort** to the patient, it is a clear **indication** that the **ring** is **enlarged**. At this **stage** the **patient** is made to **cough**. If the **impulse** is felt at the **tip** of the **finger,** it suggests an **indirect hernia**. In the case of a **direct hernia,** the **pulp** of the **finger** feels the **impulse**. But the **sensitivity** of this test is rather **low**.

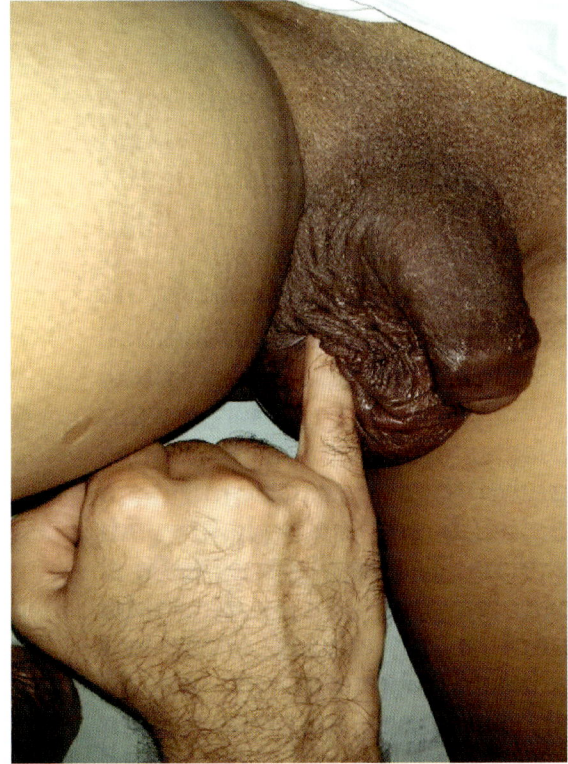

Fig. 13.4: External ring invagination test.

Q. 9. **How is the Zieman's test performed?**

This test is **useful** in **all types** of **groin hernias**, including the **femoral** hernia. After the **hernia** is **reduced**, the **index, middle** and **ring fingers** are **placed** correspondingly over the **deep ring**, the **external ring** and the **saphenous opening**. The **patient** is now made to **cough,** and depending upon **which finger** feels the **impulse** from **lateral** to the **medial** aspect, one can presume the **type** of hernia as **indirect inguinal**, or **direct or** lastly the **femoral. If** the **deep ring occlusion** and the **invagination tests** give **adequate information**, this test becomes **superfluous.**

Q. 10. **How is the tone of the abdominal muscles tested?**

In the **past,** when a **modified Bassini** or a **Shouldice type** of **repair** was being **performed regularly**, this test was an **important part** of the **clinical examination**. But presently, the **use** of a **prolene mesh** in most of the cases has made it **less important** But the **test** still needs to be **performed.** With the **patient supine** and the **elbows flexed** in **front** of the **chest**, the **state** of the **relaxed abdominal muscles** is **noted**. Now the

patient is made to **lift his head** and **upper part** of the **trunk**, and the **firm sensation** due to the **contracted muscles felt** by the **hand** signifies a **good muscular** tone. On the other hand, if the **muscles feel flabby** and **soft**, the tone is **poor**. Further multiple **Malgaigne's bulgings** will be seen in the **lower part of the abdomen** when the **tone** is **poor.** The test can also be **performed** by asking the patient to **raise both the lower limbs** with the **knee joints extended. Gravity,** in the form of **weight** of the part of the **body** raised, **provides** the **necessary resistance** to the **abdominal muscles**.

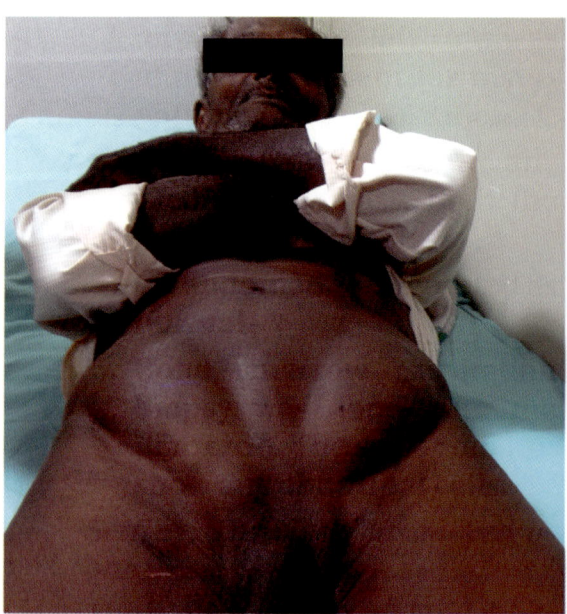

Fig. 13.5: Bilateral Malgaigne's bulgings indicating poor abdominal muscular tone.

External genitalia in the **male** is to be **examined carefully.** The male urethra is felt in the perenium. If there is a stricure, the urethra feels firm. An **associated vaginal hydrocele** will also be **revealed** during this phase of the examination.

Rectal examination is **mandatory** in **elderly males** even in the absence of **symptoms** of an **enlarged prostate**.

Examination of various systems. In the **presence of symptoms** related to the **precipitating factors** mentioned **above,** a **meticulous examination** of the **relevant systems** completes the **clinical examination.**

Diagnosis. In **most cases** the **diagnosis** is **easy**. More often than not, the **patient** is **aware** of the **condition** by the time he reaches the **hospital.**

Ultrasonography is useful to **detect** a **hernia** of **small size,** particularly in an **obese patient**. If the **surgery** is performed **laparoscopically,** the presence of a **concomitant hernia** on the **opposite side** is always **made out.** This is **important** in **children** in whom **bilateral hernias** are quite **common.** In the group of **patients where a** BHP is likely, the **post-voidal volume** of **urine** is assessed **accurately.**

When **symptoms and signs** due to **precipitating factors** are present **investigations** related to the **particular system** are required.

Q. 11. What are the complications of an inguinal hernia?

(*a*) **Irreducibility:** When a **swelling cannot** be **reduced completely** it is known as an **irreducible hernia**. Under these circumstances, **more dangerous complications** are likely to **occur** at a **later date**. The **cause** may be an **adherent omentum** or a **long loop of bowel** in a sac with a **narrow internal ring**.

(*b*) **Obstruction** is the **next stage** wherein the **lumen of the bowel** within the hernial **sac** is **obstructed,** but the **blood supply** to this **segment** is **still intact**. The **common sites** of **obstruction** are the **internal** and the **external rings**. The **bowel** tends to become **dilated** secondary to **obstruction,** and **oedematous** due to **lymphatic** and **partial venous obstruction** in the **wall** of the **obstructed bowel**. The **permeability** of the **bowel wall increases** allowing **fluid** from the **lumen** to **leak** into the **sac. Translocation** of **bacteria** makes this **fluid quite toxic. Symptoms** and **signs** of **intestinal obstruction** will be **present** at this **stage.**

(*c*) **Strangulation** is the **most dangerous** of all the **complications** of any **hernia.** The **blood supply** to the **bowel** in the **hernial sac** is **blocked** in this **complication.** It is only a **step away** from **obstruction,** and can **develop** in a **very short time.** The **veins** of the **mesentery** being **thin walled** are **compressed** in the **initial stages.** This **venous congestion aggravates** the **oedema** of the **bowel** and **leakage of fluid.** The **fluid** in the **sac** is **blood stained** and contains **both toxins** and **bacteria.** Absorption of this fluid leads to toxaemia. **High venous pressure reduces** the **tissue perfusion further.** In the **next stage,** the **arteries** in the **mesentery** are also **blocked.** Thus the **blood supply** to the bowel is lost leading to **wet gangrene** and **perforation.**

Symptoms and signs of **acute small intestinal obstruction** now become **obvious.** The patient complains of **sudden severe pain** along with **vomiting.** The **swelling** r**apidly increases** in **size.** More significantly, the **swelling** is **tense and very tender.** **Expansile impulse** on coughing is **absent. Distension** of the **abdomen** and **constipation** are **additional symptoms.** If **treatmen**t is **delayed, perforation** will occur with almost **lethal consequences.** The associated **toxaemia** or **septicaemia could be fatal** not only in **elderly patients** but also in those with **comorbid conditions** such as **diabetes** etc. **General peritonitis** will be seen only in a **small group** of patients with a **rare type** called **Maydl's hernia,** with the **gangrenous loop** being present **intraperitoneally.**

(*d*) **Richter's hernia** is a **special,** but **luckily uncommon** type of **strangulation** .In this condition, only a **part** of the **bowel,** usually along the **anti-mesenteric border** is present **inside** the **sac.** This **part** of the bowel **undergoes strangulation.** But the **symptoms and signs** of **small bowel obstruction** are **conspicuous** by their **absence.** A **high degree** of **suspicion** is **required** to make a **diagnosis.** A **previous history** suggestive of a hernia along with an **urgent ultrasonography** is very **helpful.**

(*e*) **Incarceration:** In **recent times,** this **term** has been used **instead** of **strangulation.** But traditionally, **incarceration** results from **inspissated** and **hardened faecal matter** in a loop of **large bowel inside** the **sac,** producing a **functional obstruction. Absorption** of **water** from the **contents** is **responsible** for this **uncommon complication.** A **sliding hernia** on the **left side** with the **sigmoid colon** as the **content is** the **precursor** in **most** of these **cases. Putty-** like contents that can be **indented** by **finger pressure** is said to be a **diagnostic feature.** More **often** than not, **these** patients are **explored** with a **diagnosis** of an **obstructed hernia** and the **true nature** detected only on the **operation table.**

(*f*) **Inflammation.** The **term is** used when the **contents** of a **hernial sac** undergo **inflammation.** This could be an **inflammation** of the **appendix** or the **fallopian tube and the ovary** in the female. **Sigmoid diverticulitis,** when this part of the **colon** is **inside** the **sac,**

could be another example. In addition, if the patient has **general peritonitis,** the **purulent fluid** can enter the sac and **add** to the **confusion.** The patient does **complain** of **pain** and **increase** in **size** of the swelling. The swelling is also **tender.** But it is **not tense** and the **expansile impulse** is still **present.** Examination of the **abdomen** may show **relevant findings** of **inflammation.** An **ultrasonogram,** and if time permits, a **CT scan** will help in the **diagnosis.**

(*g*) **Hydrocele of the hernial sac.** An uncommon complication, this occurs when a **plug** of **omentum blocks** the **neck** of a **complete indirect inguinal hernia.** The **fluid secreted** by the **omentum** collects in the **vaginal sac** producing a **hydrocele.** The patient has **mild dragging pain** associated with a **gradual increase** in the **size** of the swelling. A **typical history of hernia** is **available** in most **cases.** The **symptoms** are never dramatic like the situations described above. **Fluctuation** is elicited in the **scrotal part** of the **hernia** and the **firm granular omentum** is **palpable** at the **root** of the **scrotum.** In many instances **expansile** impulse may be **absent.** An **incomplete examination** may lead to a diagnosis of a **hydrocele,** and the ensuing a **scrotal approach** will cause **problems during surgery.** A **US** examination **confirms** the **diagnosis.**

Box 13.1:	Points regarding complications

- Irreducibility.
- Obstruction.
- Strangulation.
- Incarceration.
- Inflammation.
- Hydrocele of the hernial sac.

Q. 12. Is the presence of an inguinal hernia an indication for treatment?

In an **indirect hernia,** the **answer** is always **positive,** since all the **complications** described earlier are **more frequently** noted in **this type.** But the **direct one** has **few exceptions.** A **small group of patients** with **direct inguinal herniae** may be kept under **observation.** These are **elderly (+70) males** with **bilateral, small asymptomatic hernias** that **pop out** as soon as the **patient stands up,** to **disappear completely** as he **lies down.**

Q. 13. What are the operations performed for an inguinal hernia?

Herniotomy is indicated in **infants** and **young children.** The **procedure** consists of **identifying** the **hernial sac** via an **inguinal approach,** and **ligating** and **dividing** it at the **level** of the **internal ring.** The operation is based on **two anatomical facts.** The **hernia occurs** through a **patent processus vaginalis** and the **internal and external rings** are **superimposed on each other** at that **age,** with no intervening **canal** needing any **repair.**

History of surgery for **inguinal hernia** in **adults** makes very **interesting reading.** More than **200 operations** have been **described** for this **condition.** Only **two operations** stood the **test of time.** Both were **designed** to **strengthen** the weak **posterior wall** of the **inguinal canal,** and were known as **herniorraphies.** **Bassini's** and **Shouldice repairs** were **popular** for more than **100 years.** But the **recurrence rates** remained as **high** as **20%.** In addition, different **methods** of **hernioplasty** were also being **practiced.** It included the **use** of **fascia lata, skin** and **external oblique aponeurosis** with the same **objective** of **strengthening the posterior wall.** It became **clear** over a **period** of **time** that the **key** to a **successful treatment** of any **hernia is** to have a **TENSION-FREE REPAIR.** At the **present time, Lichtenstein's mesh hernioplasty** has become the **standard operation.**

Q. 14. Describe briefly Lichtenstein's hernioplasty.

An **incision** is made **parallel** and **1.25 cm** above the **medial two-third** of the **inguinal ligament**. **Skin and two layers** of the **superficial fascia** are **incised**. The **external oblique aponeurosis** is **incised along** the **direction of the incision** till the **external ring** is **opened**. The **cremasteric box** is now **exposed**. This **comprise**s of the **cremasteric muscle** and **fascia** and the **internal cremasteric fascia**. **Opening** the **cremasteric box** exposes the **contents**. In cases of **indirect inguinal hernia**, the **sac** is **anterolateral** and the **cord** is placed **posteromedially.** With **direct hernias**, the **cord** lies **in front** of the **sac**. The **sac** is identified by the **pearly white glistening appearance**. If the **sac** can be **emptied** of the **contents** by **milking movement** it is **not opened**. Otherwise, the **sac is opened** and the **contents** are **reduced**. **Adherent omentum** may have to be **separated** from the **sac** before **returning** it into the **peritoneal cavity**. The **sac** is **dissected carefully** from the **cord**. This **dissection** is continued till the **neck** of the **sac** is **reached**. The **neck** is recognised on the operation table by **three landmarks**. The neck is **narrow** especially in an **indirect hernia**. **Extraperitoneal pad** of **yellow fat** is **visible at the neck as well as the pulsations of the inferior epigastric** artery. The **neck** of the **sac** is now **transfixed, ligated and divided**. The **portion distal** to the **ligature** is **excised**. The **posterior wall** of the **canal** is **strengthened** by **placement** of a **prolene mesh**. It is placed as an **onlay mesh**, and is **anchored** to the **conjoint tendon** and the **inguinal ligament** with **prolene sutures**. A **slit** is made **laterally** for the **passage of the** spermatic cord. The **mesh acts** as a **scaffold** into which **living fibroblasts** grow **incorporating** this **foreign material** in the **body**. Since the **mesh** has a tendency to **shrink** over a **period of time**, the **mesh** should **extend** for about **three centimetres** beyond the **edge** of the **defect**. **Use** of the **mesh** has **brought down** the **incidence** of **recurrences** to about **0.2%,** and in **some hands** to even **zero**. The only **problem** associated with this **operation** is **infection**. An **infected mesh** needs to be **removed** for **control** of **infection,** thereby inviting a **recurrence**.

Q. 15. What is the role of laparoscopy in the treatment of inguinal hernia?

Laparoscopic repair is becoming a more **frequent** type of **hernioplasty.** The **defect** is approached from **within,** either **intra-abdominally Transabdominal Preperitoneal** (**TAPP**) or by the **extraperitoneal route Total Extra Peritoneal** (**TEP**). The **advantages** are that **all** the possible **defects,** namely, **indirect or direct inguinal** or even the **femoral** can be **corrected** by **placing** the **mesh** to cover all the **three defects.** In addition, a **single operation** is **curative** for **bilateral hernia.** Further, all **benefits** of **laparoscopic surgery** in general, like **less pain, shorter stay** in the hospital and **early return** to **work** are making this **operation** more **popular. Bilateral** and **recurrent** inguinal hernias are **definite indications** for this **procedure.** In a case of **recurrent hernia,** the **risk** of **damaging** the **cord structures** is **drastically reduced** by this **approach.** It is also **hoped** that in the **times to come** all **inguinal hernias** will be treated **laparoscopically.**

Q. 16. **What are the causes of recurrence in an inguinal hernia and what is the treatment?**

Despite all **advances** in field of surgery for this condition, **recurrences** do occur. The **causes** for **recurrence** can be **divided** into the following **three groups:**

(*a*) **Preoperative causes:** When a **precipitating factor** has been either **missed** or **inadequately treated** a hernia **will recur.** The **incidence** of this group has been **brought down** to a **large extent**, because most **patients** are **properly investigated** prior to **surgery.**

(*b*) **Intraoperative causes: Majority** of **recurrences** are related to **surgery.** When **herniorraphy** was the **common procedure**, the **repair** was not **tension free,** especially in a **large direct hernia,** and hence led to a **recurrence. Missing** an **additional sac** was mentioned as a **common cause.** This is **unlikely** to **occur** with the modern **laparoscopic approach.** A **portion** of the **sac** may be **retained** if the **neck** of the **sac is** not **clearly defined. Imperfect haemostasis** predisposes to **sepsis** and this is the **main culprit** these days. When the **mesh** is **removed** for **control of sepsis, recurrence** is likely to **occur.** Use of a **mesh** of **inadequate size** is also a **contributing factor**. Most **recurrences** occur in the **medial part** of the **inguinal canal.**

(*c*) **Postoperative causes:** **Inadequate convalescence** is **claimed** to be an **aetiological factor**. This is probably **true** if the **patient's work** demands **lifting heavy weights. Rest** for a period of **six weeks** is advised **after surgery,** especially for this **group.**

The **time interval** between the **first operation** and the appearance of a **recurrence** varies from a **few months** to **several years. Presence** of a **recurrent hernia** is a **definite indication** for **treatment**, since all **complications** enumerated above **occur more frequently** in this situation. A **clear bulge** at the **site** of the **scar** with **pain** is the **common mode** of **presentation.** Again, a **small sac** in an **obese person** may need **confirmation** with an **ultrasonogram.**

Q. 17. **What is the treatment of a recurrent inguinal hernia?**

Exploration via the **original incision** is **hazardous,** since there is an **increased risk** of **damaging** the **cord structures**. Therefore, a **laparoscopic** or a **preperitoneal** approach is **preferred. Placement** of a **mesh** is **mandatory.** Till **mesh** became **available, repeated recurrences** were seen **frequently.**

Box 13.2:	Points regarding causes of recurrence

- Preoperative – Missing a precipitating factor.
- Operative – Main reason.
- Missed sac – Incomplete removal of the sac – Repair under tension.
- Mesh – Inadequate size.
- Imperfect haemostasis – Sepsis – Demands removal of mesh.
- Postoperative – Inadequate convalescence.

FEMORAL HERNIA

Q. 1. **Describe the anatomy of the femoral canal.**

The **femoral canal** is a **rectangular space,** being the most **medial compartment** of the **femoral sheath.** It lies **below the inguinal ligament** and **medial** to the **pubic tubercle.** The **femoral sheath** is formed by the **fascia transversalis** anteriorly and the **fascia iliaca** posteriorly. It **covers** the **femoral vessels**. But the **medial compartment** forms the **femoral canal**. It is about **1.3 cm** in length and is usually empty. The **borders** of the **femoral ring** are as follows.

Anterior - **Inguinal ligament.**

Posterior - The **pubic ramus, iliopectineal ligament and pectineus muscle**.

Medial - **Lacunar ligament**.

Lateral - **Femoral vein.**

The **femoral ring** is covered by **fibrofatty tissue** forming a fragile **femoral septum**. It is **pierced by lymphatic vessels**. **Herniation** of the **intraperitoneal contents** through the **femoral septum** into the **canal** results in a **femoral hernia.**

Q. 2. **What is the incidence of femoral hernia?**

It is an **uncommon condition,** being responsible for only about **3%** of all hernias. It is more **common** in **women,** the reason being women have a **broader pelvis** with a **larger femoral ring**. But it is to be repeated that in **women, inguinal hernia** is more **common** than the **femoral.**

Q. 3. **What are the clinical features of a femoral hernia?**

Pain in the **groin** is the **chief complaint**. It may be **pricking in nature**. It may become **worse** on **change of posture.**

Swelling in the **groin**. Patients may present with a **painful lump**. The **size** of the swelling being **small,** the patient may **not** even be **aware** of its presence in some cases.

Most of our **patients** present with **complications**, **strangulation** being the most **frequent** one.

Q. 4. **What are the physical findings?**

A **swelling** is seen **below** the **inguinal ligament** on the **medial aspect**. It is often **small** in size being **oval** in **shape**. The **borders** are **ill defined**.

An **expansile impulse** may be felt on **coughing.** But in **obese patients** it is **difficult** to **feel** this **impulse**.

The **consistency** is **soft**. The **swelling** is usually not **reducible** since the **neck** of the sac formed by the **femoral ring** is **narrow.**

The **neck** is **below** and **lateral** to the **pubic tubercle**.

Q. 5. **What are the differential diagnoses?**

1. **Inguinal hernia:** It is often taught that though the **neck** of a femoral hernia is **below the inguinal ligament, the fundus** may **lie above the same** with the hernial **sac** assuming a **retort shape**. The **anatomical explanation** is as follows. The **membranous layer** of the superficial fascia of the anterior abdominal wall **extends** into the **thigh**. It is **attached** to the **fascia lata** (deep fascia of the thigh) along a **horizontal line drawn 2 cm below the inguinal ligament**. Hence a **large femoral hernia** does **not descend** into the **thigh,** but is forced to **turn upwards** and **laterally,** with the

fundus being **present** above the **inguinal ligament.** But in **practice** it is **very rarely seen,** since a **femoral hernia** becomes **symptomatic or complicated** much **before** this **stage** is reached.

Most often it is **easy** to **distinguish** between these **two types. Zieman's test** is also **useful** in this situation.

2. **Saphena varix:** It is a **globular swelling** resulting from **dilatation** of the **saphenous vein** close to its **junction** with the **femoral vein resulting from an incompetent sapheno femoral junction.** It may be **associated** with **varicosity** in the **limb.** It is a **soft compressible** swelling. The nature of the **cough impulse** is like a **fluid thrill.**

3. **Psoas abscess:** The **terminal part** of a **psoas abscess** may be felt as a **soft swelling** in the **medial side** of the **thigh.** But there is always a **larger component** in the **iliac region. Cross fluctuation** can be elicited **across** the **inguinal ligament.** Examination of the **lumbar spine** will **confirm** the **diagnosis.**

4. **Painful enlarged lymph node of Cloquet** may pose **problems. Presence** of a

septic focus in the **drainage area** may be **helpful. Absence** of an **expansile impulse** on coughing is a **useful sign.**

Q. 6. What are the complications?

Irreducibility: The **neck is narrow** and **many patients** present with this **complication.**

Obstruction: The **lumen** of the **bowel** present **inside the sac** is **blocked** at the **neck** leading to a **small bowel obstruction.** Patient will have a **painful swelling** in the groin with **symptoms** and **signs** of **intestinal obstruction.** A **cursory examination,** especially in **obese women,** may **miss** the **swelling** completely. In the **prescan days,** even **laparotomies** have been **performed** because a **plain X-ray** showed **air–fluid levels.**

Strangulation: Femoral hernia is the **most common type** of hernia to **develop** this life threatening **complication.** Patient has **severe abdominal pain** with **vomiting.** The **swelling** in the groin will be **very tender. Signs of obstruction** will be **present** in the **abdomen.** But a **Richter's type of strangulation** is **difficult** to **diagnose.** The swelling may be **mistaken** for an **infected lymph node or an abscess. Investigations** are often **needed** in this situation.

Q. 7. What are the investigations done in these cases?

US study: The **importance** of this study **cannot** be **over emphasised** especially in an **acute situation**. Even if there is the **slightest doubt** regarding a **hernia** it is **safer** to **order** an **US examination** rather than to **come** to **grief later**. An **enlarged lymph node** can easily be **distinguished** from the **hernial contents**.

CECT scan: It is needed when an **US study** does **not** give **adequate information**. A **small group of patients** presenting with **pain** in the groin but **with doubtful physical findings** may **benefit** from this **investigation**.

Q. 8. Is the presence of a femoral hernia an indication for treatment?

The answer is an **emphatic yes**. **Most** of our **patients** present with **complications,** thus demanding **emergency treatment**. Even those **remaining** are at **great risk** of **developing complications** because of the **narrow neck**.

Q. 9. What are the operations performed for a femoral hernia?

Similar to the **treatment** of an **inguinal hernia, surgery** for this condition has passed through **several stages**. It is **interesting** to note that even a **plug of bone** derived from the **iliac crest** was used to **obliterate the defect**. **Lockwood's low inguinal approach** has been **abandoned** due to the **limited exposure**.

Lotheissen's high inguinal operation was a **popular operation** for a long time. It **coincided** with the popularity of a **modified Bassini repair** for an inguinal hernia. It consisted of **approximating** the **conjoint tendon** to the **iliopubic tract,** thus **covering the femoral ring**. But the **limitations** were the **same**. A **tension-free repair** was **difficult** to achieve in **many patients**.

McEvedy's operation is useful for a **strangulated hernia** where **gangrenous bowel** is likely to be **present**. A **slightly oblique incision** is made about **4 cm above** the **inguinal ligament**. The **anterior rectus sheath** is **incised**. The **rectus muscle** is **retracted** exposing the **preperitoneal space**. The **hernial sac** is now **identified and opened. Gangrenous bowel** if present can be **resected**. It is **not possible** to perform **this step** with an **inguinal incision** described above. A **separate midline laparotomy** may be **needed** under these circumstances.

Mesh repair. The **availability** of the **mesh** has made a **tension-free repair** of a femoral hernia **easy**. An **inguinal incision** is made **1.3 cm** above the **inguinal ligament**. The **inguinal canal** is **opened**. An **incision** is made in the **fascia transversalis**. The **hernial sac** is **dissected** and **returned** to the **peritoneal cavity**. A **prolene mesh** is used to **cover the femoral ring**. The **mesh** is **fixed** to the **iliopubic tract** on the **medial side inferiorly**, thus **covering the defect**. **Laterally** it is **fixed** to the **inguinal ligament**. **Superiorly** it is anchored to the **conjoint tendon**.

An **alternative method** is to use the **mesh** like a **plug** to **block the femoral canal**. An **additional mesh** is used to **strengthen** the **posterior wall** of the **inguinal canal**.

Multiple Choice Questions

1. Deep inguinal ring is a defect in
   (*a*) External oblique aponeurosis
   (*b*) Internal oblique aponeurosis
   (*c*) Fascia transversalis
   (*d*) Preperitoneal fat
   Answer (*c*)

2. Which of the following is NOT a predisposing factor in development of an inguinal hernia
   (*a*) Pinhole meatus
   (*b*) Phimosis
   (*c*) Paraphimosis
   (*d*) Stricture urethra
   Answer (*c*)

3. All of the following nerves are related to the inguinal canal EXCEPT
   (*a*) Femoral branch of the genitofemoral nerve
   (*b*) Genital branch of the genitofemoral nerve
   (*c*) Ilioinguinal nerve
   (*d*) Iliohypogastric nerve
   Answer (*a*)

4. To reduce a complete inguinal hernia the patient should be supine with
   (*a*) Hips extended and internally rotated, knees flexed
   (*b*) Hips flexed and internally rotated, knees flexed
   (*c*) Hips extended and externally rotated, knees flexed
   (*d*) Hips flexed and externally rotated, knees extended
   Answer (*b*)

5. The gold standard today for inguinal hernia repair is
   (*a*) Lichtenstein's repair under local anaesthesia
   (*b*) Lichtenstein's repair under spinal anaesthesia
   (*c*) Bassini's repair under local anaesthesia

(*d*) Transabdominal preperitoneal repair (TAPP) under spinal anaesthesia

Answer (*a*)

6. Injury to the round ligament of the uterus during inguinal hernia repair produces

(*a*) Uterine prolapse

(*b*) No consequences

(*c*) Recurrence of the hernia

(*d*) Inguinodynia

Answer (*a*)

A CASE OF INCISIONAL HERNIA

Setting

- Surgical OPD.

Chief Complaint

- **Swelling** in the **region** of an **upper abdominal scar** of **1 year** duration.

History of Present Illness

- A **45-year-old man** presented to the **OPD** with the complaint of an **upper abdominal swelling** of **one year duration**. He had undergone an **elective operation 3 years ago**. He **noticed** a **small bulge** at the **site** of the **scar one year** ago. At that stage he had **no other complaints**. Over a period of **one year** the **swelling** had **gradually become bigger**. He **noticed** an **increase** in the **size** of the swelling on **coughing** or **straining** and while **passing urine**.

- He did **not** complain of **pain.**

- There was **no history** of **abdominal distension** or **vomiting.**

- His **bowel habits** were normal.

- He did not have **chronic cough** or **breathlessness.**

- There were **no urinary symptoms**.

- The **size of the swelling** had **brought** the patient to the **hospital.**

- Only **few details** regarding the **previous operation** were available. He had an **upper abdominal mass** with **dragging pain** for **2 years** prior to the **surgery**. A **CT scan** had been done and an **elective surgery** was performed a **week** after **admission. No specific advice** was given after the operation. He was totally **asymptomatic** for **2 years** after the **operation.**

- **Past and family histories** were not significant.

Occupation

- He was working as a **clerk** in a private company.

Personal History

- He was a **beedi smoker** for the last **20 years**. There was no history of consumption of alcohol or chewing paan.

- **General physical examination** was normal.

Examination of Abdomen

Inspection

- Patient in **standing position.**
- A **swelling** was **visible** in the **upper abdomen**. It was extending from **2 cm below** the **xiphisternum** to the level of the **umbilicus.** Horizontally it was extending **6 cm** on **either side** of the **midline**. The **margins** were **well defined**.
- The **shape** was a **vertical oval.** The **size** was **15 cm by 12 cm.**
- There was an **expansile impulse** on **coughing.**
- A **midline thin linear scar** was visible over the **summit of the swelling** extending from the **xiphisternum** to the **umbilicus.** The **skin** over the swelling was **stretched.**
- **No dilated veins** were seen.
- The **surface** was **smooth.**
- The **surrounding area** appeared normal.
- The **inguinal region** did not show **any bulge** on **coughing.**
- The **external genitalia** appeared normal.
- **Inspection** with the patient in **supine position**.
- There were **no changes** in the **clinical findings**.

Palpation

- The swelling was neither **warm nor tender.**

- An **expansile impulse** on **coughing** was felt during palpation.
- It was **soft** and **granular** in **consistency.** The **borders** were **well defined.**
- The **skin** was **free** from the swelling **except around the scar.**
- It was **reducible**. The patient was made to **flex** his **knee and hip joints** during the reduction. The **reduction** was **easy, complete and painless.**
- The **head raising test** revealed a **defect** in the **midline** measuring **8 cm by 4 cm** in size.
- **No mass** was **palpable** in the abdomen.
- The **tone** of the **abdominal muscles** was **good.**
- The **external genitalia** were normal on palpation.

Percussion

- The **swelling** was **dull** on percussion.

Auscultation

- **No bowel sounds** were **heard** over the swelling.
- **Rectal examination** was normal.
- **Examination** of the **respiratory system** did not show any abnormality.
- **Other systems** were **clinically normal.**

Q. 1. What was the diagnosis?

A diagnosis of an **incisional hernia** was made. The **clinical findings** would **not entertain** any other **differential diagnosis**.

Q. 2. What were the investigations done in this patient?

US abdomen: It confirmed the presence of a **large incisional hernia** with **bowel** and **omentum** as contents. **No other abnormality** was detected in the **abdomen.**

Chest X-ray was normal.

Setting: A week passes. During this period, the patient was told to **abstain** from **smoking** completely. **Chest physiotherapy** was conducted vigorously.

Q. 3. How was this patient treated?

He underwent a **mesh repair** of the hernia.

An **elliptical incision** was made to include the **scar and the umbilicus**. The **skin** including the **scar** was **separated** from the **hernial sac** taking care **not to open** the **peritoneal cavity**. The **sac** was found to have a **very thin wall**. On **either side flaps** were **raised** till the **edge of the sac**. The plane was between the **membranous layer** of the subcutaneous tissue and the **sac**. Both **omentum and bowel** could be seen **through** the **thin wall** of the sac. The **contents** were **reduced** into the **peritoneal cavity.**

The **anterior rectus sheath** was now **exposed** for about **4 cm** beyond the **edge of** the defect on all sides. The **upper limit** was at the **xiphisternum** and the dissection was carried out **beyond the level of the umbilicus**. A **prolene mesh** which would **extend 3 cm beyond the edges** of the defect was chosen for **repair**. The **mesh** was **anchored** to the **edges** of the defect with **interrupted prolene sutures**. Care was taken **not to injure the bowel** at this stage of the operation. The **edges of the mesh** were then **fixed** to the **abdominal wall** with a continuous **prolene suture 3 cm lateral** to the **first layer** of sutures. **Absolute haemostasis** was ensured at the end of the operation. **Closure** of the incision with a **suction drain** completed the operation.

The **drain** was removed **after 48 hours**. The patient as discharged on the **5th day**. He was asked to come for review 3 weeks later.

He attended the OPD after 3 weeks. The **incision** had **healed** very **well**. The **repair** appeared to be **sound**. He was advised **not** to **lift heavy weights** for **6 weeks**. He was also told to **stop smoking permanently**.

Q. 4. Define an incisional hernia.

An **incisional hernia** is **any gap** in the **abdominal wall with or without a bulge** in the area of a **postoperative scar** that can be **seen** or **felt** on **clinical examination** or detected by **imaging.**

Q. 5. What is the incidence of incisional hernia?

The reported incidence varies from **3% to 20%.** But the figures are **variable.** The **highest incidence quoted is 66%** with an average of **26%.**

Q. 6. What are the risk factors?

These can be broadly **divided into 3 groups.**

 1. **Patient factors.**

Age: The incidence is **higher after the age** of **45 years.** **Impaired wound healing** in older individuals can be explained by **delayed fibroblast migration** and **structural changes** with **reduced collagen formation.** **Comorbid conditions** are more often seen in this group.

Gender: There is some evidence to show that it is **more frequent** in **women.**

Diabetes and obesity are important risk factors.

Anaemia.

Malignancy.

Corticosteroids: It is well known that these **drugs impair wound healing.** Use of this **drug** in **combination** is **common** in **our country.** It is extremely **difficult** to obtain an **accurate drug history** from our patients. **Self-medication** with **steroids,** especially for conditions like **asthma i**s often seen.

Previous radiation though **uncommon** is a factor to be reckoned with.

Smoking has been proved to **impair wound healing.** Hence smokers have a higher incidence.

Connective tissue disorders. The **quality** of the **connective tissue** of the **anterior abdominal wall** has been shown to be **inferior** in many of these patients.

Box 13.3:	Points regarding the factors related to the patient

- Age and sex.
- Diabetes, obesity, anaemia and malignancy.
- Corticosteroids and radiation.
- Smoking.
- Connective tissue disorder.

 2. **Operative factors:** These are considered to be the **most important** of all the factors.

Incision: A **midline incision** has the **highest incidence.**

This is the most **popular incision** employed by **surgeons.** The **subumbilical midline incision** in **women constitutes** a **vast majority**. The reasons are said to be as follows.

The **linea alba** is a **less vascular** structure.

The **contractions of** the **abdominal muscles** tend to **pull the edges away** from each other.

The **fibres of the linea** are placed in a **transverse or oblique direction**. A **vertical incision cuts through** these tissues and **reduces** the inherent **strength.**

The **absence** of a **posterior rectus sheath below** the **arcuate line makes the anterior abdominal wall weaker.**

Pfannenstiel incision is frequently used by gynaecologists. But the **recti are separated** in the **midline**. Hence the **disadvantages** of a **midline incision** are **present** in this **incision.** In addition **multiple defects** are common (**swiss cheese appearance**). Further if the **exposure is not adequate**, **lateral cuts** are given on

some occasions dividing the **internal oblique** and the **transversus abdominis** muscles. If these are **not approximated properly,** an **incisional hernia** at the **lateral end** of the incision is the result.

Paramedian, transverse and oblique incisions are **less prone** for development of a hernia. But even a **muscle-splitting incision** like **McBurney's** is **not immune** from developing a hernia.

Technique: Gentle handling of all **tissues** is of paramount importance. **Too much** of **traction** tends to **reduce** the **viability** of the **tissues.**

Enterotomy: One of the **main operative problems** is an **accidental enterotomy**. **Densely adherent bowel** may easily be **injured** during the **mobilisation of the sac.** It can be **sutured immediately,** but **sepsis increases the risk of incisional hernia considerably**.

Closure: Use of **absorbable sutures** leads to a **higher incidence**. The strength of a **wound depends** on the **suture material** for the **first four weeks**. It takes about

6 months for the incision to attain 80% of the tensile strength. Hence PDS or prolene should be used for closure of incisions. The sutures are to be placed at a distance of 1 cm from each other and the lateral bites should also be 1 cm away from the edge. The total length of the suture should be 4 times the length of the incision.

Imperfect haemostasis: Extensive dissections are needed for large hernias, especially if the component separation technique is followed. Hence the chances of haematoma formation are higher despite the use of suction drains. It increases the incidence of sepsis.

3. Postoperative factors: Abdominal distension following paralytic ileus will produce increased intra-abdominal pressure and enhance the development of hernia. Again postoperative cough also increases the pressure.

The main problem will be infection. If the wound gets infected the infection will not be controlled until the mesh is removed.

Box 13.4:	Points regarding operative and postoperative factors

- Incision – Midline commonest – Subumbilical in women.
- Pfannenstiel – Subumbilical – Midline – Multiple - Lateral extensions.
- Technique – Gentle handling – Extra traction – Accidental enterotomy.
- Closure – PDS or prolene – Technique – 1 cm apart – Total length 4 times incision.
- Postop – Abdominal distension – Cough.
- Sepsis – Mesh needs to be removed – Recurrence.

Q. 7. When does an incisional hernia appear?

A wound dehiscence or a burst abdomen has become an uncommon event at the present time.

Most hernias are detected between 6 months to 2 years after the operation. But studies have shown that the separation of the wound edges takes place as early as within the first four weeks after surgery. They become clinically manifest after a period of time. 50% are detected within one year after the surgery. Later the percentage of developing a hernia is 2% every year. The figures available from our country may not present a true picture since patients tend to seek medical advice only after severe symptoms develop or development of a

complication. But a **hernia** can develop **even 10years later**. The **latter type** is said to be the result of a **connective tissue disorder** in the patient.

A **laparoscopic approach** has **reduced** the **incidence** of this condition. But it has also resulted in the appearance of an uncommon **port site incisional hernia.**

The **reluctance** of our patients to **report** till either the hernia reaches a **large size** or the **development of complications, delays the treatment** further. Havingundergone**oneoperation earlier,** this **reluctance is** to be **expected.**

Q. 8. **What are the clinical features?**

A **bulge or a swelling** in the region of the **scar.** The **size** may be **aesthetically disturbing** to the patient, especially in women, though the **Indian saree** tends to **mask** many a **subumbilical swelling.** Giant **incisional hernias** wherein most of the **bowel is outside the peritoneal cavity** is still **seen** in **our country**. An **attempt** to **reduce the contents** and **repair the hernia** may result in the **development** of an **abdominal compartment syndrome** in such patients.

Pain is a **common symptom.** It is often **colicky** and results from **partial obstruction** of **adherent bowel. Obstruction** may be the result of **adhesions** between the **bowel and the hernial sac** or **between loops of bowel.**

Attacks of **vomiting** may accompany these **episodes of pain.**

A **good percentage** of **our patients** present **with complications.**

Q. 9. **What are the physical findings?**

The patient must be made to **stand** during the first part of inspection.

A **small indistinct bulge** may be seen in the region of the **scar.** On the other hand, in some patients, a **large swelling** occupying **many quadrants** is seen, especially in the **lower abdomen**.

There is an **expansile impulse** on **coughing**.

The **margins** are distinct **except** in **obese** patients.

The **skin** over the swelling is **stretched.** The **scar** may be **broad and irregular** suggesting postoperative **sepsis.** Areas of **hyper-** or **hypo-pigmentation** are often seen.

Uncommonly in **large hernias** with an extremely **thin skin and sac, visible peristalsis** may be present.

Inspection with the **patient in supine position.**

The swelling may become **smaller in size**. But in many patients the **swelling** remains the **same in size.**

The **shape is** usually a **vertical oval.**

Hernial orifices. There may be an associated **inguinal hernia.**

External genitalia.

Box 13.5:	Points regarding the inspection findings

- Patient standing. Site and extent.
- Size and shape – Margins.
- Expansile impulse on coughing.
- Skin over the swelling – Scar – Pigmentation.
- Patient supine – Change in size.
- Hernial orifices.
- External genitalia.

Palpation: Warmth and tenderness are absent.

Size and shape: The **size** may be **larger** in **obese patients.**

Borders: On palpation the borders are usually **well defined.**

Consistency: It is most often **soft.** A **granular feel** may suggest **omentum** as one of the contents.

Skin: It is **adherent around the scar** to the underlying **swelling**, but it will be **free** in the **periphery.**

Reducibilty: Most hernias are **not completely reducible** because of **adhesions** between the **contents** and the **sac.**

Size of the defect: This has a **direct impact** on the **management. Clinically** this can be **determined** only if the **hernia is completely reducible. Having reduced the hernia,** the patient is asked to perform **the head raising test. The edges** of the **defect** can now be **distinctly felt** and the **size** can be **assessed accurately. Most** of these are in the **midline between the recti.**

Mass in the abdomen: Uncommonly, there may be a **palpable mass** in the abdomen. It may be **related** to the **original disease** for which a **laparotomy** had been done **earlier.** But it may be a **feature** of a **disease de novo.** The **nature** of the **mass** determines the **priority of treatment.**

Tone of the abdominal muscles. The **head raising** or the **straight leg raising test** will determine the **tone of the muscles.** With the **mesh being used** in most cases, **the test** has now become **less important.**

Box 13.6:	Points regarding palpation

- Site and extent – Borders.
- Size and shape – Larger than inspection in obese patients.
- Consistency – Soft – Granular – Omentum.
- Reduction – Not possible in many – Adhesions.
- If reducible – Size of defect – Muscles contracted.
- Tone of abdominal muscles.

Percussion and auscultation.

A **resonant note** indicates the presence of **bowel.** An **impaired resonance** is a common finding because of the presence of both **omentum and bowel**.

Auscultation: If **bowel sounds are heard**, the presence of **bowel** is confirmed.

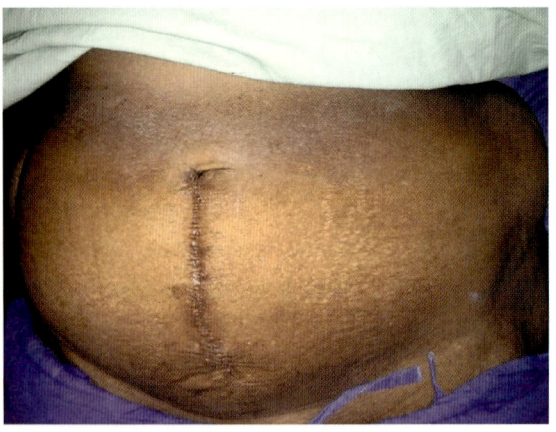

Fig. 13.6: Subumbilical incisional hernia.

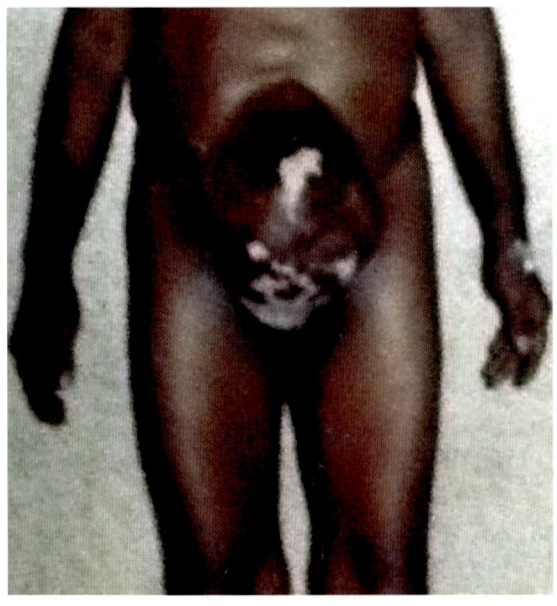

Fig. 13.7: Large incisional hernia with skin changes.

Q. 10. How is a diagnosis made in these cases?

In **most instances** the diagnosis is **easy.** The **appearance** of a **swelling** in relation to an **operative scar** is enough to identify the **hernia.** An **expansile impulse** on coughing along with **reducibility** when present, clinches the diagnosis.

The **problem** arises when an **obese patient** presents with **pain** in the **region** without an obvious **bulge** or a **swelling**. Even an **impulse on coughing** may be **difficult** to elicit in these patients. **Investigations** are **needed** under these circumstances.

Q. 11. What are the investigations?

US abdomen: It **confirms** the **diagnosis**, especially in **obese** patients with **small** hernias. It also identifies the **contents** as **omentum** or **bowel.** The study can assess the **size of the defect** even if the hernia is **not completely reducible.**

CECT scans are needed only if the **US findings** are **equivocal.** It is the **most reliable investigation** to confirm or rule out the **presence of a hernia.** The scan may also pick up **other pathologies** if they are present in the **abdomen.**

Q. 12. Is the presence of an incisional hernia an indication for treatment?

The presence of an incisional hernia is an **indication for treatment** because of the risk of **development of complications**. Some of these are **life threatening**.

Q. 13. What are the complications?

A **high percentage** of **our patients** attend the **hospital** after the development of **complications.**

As mentioned earlier, many are **irreducible** at the time of presentation.

Strangulation can occur if the **neck is small**. **Gangrenous bowel** poses problems in the **management.** Under those circumstances, the **morbidity** is **high** as are **recurrence rates.**

Obstruction will occur due to **adhesions.** If an adhesion were to cause a **twist, strangulation** and **gangrene** will follow.

Rupture: It is an **uncommon complication**, but is still seen in our country. The overlying **skin** and the **sac** become **extremely thin** before **giving way** for the intestinal loops to **protrude outside**. It is a **fascinating site** to see a lady covering the **exposed bowel** in a **plantain leaf** and **wearing a saree on top**, attending the OPD.

Box 13.7:	Points regarding complications

- Irreducibility – Adhesion between contents and sac – Between loops of bowel.
- Obstruction – Narrow neck – Uncommon – Adhesion – Common.
- Strangulation – Narrow neck – Uncommon – Twisting of a loop – Loss of blood supply.
- Rupture – Uncommon – Large hernia – Very thin skin and hernial sac.

Q. 14. What are the principles of management?

Incisional hernia is one of those conditions where the **treatment** is still **evolving.** The fact that **several procedures** are being **practiced** even today is ample **proof** that a stage of **zero recurrence** has **not** yet **been reached**.

Conservative treatment. This is advised for **patients** who belong to the **high risk** group. They usually have **morbid obesity** with **comorbid conditions** like **diabetes** or **cardiac** or severe **pulmonary disease**. Invariably the **hernia is quite large**. Such patients are advised to **wear** a custom made **abdominal corset** to have some **symptomatic relief.**

Patients with **giant incisional hernias** need special **preoperative preparation**. As mentioned earlier, they run the **risk** of developing an **abdominal compartment syndrome** immediately **after** the **operation,** which can be **fatal.** Inducing an **artificial pneumoperitoneum** to **increase the capacity** of the **peritoneal cavity** is a simple method. It may take a **couple of weeks** to attain this **objective** by gradually **increasing** the **quantum of air** introduced into the **peritoneal cavity.**

Q. 15. Describe the operations done for an incisional hernia.

Open surgery. Several operations have been described for the relief of this condition. The **success rate** of any operation can be **assessed** only if the patients are **followed** up for **10 years.** Many **popular operations** of the **past** are **no longer practiced** because of the **high rates of recurrence.** The **advent** of the **mesh** and **laparoscopy** has made a **significant difference** in the management of this condition.

It was **realized very early** that **bringing the edges** of the **defect together** even **without any tension,** was an **inadequate procedure.** The **poor quality** of the **tissue** made **recurrences inevitable.** Hence **placement** of a **mesh** is an **integral part** of **most of the operations** practiced at the present time.

Onlay mesh repair. It is used when the **edges of the defect** can be **approximated without tension (gap less than 3 cm).**

This is useful for **subumbilical hernias.** The **adherent scar** is **separated** from the **hernia sac** by careful dissection. One should **avoid opening** the **peritoneal cavity.** Much more important is to **avoid** an **accidental enterotomy,** which can increase the **postoperative morbidity.** The **scar is excised.** The **hernial sac** is dissected free **on all sides.** It is then **inverted back** into the **peritoneal cavity** with the **contents.** The **edges** of the gap are now **clearly defined.** **Interrupted prolene sutures** are used to **approximate the edges.** A **second layer** may be used to **invert** the **first** one to act like a **buttress.** A **prolene mesh** is now placed over the **area (onlay repair)** and **anchored** with **interrupted prolene sutures at the midline.** A **second layer of sutures** are used to **fix the mesh** at its edges to the abdominal wall. These sutures are to be placed a minimum of **3 cm beyond** the **suture line** on the midline.

A **modification** is required if the **gap is large**. It is more often seen in the **upper abdomen** since the **rigid costal margin prevents** a **tension-free approximation**. Once the **hernial sac** is **inverted no attempt** is made to bring the edges together. A **large mesh** is placed **over the defect** to cover an **area 3 cm to 4 cm** beyond **the edges**. The **mesh** is **fixed to the edges** of the **defect** with interrupted **prolene sutures**. A **second layer of sutures anchors** the **edges of the mesh** to the **healthy abdominal wall.** This needs **extensive dissection** of the **anterior abdominal wall.**

Both **these operations** have given **good results**. The inherent **disadvantage** in the use of the mesh is **sepsis**. If the wound is **infected,** the **morbidity is high**. Unless the **mesh is removed**, this infection will **not be controlled** and a **recurrence** becomes a **certainty.**

Preperitoneal placement of the mesh (Stoppa procedure). It is useful for **lower abdominal hernias**. A **large preperitoneal space** is created by **blunt dissection** after the **hernial sac** has been **dissected**. A **mesh** is now **placed** in this **space** extending from the **pubis to the umbilicus vertically** and **laterally** till the **iliac crests**. **No** attempt is made to **fix** this **mesh** in place. The **positive intra-abdominal pressure** is said to **maintain** this **mesh in its position.** The operation is **technically difficul**t, but **covers the lower half** of the **anterior abdominal wall** adequately. Hence the **recurrence rates** are very **low.**

Component separation technique. (Ramirez operation). The **advantage** as it was originally described was that it was a **meshless repair**. It is **primarily** used for **large upper abdominal hernias,** especially in **men**. The **hernial sac** is dissected and **inverted** into the peritoneal cavity like in **any other procedure**. The **lateral skin flaps** are **raised** till the **anterior axillary line**. The **external oblique aponeurosis** on **either side** is **incised** at this **level**. The **flap** containing the **external oblique** and the **recti** is **separated** from the **internal oblique** on both sides and **mobilised medially**. It is now **possible** to **bring the edges** of the **defect together without tension.**

A **gap of 10 cm** size can be **repaired** in this fashion. The **two medial flaps** are **approximated** in the **midline** with **interrupted prolene sutures**. The **lateral edge** of the **external oblique** is **anchored** to the **deeper layers** with **interrupted sutures**.

Recent **modifications** incorporate a **mesh** in this repair. An **onlay mesh** is **fixed** on the **midline suture line. Laterally two meshes** are placed on the **internal oblique** at the **edges** of the **separated external oblique** to **strengthen** the **abdominal wall.**

The operation is not very **popular** because it involves **extensive dissection** of the **abdominal wall**. It is a **time consuming** operation. **Haematoma** and **flap necrosis** are the common **postoperative complications**. In addition once a **mesh** is **used** the **advantage** of a **meshless repair** is **lost.**

Q. 16. Describe briefly the laparoscopic repair of an incisional hernia.

Laparoscopic repair of incisional repair is the **most popular operation** for this condition. The **hernia** is approached from within the **peritoneal cavity**. The **contents** are **reduced** under **vision. Adherent omentum** is released. A component **mesh**

with an **inner layer of vicryl** and an **outer layer of prolene** (**sandwich mesh**) is used to **cover the defect (inlay placement)**. The **mesh** should **extend 3 cm to 4 cm** beyond the **edges of the defect**. The **mesh** is anchored in **place** with the help of **tackers. Transfascial sutures** are a **less expensive** method of **mesh fixation**. A **prolene mesh** is **not used** in this **location. Bowel** is likely to get **adherent** to the **mesh**. It may result in **intestinal obstruction**. If the **bowel wall** is **eroded**, a **faecal fistula** will be the result. It is the **most dreaded complication** following a mesh repair. **Biological meshes** are now available. They **avoid** most of the **problems** associated with the **conventional mesh**. But they are **more expensive**.

The following are the **advantages** of this approach.

The **dissection** is **minimal.** The approach **avoids** the **previously operated area.** The problems of **identifying** the **proper tissue planes** are **absent**. The **risk** of **infection** is **reduced.**

Reduction of contents is **easier** as compared with the open surgery.

Multiple defects (common following a **Pfannenstiel** incision) are **easily identified**.

A **large mesh** can be used to cover **all the weak areas**.

The **main disadvantage** is that the chance of **accidental injury to the bowel** is higher in this approach. The **cost** of the **sandwich mesh** may be **too high** for many of our patients. **Port site hernias** have been described following this operation.

Despite all these developments, the **recurrence rate** has **not** yet touched **zero**. The figures quoted at the present time range between **3% and 20%.** It is likely that in **future** most incisional hernias will be **repaired laparoscopically**. In addition **better understanding** of the **aetiological factors** including the **biological aspect** should **help in reducing** the **incidence** of these hernias.

Box 13.8:	Points regarding surgical treatment

- Onlay repair – Defect 3 cm or less – Lower abdomen.
- Approximation of the edges – Onlay mesh – 3 cm to 4 cm beyond the suture line.
- Defect larger – Onlay mesh – Fixed to the edges – Edge of the mesh anchored – 3 cm to 4 cm away.
- Stoppa operation – Lower abdomen – Preperitoneal placement of the mesh.
- Lower half of the abdomen – Low recurrence rates.
- Component separation – External oblique flap mobilised by lateral division.
- Closure in midline – Defect of 10 cm size – Covered.
- Lengthy operation – extensive mobilization – haematoma and flap necrosis

Box 13.9:	Points regarding laparoscopic repair

- Popular – Minimal dissection – Sepsis less common.
- Multiple defects – Identified.
- Size of defect – Not significant – Large mesh to cover weak areas.
- Component mesh – Ideal – Fixed with tackers or transfascial sutures.
- Prolene mesh not used – Adhesions – Obstruction.
- Bowel erosion – Faecal fistula.
- Accidental enterotomy.
- Cost of the mesh.
- Port site hernia.

Q. 17. Describe the clinical features of an umbilical hernia in an infant.

The **umbilical defect** is present in the **foetus** for the passage of the **umbilical vessels.** This usually **closes spontaneously** within a **few months** after **birth**. The mother may bring the **child** with a **complaint of a swelling** in the **umbilical region**. Most are **easily reducible**. Following **reduction**, a **small defect** is felt **directly** under the **umbilical scar.**

Q. 18. What is the treatment?

These children can be **observed** till the age of **four years** since **most defects** tend to **close spontaneously**. Complications like **strangulation** demand **treatment**. Again a **large hernia** may need **treatment** at a **younger age. Strapping** with or without a **coin** is **no longer practiced**.

Repair of the defect is the **procedure** needed for these children. A **subumbilical incision** is made and the **sac** is **exposed**. The **contents** if any are **reduced**. The **defect** is closed **transversely** with a **prolene sutures**. The umbilical **skin** is **fixed** to the **abdominal wall** to **reproduce** the **depressed appearance**.

Q. 19. Describe the features of an umbilical hernia in an adult.

Most of these are **paraumbilical** hernias due to a **defect** in the **linea alba,** just **above** the **umbilicus**. But in **women**, the **defect** may be **subumbilical**. **True umbilical hernia** persists in a **few adults**. A **button** of **the greater omentum herniates** through a small **defect** when the **patient strains**. They are **asymptomatic** and **do not need** any **treatment**.

Paraumbilical hernias can assume a **large size**. The **umbilicus** is **displaced** usually **downwards**. It can cause **dragging type** of **pain**. It is also liable for the **complications**

described in relation to **other hernias**. Hence it **needs treatment**.

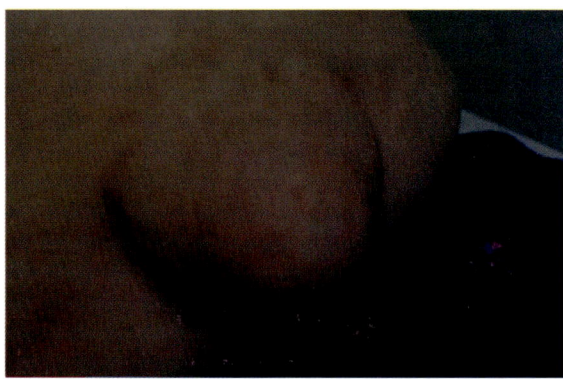

Fig. 13.8: Large paraumbilical hernia.

Q. 20. What is the treatment for a paraumbilical hernia?

Mayo's operation comprising of **double breasting** the **anterior rectus sheath** to **cover the defect** was a **popular operation** in the **past**. But the **cause** for **herniation** is probably the **poor quality** of the **connective tissue** in the **anterior abdominal wall**. Hence a **mesh** is used to **cover the defect** at the **present time**. The **principles** are the **same** as for an **incisional hernia**.

Q. 21. What is a fatty epigastric hernia and how is it treated?

A **fatty epigastric hernia** is the result of **herniation** of **extraperitoneal fat** through a tiny **defect** in the **linea alba.** These **small openings** are meant for the **passage of blood vessels** supplying the **subcutaneous region** and the **skin.** This **hernia** is **unique** in that it does **not have** a **peritoneal sac.** Over a **period of time** some of them **enlarge** to become a **true epigastric hernia**. It has a **sac** filled usually with **greater omentum.**

The hernia appears as a **small midline swelling** between the **xiphisternum** and the **umbilicus**. It is **painful and tender. Expansile impulse** may be **difficult** to elicit because of the **small size.** They are **not reducible**. Occasionally they **simulate** the symptoms of **acid peptic disease (APD).** An **endoscopy** is needed to **rule out APD.**

Since a **fatty epigastric hernia** is **symptomatic,** it needs **treatment.** A **small incision** is made **over the swelling**. The **defect** in the **linea alba** is slightly **enlarged** to **return** the **fat** to the **extraperitoneal space**. The **defect** is **closed transversely** with **interrupted prolene sutures.** A **large epigastric hernia** is treated like a **paraumbilical hernia** with a **prolene mesh.**

■■■

Hydroceles

14

A CASE OF VAGINAL HYDROCELE

Setting

- Surgical OPD

Chief Complaint

- **Swelling** of the **right side** of the **scrotum** of **5 years** duration.

History of Presenting Illness

- A **28-year-old male** patient presented to the OPD with complaints of a **swelling** in **the right side** of the **scrotum,** which was **initially small** to begin with and had **gradually increased** in **size** over a period of **5 years. Pain** was **rarely present,** and when present was **dull** in nature or associated with **a heavy dragging** sensation **down** the **scrotum.** However, the feeling of **discomfort** had been **increasing** since past **few days**.

General Physical Examination

- No **abnormality** could be identified on general physical examination.

Local Examination

Inspection

- At the time of **inspection**, the patient was asked to stand and cough.
- There was **no bulge** in the **groin, thereby ruling out** an associated **inguinal hernia.**
- **Side:** The **scrotal swelling** was **unilateral** and present on the **right side.**
- **Size:** The swelling appeared to be **the size** of a **large orange**.
- **Shape:** The swelling appeared **oval** in shape.

- **Skin** over the swelling was **stretched**, as shown by the **loss of scrotal rugosities**.
- **Surface** was **smooth**.
- **Dilated veins** were present over the **swelling**. These were probably the **result** of the **stretching of the skin**.
- **Shift** of the **median raphe** to the **left side** was observed.
- The **penis** was **deviated** to the **left side**.

Palpation

- The **swelling** was neither **tender** nor **warm**.
- Shape and size. It was oval in shape measuring 8 cm and 5 cm in size.
- It was **possible** to **get over** the **swelling** proving that it was a **scrotal swelling** (Fig. 14.1).
- **Consistency** was **soft.**
- **Fluctuation** was **positive** (Figs 14.2 and 14.3).
- **Transillumination** was **positive**.
- **Testis, epididymis and spermatic cord** could be **palpated** and they all appeared to be **normal**.
- There was **no hydrocele** on the left side.
- The **scrotal skin** was **thinned** out and **stretched**.
- **Examination of the abdomen** did not reveal **enlarged pre- and para-aortic lymph nodes.**
- **Inguinal lymph nodes were not palpable**.

Box 14.1:	Points to be noted in history of present illness

- Swelling of the scrotum: Unilateral or bilateral.
- Duration: Several years.
- Rate of growth: Very gradual.
- Pain: Absent in most cases.
- Dragging sensation in large hydroceles.
- History of fever with chills: Filariasis.
- History of trauma: It may be related to minor trauma. Major trauma may lead to haematocele.
- Chronic cough: This may be suggestive of tuberculosis.

Box 14.2:	Points to be noted on inspection

- Rule out hernia
- Side: Unilateral or bilateral
- Size and shape: Size, variable; shape, oval
- Skin over the swelling: Stretched; presence of dilated veins
- Shift of the median raphe
- Deviated and buried penis

Box 14.3:	Points to be noted on palpation

- Warmth and tenderness
- Getting above the swelling to prove a scrotal swelling
- Size and shape
- Consistency: Soft or firm
- Fluctuation (Most important sign)
- Transillumination
- Identification and palpation of testis
- Palpation of epididymis
- Palpation of spermatic cord
- Scrotal skin: Thickening, sinus

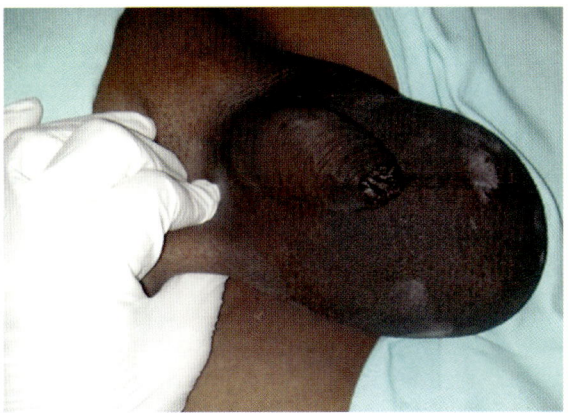

Fig. 14.1: Palpation showing that it is possible to get above the swelling, thereby revealing the scrotal nature of the swelling.

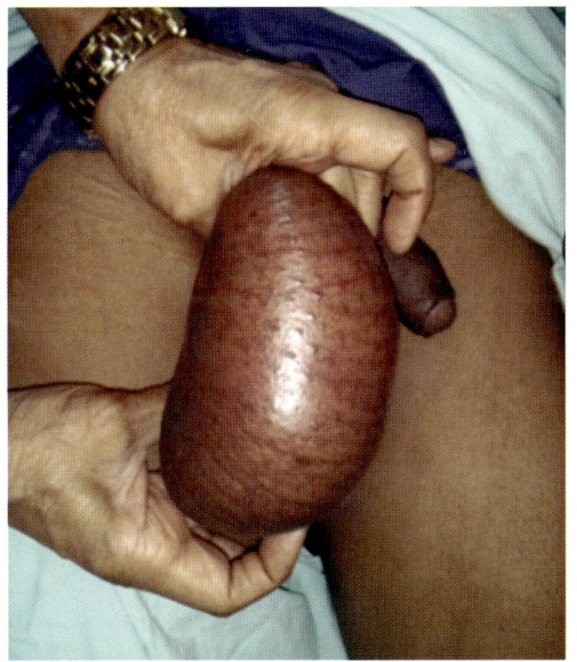

Fig. 14.2: Fixing of swelling before eliciting fluctuation.

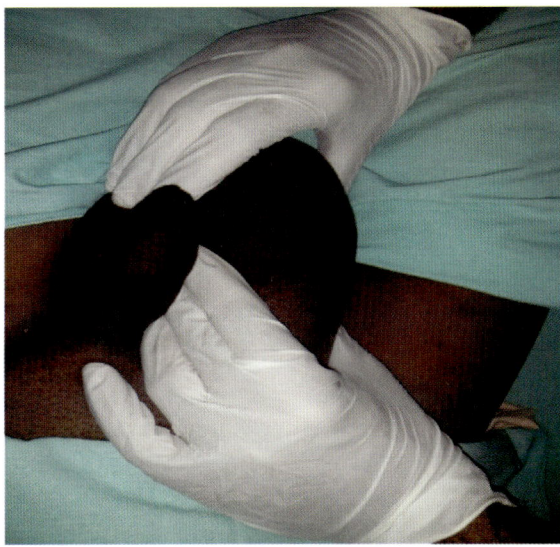

Fig. 14.3: Fluctuation elicited in two directions at right angles to each other.

Q. 1. What was the clinical diagnosis?

The **diagnosis** was an **idiopathic primary vaginal hydrocele.** It was **possible to get above the swelling** proving that the **swelling was purely scrotal in nature. A positive fluctuation** confirmed the **diagnosis.** A **positive transillumination** test **strengthened** the **diagnosis. Since the testis and epididymis** were **normal, a diagnosis** of **idiopathic hydrocele** was made.

Q. 2. What were the treatment options available for this patient?

(*a*) Surgery

(*b*) Aspiration

(*c*) Sclerotherapy

(*d*) Aspiration followed by surgery

(*e*) None of the above

The **correct answer** was (*a*)

In this case, the **patient** was facing **extreme physical discomfort** so **surgery** was chosen as a **treatment option**. There was **discomfort** due to the **enlarged size** of the **scrotum**. The **patient** also was experiencing a **heavy dragging sensation.** There was also a **risk** of **developing complications** at a **later date**.

Setting: **The clock moves forward by one week.** The **patient** was posted for **surgery.**

Q. 3. **What was the operation performed in this patient?**

Subtotal excision of the **parietal layer** of the **tunica vaginalis** was **performed.**

Q. 4. **What is a vaginal hydrocele?**

A **small quantity** of fluid is **always present** in the **vaginal sac**, acting as a **shock absorber** to **prevent injury** to the **testis.** A **vaginal hydrocele** occurs due to a **collection** of a **large quantity** of **fluid** between the **two layers** of the **tunica vaginalis.** If the **aetiology** cannot be **determined,** they are known as **primary** or **idiopathic**

hydroceles. It could be **due** to either **excessive secretion** or **failure** of **absorption** of the **secreted fluid. Secondary hydroceles** result from a **disease** of **the testis or epididymis**.

Q. 5. **What is fluctuation? How is fluctuation elicited?**

Fluctuation is **the sign** to **diagnose** a **hydrocele**. This **sign** is based on the **fact** that when **pressure** is **applied** to a **fluid medium**, it is **distributed uniformly** in all **directions.** It is **important** to **fix** the **swelling** properly **before** eliciting this **test.** The next step is to **perform** the test in **two directions** at right angles to each other. Figs. 14.2 and 14.3 demonstrate this method.

Q. 6. **What is transillumination? How is it elicited?**

Transillumination is the **next stage** of **examination.** In this test, a **source of light** is held **below** the **scrotum** to see if the **fluid inside** the **sac** is **clear** or **not.** One should **avoid placing** the **torch** on the **posterior** and **inferior surface** of the **swelling,** because of the **location** of the **testis.** If the **test** is **positive**, it **strengthens** the **diagnosis.** But **transillumination test** may be **negative** under the following circumstances:

(*a*) The **scrotal skin** is **thick** as is **commonly** seen in **filarial hydrocele**.

(*b*) The **parietal layer** of the **tunica vaginalis** is **thick** preventing the **transmission of light**, as is seen in many **longstanding hydroceles**.

(*c*) **Contents** may **not** be **clear** as in a case of **chylocele**.

Q. 7. Under what circumstances will the testis and epididymis be palpable in a case of vaginal hydrocele?

If the **hydrocele** is **soft and small** in **size** these structures **will be palpable**. In patients with **tense** and **large hydroceles**, it is **not possible** to **feel** these **structures**.

Q. 8. How is testis and the epididymis identified in a case of hydrocele?

The **testis is located in the posteroin-ferior part** of the **hydrocele sac. It is felt** as a **longitudinally oval structure. The surface** will be **smooth** and the **consistency soft.** The **most important clinical sign** is **testicular sensation.** It is **not the pain felt in the region** during **palpation. It is described** as **a sickening sensation felt** around the **umbilicus** when **gentle pressure** is **applied** to the **testis.** The **umbilical site** is **because** of **referred pain.** The **epididymis** is **felt** as a **hood** at the **top** of the **testis.** It is **soft** and has a **smooth surface.**

Q. 9. What is the importance of the position of the penis in a case of vaginal hydrocele?

Unilateral hydroceles cause **deviation** of the **penis** to the **opposite side.** This has **no clinical significance.** But the **penis** may be **buried** in cases of **large hydroceles.** A **wrongly placed incision** may **include** the **penile skin** also**.** Hence **care** should be taken to **avoid** this **mistake** while **making** the **incision.**

Q. 10. Why is palpation of lymph node important in these cases? When are inguinal lymph nodes enlarged?

Since the **lymphatics** of the testis **drain** into the **pre-aortic** and **para-aortic nodes, palpation** of the **abdomen** around the **umbilicus** may reveal a **nodal mass** in a case of **testicular malignancy.** The **deep** and **retroperitoneal location** of the **mass** makes it **difficult** to **palpate,** unless there is a **massive enlargement.**

Inguinal lymph nodes are **enlarged** only when a **malignant tumor** of the **testis involves** the **scrotum,** or **surgical intervention** has been **performed** in the **inguinoscrotal**

region **earlier disturbing** the **normal lymphatic flow**, like an **orchidopexy** or a **hernia repair**.

Q. 11. **How are secondary hydroceles distinguished from the primary variety?**

Secondary hydroceles as mentioned earlier are **secondary** to the **diseases** of the **testis** or **epididymis**. In most cases of **secondary hydroceles**, the **following findings** are useful to **distinguish** between the **two types**.

(*a*) **The size is small**. The only **exception** is **filariasis**.

(*b*) The **testis** and the **epididymis** are **palpable**. The **abnormal clinical findings** in the **testis** and the **epididymis** will **help** to arrive at a **correct diagnosis**. In **malignancy**, there will be an increase in the **size**, the **surface will be irregular** and the **consistency** will be **hard**. Most **importantly**, **testicular sensation** will be **lost**.

Tuberculosis primarily involves the **epididymis**. It will be **hard and craggy**. The **vas deferens** will be **beaded** due to the **presence** of **tubercles** along the structure. **Late cases** may have a **sinus** with **undermined edges** on the **posterior aspect** of the **scrotum**.

Filariasis causes an **increase** in the **size** of the **testis** and **epididymitis** due to **chronic inflammation**. The **surface** will be **smooth** and the **consistency firm**. **Testicular sensation** will **be present**. The **scrotal skin** may be **thickened**. **Inguinal lymph nodes** are often **enlarged**.

Q. 12. **What are the investigations performed in cases of hydroceles?**

In most cases, the **clinical findings** are **adequate** to **arrive at a** diagnosis. If there is any **doubt as to the cause**, an **ultrasound examination** of the **scrotum** will be extremely **useful**. Even if there is the slightest **suspicion** about **malignancy**, this **examination** is **mandatory**.

Q. 13. **What are the indications for treatment?**

The most **common** indication is the **physical discomfort** resulting from an **enlarged scrotum**. **Dragging pain** may be another **reason**. The **risk** of **complications** is an additional **indication**. But all the **complications** are very **uncommon**.

Q. 14. **What are the complications of a vaginal hydrocele?**

(*a*) **Infection**. **Infection** reaches the **hydrocele sac** via the

lymphatics of the **cord** converting it into a **pyocele.** The **septic process** can **spread** to involve the **testis** resulting in its **loss.**

(*b*) **Trauma:** An **enlarged scrotum** is more **prone** for **trauma**, leading to either a **rupture** of the **vaginal sac** or formation of a **haematocele.** **Haematocele** is likely to cause **pressure atrophy** of the **underlying testis.** **Haematocele** is **difficult** to **distinguish** from **malignancy** since **some patients** with **malignancy** may give a **history** of **previous trauma**. An **US examination** will settle the **problem**.

(*c*) **Pressure atrophy** of the testis. **Longstanding hydroceles** are known to cause **pressure atrophy** of the testis by the constant **hydrostatic pressure** of the **fluid** in the sac.

(*d*) **Calcification: Calcification** of the **parietal layer** has been reported in **hydroceles** of **several years duration**. Since **the swelling** feels **hard,** a doubt of **malignancy** may arise in the clinician's mind. **Ultrasonology** is useful in identifying the **calcification.**

(*e*) **Hernia of hydrocele sac. Hernia** of the **hydrocele** sac occurs when there is a **defect** in the overlying **internal spermatic, cremasteric** and **external spermatic fascia,** and **the parietal layer** comes to occupy **the subcutaneous plane** due to **herniation** through these **defects.** This is an **inconsequential complication**.

Box 14.4:	Points regarding complications

- Infection.
- Trauma leading to haematocele.
- Pressure atrophy of the testis.
- Calcification.
- Hernia of the hydrocele sac.

Q. 15. **What are the surgical options available in a case of vaginal hydrocele?**

(*a*) Eversion of the sac.

(*b*) Partial excision with eversion.

(*c*) Subtotal excision.

(*d*) Lord's plication.

Elderly patients with **small hydroceles** can be kept under **observation.** These need to be **treated** only if the **size** becomes **larger** or any of the **complications** mentioned above **develop** over a period of **time.**

(*a*) When the **hydrocele sac** is **small** in **size** and the **wall is** thin, a **simple eversion** will **suffice.** In this **procedure,** through a **scrotal incision**, the **hydrocele sac** is **opened** along the **anterior wall**, and all the **fluid** is **drained**. The **parietal layer** is then **everted behind** the **testis** by **few sutures**. The **success** of this **operation** depends on the **following factors**. The **fluid** that is **secreted** by the **layers** of the **tunica vaginalis** is **absorbed** by the **scrotal lymphatics**. Again, as the **smooth lining** of this **layer,** which is **primarily** of **mesodermal origin**, comes into **contact** with the **rough scrotal tissue,** a process of **gradual denudation** takes place, **reducing** the **volume** of **fluid** that is **secreted.**

(*b*) **Partial excision with eversion**. If the **size** of the sac **is large**, and the **sac wall thin**, the **peripheral portion** of the **parietal layer** is **excised**. The **remaining part** is **everted** behind **the testis**.

(*c*) The **most common procedure** is **subtotal excision** of the **parietal layer**, also called as **radical cure**. **Most** of this **layer** is **excised**

leaving a **thin rim** around the **testis**. This is **indicated** when the **size** of the sac is **large** and the **layer** is **thick**. A **complete excision** of the **tunica vaginalis** is **never done** since the **visceral layer** is **firmly adherent** to **the testis**.

(*d*) **Lord's plication** is **performed** in **large hydroceles** with a **thin sac**. The **operation** consists of **plicating** the **parietal layer** around the **testis** by properly **placed stitches**. The **advantage** of this **operation** is the **minimal dissection** required, thereby **reducing** the **risk of haematoma formation**.

Complications following these operations are **uncommon. Imperfect hemostasis** leading to the **formation** of a **hematoma** that gets infected has been described. **Severe sepsis** may lead to **loss of testis.**

Q. 16. **What are the other modalities** of **treatment available in a case of a hydrocele?**

Aspiration:

In this procedure, the **hydrocele fluid** is **aspirated** to **reduce** the **size** of the **swelling.** The **site** chosen for **insertion** of the

needle should be **fluctuant** and preferably **transilluminant**, to **avoid injuring the testis.** The **fluid** is **yellow** or **amber coloured** and it **shimmers** in **reflected light** due to the presence of **doubly refractile cholesterol crystals.** This **procedure** gives only **temporary relief** since the **fluid** will **recollect** again. Therefore, the **indications** for aspiration are as follows:

(*a*) The patient desires a **temporary postponement** of the **operation.**

(*b*) The patient has **severe systemic disease** like **cardiac, renal or hepatic**, **contraindicating** any **surgical procedure.**

Complications described after aspiration include **infection** and **injury** to the underlying **testis.**

Sclerotherapy:

This has been described as an **adjuvant procedure** following **aspiration** to **prevent recurrence.** It is **performed** only if the **size** of the sac is very **small** and **wall is thin.** Once all the **fluid** has been **emptied,** a **sclerosing agent** like **tetracycline** is introduced into the **cavity, inducing** an **aseptic**

inflammation that **binds** the two **layers** of the **tunica together,** **preventing recurrence.** Though mentioned in the literature, this is an **uncommonly performed procedure.**

Box 14.5:	Points regarding treatment
Treatment modality	**Features**
• Surgical options	• Eversion of the sac. • Partial excision with eversion'. • Subtotal excision (Radical cure). • Lord's plication.
• Aspiration	• Temporary relief. • Postponement of surgery. • Contraindications for surgery.
• Sclerotherapy	• Induction of fibrosis by aseptic inflammation.

Q. 16. Describe the anatomical classification of hydroceles?

In **addition** to the common type of **vaginal hydrocele** described earlier, **depending** on the **location** of the **fluid,** the following **anatomical varieties** are seen in clinical practice.

(*a*) **Congenital hydrocele (infantile inguinal hernia):** In this condition, the **processus vaginalis** remains **patent,** allowing the **peritoneal fluid** to **trickle**

down from the **peritoneal cavity**, into the **vaginal sac.** Commonly seen in **children,** the **mother complains** that the **scrotum** appears to be **normal** in **size** in the **morning** but **tends** to become **bigger** by **evening**. Examination reveals a **moderate-sized inguinoscrotal swelling**. When the child is made to **cry** or **cough** there is an **impulse** in the nature of a **fluid thrill** rather than an **expansile one**. **Treatment** consists of a **herniotomy** followed by **aspiration** of the fluid in the sac.

(*b*) **Infantile hydrocele:** Here the **communication** of the **processus vaginalis** with the **peritoneal cavity** is **closed off** at the **internal ring**. But the **remaining portion** remains **patent** allowing the fluid from the vaginal sac to **extend** along the **inguinal canal** until the **internal ring**. The disease need **not be seen** during **infancy** exclusively. **Treatment** demands an **inguinoscrotal approach** with **subtotal excision** of the **sac,** taking care **not** to **damage** the structures of the **spermatic cord.**

(*c*) **Encysted hydrocele of the spermatic cord:** The **processus vaginalis** is closed **both** at the **upper** and **lower ends** along the **spermatic cord**, resulting in **collection** of **fluid** in the **central portion**. Thus, a **globular swelling** is seen in the **upper part** of the scrotum. On **palpation,** the **swelling** is felt to be **independent** of the **testis**. It is **fluctuant** and **brilliantly transilluminant.** It has **transverse mobility**, along **with** the **spermatic cord**. But this is **abolished** when **downward traction** is **applied** to the **testis.** This **traction test confirms** the **diagnosis. Excision** is the choice of **treatment, without damaging t**he structures of the **cord.**

(*d*) **Abdomino scrotal** or **hydrocele en bisac:** A **rare type** of hydrocele, this has **two components**—one in the **retroperitoneal region above** the inguinal **ligament** and the other in the **scrotum. Cross fluctuation** can be **demonstrated** between the **two.** Commonly **mistaken** for an **inguinal hernia** with an **associated hydrocele,** ultrasonogram is useful in **differentiation.** The **abdominal sac** is **excised completely** and a **subtotal excision** is performed for the **scrotal** part via an **inguinoscrotal incision**. The **genesis** of this type has **not** been completely **understood**. It could be due to **sequestration** of a **portion** of the **processus vaginalis retroperitoneally** during the **descent** of the **testis** from the **abdomen** to the **scrotum.**

Box 14.6:	Points regarding the anatomical classification

- Congenital hydrocele.
- Infantile hydrocele.
- Vaginal hydrocele.
- Encysted hydrocele of the cord.
- Abdomino scrotal hydrocele.

Multiple Choice Questions

1. CROSS FLUCTUATION is elicited in
   (a) Hydrocele of Tunica Vaginalis
   (b) Hydrocele of Canal Of Nuck
   (c) Congenital Hydrocele
   (d) Hydrocele En Bisac
   Answer (d)

2. A Herniotomy is the Treatment of choice for
   (a) Hydrocele of Tunica Vaginalis
   (b) Hydrocele of Canal Of Nuck
   (c) Congenital Hydrocele
   (d) Hydrocele En Bisac
   Answer (c)

3. The Correct method of the surgical procedure for a Hydrocele of the Tunica Vaginalis is
   (a) Subtotal Excision with Eversion of the sac
   (b) Total Excision with Eversion of the sac
   (c) Subtotal Excision with Inversion of the sac
   (d) Total Excision with Inversion of the sac
   Answer (a)

4. The layer of the scrotum which is partially excised during a surgical procedure for a Vaginal Hydrocele is
   (a) Tunica Albuginea
   (b) Visceral Layer of the Tunica Vaginalis
   (c) Parietal Layer of Tunica Vaginalis
   (d) Tunica Vasculosa
   Answer (c)

TRUE/FALSE

1. A Hydrocele of the Tunica Vaginalis can be fluctuant but need not be Transilluminant.

   Answer: TRUE

2. A Hydrocele which communicates with the peritoneal cavity is called an Infantile Hydrocele.

   Answer: FALSE

3. The surgical treatment for a congenital hydrocele is a HERNIOTOMY.

   Answer: TRUE

4. Sclerotherapy is an accepted treatment modality for a Hydrocele.

   Answer: TRUE

5. The fluid of a Vaginal Hydrocele clots immediately on stasis.

   Answer: FALSE

6. It is possible to GET ABOVE THE SWELLING in an Infantile Hydrocele

   Answer: FALSE

■■■

Testicular Tumours

15

A CASE OF SEMINOMA OF THE TESTIS

Setting

- Setting Surgical OPD

Chief Complaint

- **Swelling** in the **left side** of the **scrotum** of **6 months duration**.

History of Present Illness

- A **28-year-old man** presented to the OPD with the **complaint** of a **swelling** in the **left side** of the **scrotum** of **6 months duration**. The swelling was **small** initially, but has **increased rapidly** over the **last six weeks**.
- He felt **a heavy sensation** in that region especially on **standing** for a **long time**. There was **no pain**.
- There was **no history** of **trauma.**
- He did **not** complain of **fever** with **chills** and **rigor.**

- He did **not** have any **respiratory symptoms**.
- There was **no** history of **back pain**.
- There was **no** history of **loss** of **weight** or **appetite.**
- **Personal, family and past histories** were insignificant.

Treatment History

- He had **consulted** his **family physician** who made a **diagnosis** of **hydrocele,** and **advised him** to **undergo an operation**.
- **General physical examination** showed a healthy individual. There was no pallor, jaundice or oedema of the ankles.

Local Examination

Inspection

- **Patient was in standing position**. He was made **to cough**. There was **no bulge** in the **groins** ruling out an **associated inguinal hernia**.

- **Patient supine**. A **swelling** was seen in the **left side** of the **scrotum.**
- It was **oval** in shape measuring **18 cm by 10** cm in **size**.
- The **margins** were **distinct.**
- The **skin** over the **swelling** was **stretched. No dilated veins** were seen.
- The **median raphe** was **shifted** to the right side.
- There was **no deviation** of the **penis.**

Palpation

- It was **possible** to **get above** the **swelling.**
- The swelling was **not warm or tender.**
- The **size** and **shape** were **confirmed** on palpation. The **borders** were **well defined**.
- The **consistency** was **firm.**
- **Fluctuation** was **positive. Transillumi-nation** was **negative.**
- The **testis** was **palpable**. It was larger in size as compared to the opposite side. It was **not tender**.
- The **size** was **15 cm by 10 cm**. The **shape** was **oval.**
- The **surface** was **smooth.** The **consistency** was **firm**.
- **Testicular sensation** was **absent.**
- The **epididymis** was palpable and **normal.**
- The **spermatic cord** was **thickened.**

- The **scrotal skin** was **normal.**
- The **right testis** was **palpable** and **normal.**
- There was **no hydrocele** on the **right side.**

Examination of Abdomen

- **Pre-** and **para-aortic lymph nodes** were **not palpable.**
- There was **no hepatomegaly.**

Examination of Inguinal Region

- A few **soft inguinal nodes less** than **1 cm** in **size** were **palpable** on **both sides.** They were **discrete** and **nontender.**
- **Examination of the supraclavicular region** did **not** reveal any **palpable lymph nodes.**
- **Examination** of the **respiratory system** was **normal.**
- There was **no tenderness** along the **spine.**

Q. 1. **What was the clinical diagnosis?**

The **diagnosis** was a **testicular tumour** probably a **seminoma with a secondary vaginal hydrocele.** The **points** in **favour** of the **diagnosis** were as **follows.**

It was **possible to get above** the **swelling,** proving that it was **a scrotal swelling.** The **fluctuation test** was **positive** confirming the **presence** of a **hydrocele.**

A **testicular tumour** was **detected** by **the loss** of **testicular sensation.**

A **seminoma** was **likely** because the **testis** was **enlarged,** the **surface** was **smooth** and the **consistency** was **firm.**

Q. 2. What were the investigations done in this patient?

US study. It showed an **enlarged testis** having a **homogenous appearance** of **low echogenicity.** **Colour Doppler** study showed **increased vascularity.**

US abdomen showed enlarged **pre-** and **para-aortic lymph nodes.**

CT abdomen confirmed the presence of **enlarged pre-and para-aortic lymph nodes.**

Tumour marker study: Serum AFP, Beta fraction of HCG and lactic acid dehydrogenase levels were within **normal limits.**

FNAC of **tumour** in the **testis** was done under **US guidance.**

Setting: A week passes.

FNAC: The **report** was **seminoma.** The **smear** showed **uniform sheets** of **round eosinophilic cells** with **prominent nucleoli.**

Q. 3. What was the treatment strategy planned for this patient?

He was told that he **needed** an **orchidectomy.** It took **some time** to **convince** the **patient** about the **seriousness** of the **disease** and the **possible metastatic spread** to **vital organs.** It is to be **remembered** that the **patient** came to the **hospital** for a **simple procedure** like **surgery** for **hydrocele.** He was also **told** about the **need** for **postoperative chemoradiation.**

Q. 4. What was the operation performed on this patient?

The patient **underwent** a **high orchidectomy.** An incision was made **above** and **parallel** to the **inguinal ligament.** The **inguinal canal** was **opened.** The **spermatic cord** was identified, **ligated and divided** at the level of the **internal ring.** The entire **cord** along with the **testis** containing the **tumour** was **removed.**

Q. 5. What was the histopathology report?

The tumour was reported as a seminoma.

Q. 6. What was the postoperative treatment?

He underwent **concurrent chemoradia-tion.** The **drugs** used for chemotherapy included **carboplatin, vincristine and bleomycin.** In addition, **EBRT** was used to **control** the **pre- and para-aortic nodes.** The **response** to **treatment** was very **satisfactory.**

Q. 7. What could be the possible outcome for this patient?

The **prognosis** should be **very good.** **Seminomas** are **highly radiosensitive**

tumours. The **addition** of **chemotherapy** should **reduce** the chances of **recurrence** in the **retroperitoneal nodes** as well as the **development** of **metastatic disease**.

Q. 8. What is the incidence of testicular tumours?

Testicular tumours are responsible for only **one percent** of all **malignancies**. But unfortunately they are the **second-most common cause of death** in **men** between the ages of **20 and 40 years**. **Trauma** has the dubious **distinction** of being in the **top of the list**. An **increase** in the **incidence** has been **described in the Western countries** over the last few decades. **90%** of these are **germ cell tumours**. A **deregulation** of the **pluripotent fetal germ cells**, probably **caused** by **genetic abnormalities,** is said to be the most **important aetiological factor**.

Q. 9. What are the risk factors in relation to testicular cancers?

Testicular dysgenesis syndrome, which includes **cryptorchidism** and **undescended testis,** is considered to be the most important **risk factor**. The **risk persists** even if an **orchidopexy** has been performed at a **young age**. But the **advantage** is that the **diagnosis** is much **easier** in a **scrotal testis**. The **contralateral testis** is also more **prone** for **malignancy**, thereby **strengthening** the **genetic theory**.

Klinefelter's syndrome.

Family history of testicular tumours among **first degree relatives**.

Box 15.1: Points regarding risk factors
• Deregulation of pluripotent fetal germ cells – Main factor.
• Testicular dysgenesis syndrome – Cryptorchidism, undescended testis.
• Klinefelter's syndrome.
• Cancer among first degree relatives.

Q. 10. How are germ cell tumours classified?

It is necessary to **understand** the **pathology** of these tumours because their **biological behavior** differs, and therefore the **treatment** as well as the **outcome** also will be **different.** The following are the **main types** seen in clinical practice.

1. **Seminoma**
2. **Teratoma**
3. **Choriocarcinoma**
4. **Yolk sac tumour (rare)**

Seminoma: This is the **commonest** type of malignancy **(50%). Cut sections** show a **lobulated homogenous** mass, varying from **gray** to **pink** in **colour**. These tumours are subdivided into 3 groups **microscopically.**

The **classic** variety is responsible for **85%** of tumours. **Sections** show **monotonous sheets** of **large eosinophilic cells** with **abundant cytoplasm** and **round hyperchromatic nuclei** with **prominent nucleoli.**

Anaplastic group (3%). Sections show **more than 3 mitotic figures** per **high power field.**

Spermatocytic (5%): Microscopy shows **well-differentiated cells** resembling **secondary spermatids.** These tumours are seen in **elderly males** and have a **good prognosis.** The tumour has a **pale gray, mucoid** and **oedematous appearance.** The main features on **microscopy** are **nodules** of **cells** with **spaces** filled with **fluid. Giant cells** are **common. Stroma** is **minimal.** About **6%** of these patients show a **sarcomatous component** with plenty of **undifferentiated cells,** and they are **more aggressive** tumours with a **poor outcome.**

Spread of these tumours occurs primarily via the lymphatics. The **retroperitoneal nodes** are commonly involved. The **pre-and para-aortic groups** are **mainly involved.** A group of **lymphatics accompanying** the **vas deferens** can **carry malignant cells** to the **common iliac group** of **nodes** as well. Later the tumour can **spread** to the **mediastinal** and **supraclavicular nodes. Blood spread** is **uncommon.**

Teratoma well differentiated (Mature teratoma). These are **uncommon tumours (5%).** Macroscopically the tumours are **large in size,** being **multinodular** and having a **variable consistency. Cut sections** have a **heterogeneous** appearance with **solid, cartilaginous** and **cystic** areas. **Histopathology** reveals **tissues** developed from **ectoderm, mesoderm and endoderm.** The tumour can **spread** both by the **lymphatic** and **haematogenous** routes. **Lymphatic spread** leads to enlarged **retroperitoneal nodes. Blood spread** gives rise to **secondaries** in the **lungs, liver** and **central nervous system.**

Teratoma undifferentiated (immature teratoma). This type is biologically **more aggressive,** and hence the **recurrence rates** are **high. Histopathology** shows **primitive cells** derived from all the **three varieties** of the **pluripotent germ cells. Mixed cellularity** along with a **high percentage of mitosis** is the feature of an **undifferentiated teratoma.**

Choriocarcinoma: This is a **rare** type of germ cell tumour. Pure choriocarcinomas are rare (1%). Frequently, cells seen in **nonseminomatous type** of tumours are **present** in addition to the typical microscopic appearance of a choriocarcinoma. Hence it is sometimes graded as **teratoma trophoblastic**. Often the **metastatic disease** is **detected first**, only to unveil the **primary tumour** in the **testis afterwards**. Macroscopically the **testis** may be **normal** in size or it may be **slightly enlarged**. Cut sections show abundant **haemorrhage** with areas of **necrosis.** The periphery shows **grayish viable tissue**. Histologically, the tumour is composed of two types of cells. They are the **syncytiotrophoblasts** and **cytotrophoblasts.** The former are **large multinucleated cells** with **vacuoles** in the **cytoplasm.** They have **pleomorphic smudged nuclei.** The **cytotrophoblasts** are **small to medium** in size with **clear cytoplasm** along with **mild** to **moderate pleomorphism**. The background shows **extensive haemorrhage** and **necrosis**. **Blood spread** is **very common** though **lymphatic spread** can also occur.

Box 15.2:	Points regarding pathological types

- Seminoma-50% – Homogeneous – Gray or pink cut section.
  - Micro 3 subtypes – Classic - 85%.
- Large cells with round hyperchromatic nuclei and prominent nucleoli.
  - Anaplastic – 3% – More than 3 mitotic figures per HPF.
  - Spermatcytic-5% – Elderly males – Sec spermatids
- Teratoma differentiated – Cells from all 3 germ layers.
  - Undifferentiated – Primitive germ cells – Pleomorphism.
- Choriocarcinoma – Haemorrhage and necrosis.
- Syncytiotrophoblasts – Multinucleated giant cells – Vacuoles in cytoplasm.
- Cytotrophoblasts – Round small to medium size – Moderate pleomorphism

Q. 11. What are the clinical features of testicular cancers?

In the **absence** of **specific clinical features**, a **delay** in **diagnosis** is very **common**. The **common feeling,** even in the **educated class** is to consider **any scrotal swelling** as a **hydrocele.**

Symptoms:

1. **Age: Seminoma** is seen in the age group of **15 to 35 years** and **teratoma** a **decade later**. **Spermatocytic seminoma** occurs in **men** over **60 years** of age.

2. **Swelling** of the **scrotum** is the most **frequent complaint.**

Since **hydroceles** are **very common**, the **patient** and occasionally the **clinician** too, tend to **miss** the **malignancy**. A **recent rapid increase** in **size** of the swelling may bring the **patient** to the **hospital**.

3. A feeling of **heaviness** or **dragging sensation** in the **scrotum** is felt by some patients. **Pain** develops only in **later stages.**

4. A **small group** of patients present with a **clinical picture** simulating a case of **epididymo orchitis** (described as a **hurricane type** in the past). They have **severe pain** radiating **down** the **scrotum** of a **short duration**, along with **swelling** and **tenderness** in the **testis**. The **cord** appears to be **thickened**. Since **filariasis** is **endemic** in **several parts of our country** and **epididymo orchitis** is a common **manifestation** of the **disease, the chances** of **missing the diagnosis** in this group is very **high.**

5. **History of trauma:** Patient may **attribute** all his **symptoms** to a **history** of **trauma,** usually **minor** in nature. But it is **very likely** that **trauma** brings the **attention** of the **patient** to a **pre-existing tumour**.

6. **Gynaecomastia** is seen in a small number of patients.

7. **Symptoms due to metastases**

   (*a*) **Dragging pain** in the **flanks, back and abdomen** is due to a **large abdominal mass.**

   (*b*) **Swelling** in the **neck** resulting from **supraclavicular lymphadenopathy**.

   (*c*) **Respiratory system: Cough** with **chest pain** and haemoptysis are due to **secondary deposits** in the **lung.**

   (*d*) **Uncommonly, patients** may present with **secondary deposits** in the **CNS** or **skeletal system.**

To conclude, **testicular malignancies** belong to **that variety** of tumours, wherein **symptoms** due to the **primary tumour** are **nonspecific** and **symptomatic secondaries** may **manifest early,** and only a **diligent physical examination** along with the **necessary investigations** will help to clinch the **correct diagnosis.**

Box 15.3:	Points regarding symptoms due to testicular cancer

- Swelling of the scrotum – Duration months. Recent rapid increase in size.
- Dragging or heavy sensation. Pain late symptom.
- Picture resembling epididymo orchitis.
- Pain in the flanks or back – Large abdominal mass.
- Respiratory symptoms.
- Swelling in the neck – Supraclavicular nodes.
- Rarely CNS or skeletal symptoms.

Q. 12. What are the clinical signs in these cases?

Examination of the scrotum.

1. **Unilateral swelling** of the **scrotum** is observed in most cases.

2. The **overlying skin** is **stretched.**

3. On **palpation**, a **small secondary hydrocele** is often **present.**

4. The **testis** is **palpable and enlarged. Choriocarcinoma** may present with a **testis** of **normal size**.

5. The **surface is smooth** in **seminoma** but **irregular** in a case of **teratoma.**

6. The **consistency** is **firm** or **hard** in **seminoma** and is **variable** in **teratoma.** It could be **soft** in **choriocarcinoma**.

7. The **most important sign** is **loss of testicular sensation**

due to **infiltration** of the **nerves** by the growth of the **tumour**. **Testicular sensation** is **defined** as a **sickening sensation** felt **around the umbilicus** when **pressure** is applied to the **testis (referred pain)**.

The **overlying skin** is **free,** except in **patients** who have undergone **previous scrotal surgery**.

8. The **spermatic cord** is **thickened** due to **spread** of **tumour** cells along the **lymphatics** or the **vas deferens**.

Examination of regional lymph nodes. Testicular lymphatics primarily drain into the **pre-** and **para-aortic nodes**, since **these vessels** accompany the **testicular veins**. The **right testicular vein** empties into the **inferior vena cava** and the **left** into the **left renal vein**.

1. The **pre-** and **para-aortic nodes** are palpated in the **central part** of the **abdomen.** Since they are **deeply placed**, they are likely to be **missed** until they assume a **large size**. When palpable, the **mass** is **retroperitoneal**, **firm**-to-**hard** in consistency with a **nodular surface** and **fixed.**

2. In addition, the **common iliac nodes** may be **enlarged** due to **spread** of the tumour along

lymphatics accompanying the **vas deferens**.

3. The **inguinal nodes** are **enlarged** under the **following** exceptional **circumstances** only.

   (*a*) **Infiltration** of the **overlying scrotal layers**. This is an **uncommon finding**, except when **previous surgery** has been performed.

   (*b*) **Previous inguinal surgery** for **undescended testis** or **hernia** or a **varicocele disturbs** the **normal lymphatic flow** allowing the **tumour** to **spread** to **inguinal nodes**.

Clinical features due to distant metastases.

1. **Palpable supraclavicular lymph nodes**. In an **asymptomatic young man**, if **this node** is detected, one of the **primary malignancies** to be **searched** for is **always** the **testis**. The **nodes** are **firm-to-hard** in consistency. They are **mobile** in the early stages, but are **fixed later** due to **extracapsular spread**. **Tumour cells** reach this **group** via the **mediastinal route** and hence **both sides of the neck** need to be **examined** carefully.

2. **Examination of the chest** may **not detect secondaries** in many instances. **Signs of consolidation** are suggestive of **metastatic disease**.

3. **Bony metastases** are **rare.** If they are **present,** the patient may have **pain** and **tenderness** along these **sites.**

4. **Signs** due to **secondaries** in **CNS.**

Box 15.4:	Points regarding clinical signs in these cases

- Unilateral swelling of the scrotum – Small secondary Hydrocele – Testis palpable.
- Testicular sensation lost.
- Seminoma – Testis enlarged – Smooth – Firm
- Teratoma – Testis enlarged – Irregular surface – Variable consistency.
- Choriocarcinoma – Size often normal – Soft.
- Abdominal Mass – Retroperitoneal nodes.
- Supraclavicular nodes.
- Signs due to secondary deposits in CNS or skeletal system.

Q. 13. What are the investigations needed in a case of testicular cancer?

US study: Examination of the **scrotal contents** by **ultrasound** is the most **useful investigation** to diagnose **malignancy**. It has a **sensitivity of 100%.** The appearance in **seminoma** is that of a **homogeneous hypoechoic intratesticular mass. Mature teratoma** on ultrasound, tends to be cystic with **heterogeneous echoes** in the **fluid. Solid components of varying echogenicity** are also seen, some with **posterior shadowing**. **Undifferentiated teratomas** have **solid areas** of **mixed echogenicity** with areas of **haemorrhage. Cystic areas** are **uncommon. Choriocarcinoma** shows areas of **haemorrhage** and **necrosis.**

Ultrasound is also **helpful** to identify a **tumour** in the **testis** when **patients** present with an **abdominal mass** of **lymph nodes** or **supraclavicular lymphadenopathy**, in the **absence** of **local symptoms** and **signs**. The **testis** may be in the **scrotum** or **ectopic** in position. Again in the group **simulating** a picture of **epididymo orchitis, ultrasound** is **diagnostic**. In addition, the state of the **opposite testis** can also be assessed. It must be stressed that this **investigation** is mandatory when there is the **slightest doubt** regarding a **malignancy** in the **testis.**

Ultrasound examination of the abdomen. It may reveal **enlarged pre- and para-aortic** as well as **iliac nodes. Large mass** of nodes can **compress** the **ureters** leading to **bilateral hydronephrosis.**

CT scan has become the **most reliable investigation** in this disease. **CT** of the **abdomen** may reveal **more nodes** especially those **less than 1 cm. in size.** In addition, the **architectural changes** are **better** made out on **CT** compared to **ultrasound.**

CT chest will show **enlarged mediastinal nodes** as well as **secondaries** in the **lung** and is far **superior** to a routine **chest X-ray**. If **CNS symptoms** are present, especially in a **choriocarcinoma,** a **CT** of the **brain** is warranted.

Tumour markers.

(*a*) **Serum Alpha Feto Protein:** It is a **glycoprotein synthesized** in the **liver** and **yolk sac** during **pregnancy**. Hence the **prefix "feto"** is used to describe this **tumour marker**. The word **alpha** is **derived** from its **electrophoretic characters**. The **levels** are **normal** in a **seminoma**. In **teratomas** the **levels are high,** since **AFP** is **secreted** by the elements of the **yolk sac** present in the **tumour.**

(*b*) **Beta fraction of HCG:** This tumour marker reaches a high **concentration** during **pregnancy**. This **tumour marker** is **secreted** by the **syncytiotrophoblast** cells found in **choriocarcinoma.** Hence it is mostly **raised in** patients with **this type of** tumour.

(*c*) **Lactic acid dehydrogenase:** It is a **nonspecific tumour marker** and is found to be **raised** in many **other cancers**. In patients with **nonseminomatous cancers, raised levels,** along with **high levels of AFP** and/or **HCG** indicate the **presence** of **metastases.**

All these **tumour markers** are more useful in **assessing** the **prognosis. Normal levels do not rule out** a diagnosis of **malignancy. Return** of **raised levels to normal** indicates that the **treatment** has been **effective. Increased levels** in the **post-treatment period** suggest the development of **metastatic** or **recurrent disease,** even in the **absence** of any **clinical findings.**

Biopsy: A **trans scrotal FNAC,** preferably under **ultrasound guidance,** is now the **accepted** mode of **investigation** to **prove the diagnosis.** In the **past,** an **inguinal exploration** was **advised,** due to the **fear** of **spread of the tumour** caused by a **breach** in the **tunica albuginea** by the **FNA needle.** But this hypothesis is **no longer valid. Biopsy** will help us not only to **diagnose malignancy,** but also to identify the **pathological type,** because the **treatment** and the outlook **differ** depending on the **type** of the **tumour.**

Box 15.5	Points regarding investigations

- US testis. Seminoma – Homogeneous – Hypoechoic.
- Teratoma differentiated – Cystic – Solid elements – Posterior shadowing.
- Teratoma undifferentiated – Solid – haemorrhage.
- Choriocarcinoma – Haemorrhage with necrosis.
- CT abdomen. More nodes – Structural changes.
- CT chest – Mediastinal nodes.
- Tumour markers – AFP – Teratoma.
- β–HCG – Choriocarcinoma.
- LDH – Nonspecific.
- FNAC

Q. 14. How are testicular tumours staged?

The classical **TNM classification** can be simplified into **three stages.** These stages will **influence** the **treatment** and the **prognosis.**

Stage I: The tumour is **restricted** to the **testis. Depending** upon the **extent** of **spread** into the **adjacent structures,** this **stage** is further **divided into 4 subtypes.** For example, **T4** indicates **involvement** of the **scrotum** needing an **extended local surgery** and an inguinal node dissection.

Stage II: In this stage the **pre- and para-aortic nodes** are involved. Further, if the **nodes** are **more** than **5 in number** or the **size more** than **2 cm** the **outlook is poor.**

Stage III: This stage implies **spread beyond** the **retroperitoneal (RP) nodes**.

This **staging** is based not only on **physical examination,** but also on **imaging studies** and the **levels of tumour markers.** If the **tumour markers** are **high,** even a **stage II tumour** is **upgraded** to the **third stage.** Patients in **stage II and III** can be further **stratified** into a **favourable** or an **unfavourable** group. Patients with **RP nodes** and **secondaries** in the **lung** with **low levels** of **tumour markers** fall into the **favourable group.** The **other group** consists of patients with **secondary deposits in liver, bone and brain,** in **addition** to the **lung,** and associated with **high levels** of **tumour marker.**

Box 15.6	Points regarding staging of testicular cancers

- **Stage I:** Tumour confined to testis – 4 subtypes TI to T IV.
- **Stage II:** Enlarged RP Nodes.
- **Stage III:** Spread beyond RP Nodes.
- Level of tumour markers –
  - Low – Favourable.
  - High – Unfavourable.

Q. 15. What are the treatment strategies?

The **first step** in the **treatment** is a **high orchidectomy.** The **entire spermatic cord** along with the **testis** is **removed** in this **operation. Testicular cancers** are an **exception** to the **general principles** of **treating cancers.** A **radical surgery is performed** for the **primary tumour irrespective** of the **stage** of the **disease.** It **reduces** the **tumour burden.** It also provides **enough tissue** for not only **histopathology,** but also for **immunohistochemistry** and possible **genetic studies.**

The **further stages** of **treatment depend** on the **type of tumour.**

Seminoma: Seminoma is a **highly radiosensitive tumour.** For stage I disease, **EBRT** to the **RP nodes** is **adequate.** But **recurrences** may occur especially in the **unfavourable group.** Hence for **patients** with **stage I (unfavourable)** and for stage **II and III patients combined modality** offers the **best results. Concurrent chemoradiation** is planned for these **patients.** The **chemotherapy regime** consists of **Carboplatin, Vincristine and Bleomycin.** It is combined with **EBRT** for the **RP nodes,** the dose being **30 to 35 Gy. Prophylactic radiation** to the **mediastinal and supraclavicular nodes (mantle field)** is **no longer practiced,** for the risk of inducing **pulmonary fibrosis.** The **drugs** used as **second line** of **chemotherapy** for **recurrent** or **metastatic disease** include, the **taxanes** along with **vinblastine, ifosfamide and gemcitabine.**

Nonseminomatous tumours: The **initial treatment** is a **radical inguinal orchidectomy.** This is followed by a **course** of **chemotherapy** as per the schedule mentioned above. The availability of **Cisplatin group** of compounds has made a **profound difference** in the **outcome** of **this group** of patients. **Radiotherapy** has **no place** in the treatment because these tumours are **highly radioresistant.** Patients in **stage I and II** do **well** with this regime. But **recurrences** are **more common. Recurrences** in the RP nodes or **nodes persisting** after **chemotherapy** need a **radical retroperitoneal lymph node dissection (RPND).** The availability of **laparoscopy** and the **improvement** in the **technique** with the **nerves** being **protected** has **reduced** the complication of **impotency** and **urinary problems considerably.** But as mentioned earlier, **distant metastases** do occur at a **later date** and may need **second line** of chemotherapy. But the **outlook** is **poorer** when compared with a seminoma.

Choriocarcinoma: The **treatment regime** is the **same** as for a **teratoma. Taxanes and Ifosomide** are **more frequently used.** But the **response rates** are **lower. Blood borne metastases** are very **frequent. Haemorrhage** into the **secondary deposits** is often **life threatening.**

Box 15.7	Points regarding the treatment

- High inguinal orchidectomy for all patients.
- Seminoma – Concurrent chemoradiation.
  - Carboplatin, Vincristine and Bleomycin.
  - EBRT to RP nodes – 30 to 35 Gy.
- Teratoma – Chemotherapy – Same as above.
  - RPND – Nerve-sparing technique – Less morbidity.
  - Secondary line of chemotherapy drugs.
- Choriocarcinoma – Chemotherapy with standard or more powerful drugs.

Q. 16. What is the prognosis in testicular cancers?

Spermatocytic seminomas have the **best prognosis. Early stages of seminomas** are **curable diseases** because they **respond very well** to **chemoradiation.** The **five year disease-free interval** is about **95%. Teratomas** are basically **more aggressive** tumours. Patients with a **mature variety** belonging to an **early stage** do **well** with **chemotherapy,** the **survival rate** reaching the **same level** as that of a **seminoma.** The **immature variety** has a **poorer outlook. Choriocarcinomas** are the **most aggressive** and hence the outcome is **very poor.**

A CASE OF CARCINOMA OF THE PENIS

Setting

- Surgical outpatient department.

Presenting Complaint

- A **nonhealing ulcer** in the **penis** for the last **six months**.

History of Present Illness

- This **52-year-old man** had come to the outpatient department with an **ulcer** in the **glans penis** of **six months** duration. He had noticed a small **blister** which had **burst open** resulting in an **ulcer**. The ulcer had been **gradually increasing** in size. The patient did not complain of any **pain**. There was a history of **foul smelling discharge** from the ulcer. There was no episode of **bleeding** from the ulcer. Patient did **not** have any **urinary symptoms**. He had **not** lost any **weight** during the last six months.

Past and Personal History

- The patient did not give any past history of **phimosis**. There was no history of exposure to **sexually transmitted disease** in the past.

General Physical Examination

- There was **no** significant **abnormality** on general examination.

Local Examination

Inspection

1. **Site and extent:** Inspection revealed a **proliferative ulcer** situated at the glans penis. It was seen on the **dorsal aspect** extending on to both **lateral sides.**
2. **Size:** The ulcer measured 4 cm by 4 cm in size.
3. **Shape** was circular.
4. **Floor:** The floor showed plenty of **slough** with **reddish nodular** tissue. The **floor** appeared to be **raised** in relation to the surrounding area.
5. **Margins:** The margins were **irregular.**
6. There was a **foul smelling discharge** from the ulcer.
7. **Surrounding area:** The **urethral orifice** was **normal.** The distal part of the **shaft** of the penis appeared **swollen**.

Palpation

1. The area around the ulcer was not **warm.** The ulcer showed minimal **tenderness.**
2. The **edges** of the ulcer were **raised and everted**.
3. There was marked **induration** at the base, which was formed by the **glans penis.** The induration was **extending** into the **shaft** for about **2 cm** from the **corona glandis.**

4. **Palpation** of the **urethra** did not show any abnormality.

5. **Testes** on both sides could be **palpated** and were **normal.**

6. **Palpation of inguinal lymph nodes.** On the **right** side **multiple** lymph **nodes** were palpable. They belonged to the **superficial horizontal** group. The largest node measured **2 cm** in size. They were **hard, nontender**, **mobile** and **discrete**. **External iliac** nodes were **not palpable.**

7. Palpation of the left inguinal region did not reveal any lymphadenopathy. External iliac nodes were not palpable.

8. Examination of **other systems** did not reveal any abnormality.

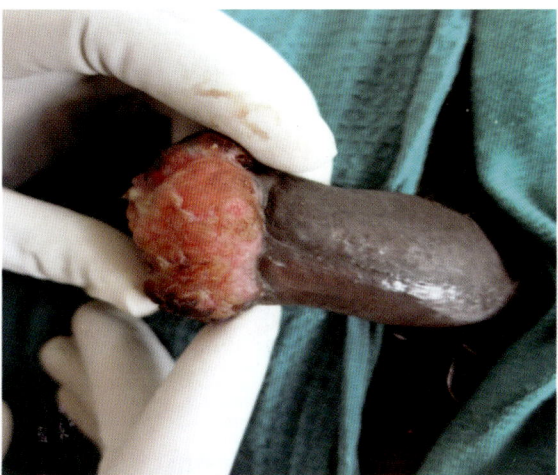

Fig. 15.1: Proliferative ulcer in the glans penis.

Box 15.8	Points to be noted in history

- Ulcer – Mode of onset – Rate of growth. Pain
- Discharge – Foul smelling – Blood stained.
- Difficulty in micturition.
- Swellings in the inguinal region.
- Previous history of phimosis or STD.

Box 15.9	Points to be noted on inspection

- Ulcerated growth in the glans penis – Corona – Common site.
- Site and extent – Size and shape.
- Floor – Slough and reddish nodular tissue.
- Elevated or excavating type of floor.
- Foul smelling discharge – Blood stained.
- Margins – Regular or irregular.
- Urethral meatus – Normal.
- Surrounding area – Swelling – Extension to the shaft.

Box 15.10	Points to be noted on palpation

- Warmth and tenderness.
- Edges – Raised and everted.
- Base – Induration – Confined to glans – Extension to shaft.
- Late stages – Local fixity to the pubic bone – Rare.
- Palpation of the urethra.
- Inguinal lymph nodes – Both sides – Number, size and shape, consistency and mobility.
- Bilateral external iliac nodes.
- Examination of the abdomen – Essentially normal.

Q. 1. What was the clinical diagnosis?

The diagnosis was **carcinoma of the penis**. It was based on the presence of a **proliferative type** of ulcer with **raised and everted edges** as well as **induration.**

Q. 2. What other conditions can present with an ulcer in the penis?

The following three conditions can manifest with an ulcer in the penis: a **primary chancre** due to syphilis, **granuloma venereum** and a transitory ulcer in **lymphogranuloma inguinale**. All these are rather uncommon at the present time.

Q. 3. **What were the investigations?**

Multiple **edge biopsies** were done. The report was a **well-differentiated squamous cell carcinoma**. **Ultrasound** of the **left inguinal** and both **iliac** regions did not show **any lymphadenopathy**. **Chest X-ray** was normal. **Renal function tests** were normal. **Ultrasound** of the **abdomen** was normal.

Box 15.11 The necessary investigations
• Multiple edge biopsy – Squamous cell carcinoma – Broder's classification.
• US abdomen – Nonpalpable inguinal and external iliac nodes.
• FNAC of inguinal nodes – Limited value.
• Chest X-ray – Normal.
• Renal function tests.

Q. 4. **What are treatment options for the primary tumour for this patient?**

(*a*) Circumcision.

(*b*) Partial amputation of the penis.

(*c*) Total amputation of the penis.

Answer. (*c*).

Setting: A few days later the patient was posted for surgery.

Q. 5. **What was the operation of choice for this patient?**

Total amputation of the penis was the best operation. Once the **shaft** was **involved**, the **entire penis** had to be removed; since anatomically the **shaft** showed signs of involvement, thus allowing the **malignant cells** to **spread** within the **corpora cavernosa**, which consists of **blood-filled spaces** with **free communication** between them. Following **removal** of the **penis,** the **bulbous urethra** was implanted in the perineum as a **perineal urethrostomy**.

Q. 6. **Describe briefly the steps of total amputation of the penis**.

The nature of the operation should be **explained in detail** to the patient since loss of the organ leads to great **psychological distress**. He needs to be assured that plastic **surgical reconstruction** is **feasible**. Since many belong to the **older age** group, the demand for **reconstruction** is very **low**. The main principles of the procedure are as follows. A segment of the **urethra 4 cm** in length (bulbous portion) is **dissected** from the **corpora**. The **penis** is then removed by dividing the **suspensory ligament** and the **corpora** from the **pubic bone**. The **superficial** and **deep vessels** are **ligated** to obtain absolute haemostasis. The **urethra** is implanted as a **perineal** urethrostomy for passage of urine.

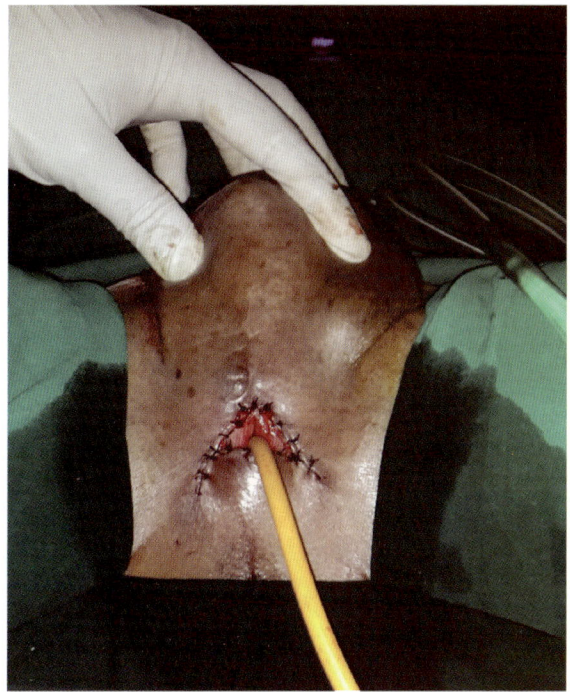

Fig. 15.2: Perineal urethrostomy following a total amputation of the penis.

If the **indications** for the operation are **strictly adhered** to, the incidence of **local recurrence** is **very low**.

Q. 7. How were the secondary lymph nodes treated in this patient?

The role of **FNAC** in the management of these nodes is **limited**. A **negative** report does not always **rule out malignancy**. The clinical findings of **hard mobile** nodes suggested **malignancy.** They were treated by an **ilioinguinal radical lymphadenectomy**. Through a horizontal **S-shaped** incision made at the **groin crease**, the **following structures** were **removed en bloc**. They included the **fat, fascia and the lymph nodes** in the **femoral triangle**. The lymph nodes excised were the **superficial horizontal** and **vertical groups** as well as the **deep inguinal** groups, including the **node of Cloquet** located within the femoral canal. In addition, the **femoral sheath** and the **terminal portion** of the **long saphenous vein** were excised. Exposure of the **external iliac region** was obtained by **division of the inguinal ligament**. The **external iliac lymph nodes** and the surrounding fat in relation with the **external iliac vessels** were removed.

Q. 8. What are the common postoperative complications?

The postoperative complications include **skin necrosis, lymphorrhoea** and **lymphoedema** of the lower limb. The risk of **femoral blow out** leading to **exsanguinating bleed** is **reduced** by **covering** these **vessels** by a **sartorius transposition flap**. In properly selected cases, **preservation** of the **long saphenous vein** is being practised. This has been shown to be as **effective** as the standard **operation** as far as the **prognosis** is concerned. But the **postoperative morbidity** of **lymphoedema** is **less** following this modification.

Q. 9. What is the prognosis for this patient?

Squamous cell carcinomas are **locoregional cancers**. **Spread beyond** the **external iliac nodes** is **uncommon**. Hence a **total amputation** of the penis along with a **radical lymphadenectomy** should give a **good prognosis**. Presence of **enlarged external iliac nodes** is the only **unfavourable factor** in this patient.

Q. 10. How does phimosis cause an increase in the incidence of penile cancers?

Bacterial action on the **desquamated epithelium** results in the formation of **smegma,** which tends to accumulate in the preputial sac and acts as a **chemical carcinogen** leading to cancer.

Q. 11. What are the causes of acquired phimosis in an adult?

Diabetes and **subpreputial cancers** are the causes for **acquired phimosis. Diabetes** is much more **common.** Repeated attacks of **balanoposthitis** cause

the formation of **adhesions** between the layers of the prepuce, leading to the development of **phimosis.** The prepuce appears **oedematous** and **macerated.** The **preputial opening** has a typical appearance with **multiple cracks.**

Q. 12. Can this cancer be prevented?

Religious circumcision is being performed either at the **neonatal stage** or during early childhood by certain communities; this can **prevent** this **cancer.**

Q. 13. Why is cancer penis common in the lower strata of society?

Poor personal hygiene leading to **accumulation of smegma** is the main reason for this increased incidence.

Q. 14. Why do most of our patients report at an advanced stage of the disease?

There is an **innate shyness** on the part of the patient to come to the doctor in this situation. Again there is a fear that a **diagnosis of STD** may be made casting aspersions on the **moral status** of the patient. Hence a vast majority of our patients come at a **stage** where the cancer has already infiltrated the **shaft** of the penis and with **enlarged nodes**.

Q. 15. What is a subpreputial cancer and how does it differ from the common variety?

In the presence of **phimosis,** the **growth** is covered by the **preputial skin.** The patient complains of **foul smelling discharge** from the preputial orifice. On palpation, induration is felt under the **prepuce.** Hence a **careful examination** is necessary. The **extent** of induration depends on the **size** of the tumour. At a **later stage,** the cancer can spread to involve the **corona glandis** and the **glans penis.**

Q. 16. How is subpreputial cancer diagnosed?

A **dorsal slit** of the prepuce is performed under local anaesthesia. The **growth** is now **visualised.** The **size and the extent** of the cancer can be accurately assessed. **Edge biopsy** confirms the **diagnosis.**

Q. 17. What are the common premalignant conditions?

(*a*) **Leukoplakia** is characterised by the presence of **solitary or multiple whitish plaques** involving the **prepuce** or **glans penis.**

(*b*) **Balanitis xerotica obliterans.** It is a **chronic inflammatory condition** of **unknown aetiology.** It results in an **indurated plaque** in the **glans** often leading to **meatal stenosis.**

(*c*) **Paget's disease** appears as a **reddish nonhealing ulcer** in the glans. **Biopsy** is always needed to rule out **malignancy.**

(*d*) **Queyrat's erythroplakia. (eryth-roplasia)** is grouped by many as **cancer in situ** and included under **Bowens disease.** It appears as a **single or multiple reddish** patches with **encrustation and scaling. Itching** is a common symptom.

(*e*) **Buschke Lowenstein tumour** is a **large exophytic** mass present in the **prepuce.** It may show **malignant features** in some instances, but **does not metastasise.**

Q. 18. What is the role of sentinel node biopsy in carcinoma of the penis?

It is indicated when **inguinal lymph nodes** are not detected either by **clinical examination** or by **ultrasound.** The **rationale** behind this procedure is as follows. **Sentinel nodes** are **first group of nodes** to be infiltrated by **malignancy.** If they do **not show** any evidence of **metastases,** a **lymph node dissection** can be **avoided.** Thus the **morbidity** associated with this procedure like **refractory lymphoedema** can be **prevented.**

Q. 19. Describe the procedure of a sentinel node biopsy.

The **sentinel node** is identified by the use of a **dye** as well as a **radioactive isotope. Methylene blue** and **radioactive sulphur colloid** are injected **into and around the tumour.** The **inguinal region** is examined for **radioactivity** with a handheld **gamma camera. If high activity** is detected, an **incision** is made in the **inguinal region.** Presence of **blue** coloured nodes with **high radioactivity** suggests **metastatic nodes.** These nodes are **excised** and sent for **frozen section** examination. If the test is **positive,** a **radical surgery** is performed. A **negative report** needs only **observation.** The procedure is usually **combined** with the **surgery** for the **primary tumour.**

Q. 20. Which are the other cancers where sentinel node biopsy is being practised?

Malignant melanoma and **carcinoma of the breast** are the other two cancers where **sentinel node biopsies** are performed.

Q. 21. What is the treatment of a subpreputial cancer?

Cancers confined to the **prepuce** are treated by circumcision provided a **2 cm clearance** can be obtained beyond the **edge of induration** by this procedure. Otherwise these patients need **a partial amputation.**

Q. 22. What is the indication for a partial amputation of the penis?

The **growth** must be confined to the glans penis. In addition after **division** of the **shaft 2 cm beyond the edge of induration,** the remaining **stump** should at least be **2 cm to 3 cm** in **length.** A **shorter stump** would cause the **urinary stream** to trickle down the **scrotum** leading to **ammoniacal dermatitis,** making the **patient miserable.** Such patients end up with a **total amputation.**

Q. 23. What are the advantages of a partial amputation?

Psychologically, the operation is **less traumatic** to the patient. A **total amputation** would mean **loss of manhood,** which may not be acceptable to some patients. **Successful sexual intercourse** has been reported after a partial amputation.

Q. 24. What is the indication for total amputation of the penis ?

Cancers involving the shaft of the penis need this amputation. Unfortunately this is the most common surgical procedure in our country.

Q. 25. What are the causes for the enlargement of inguinal nodes in these cancers?

Inguinal lymph nodes could be **enlarged** either due to **infection** or **infiltration. Infected nodes** are found in about **20%** of the patients. They are **soft and tender**. They respond to **antimicrobial therapy**. If the lymph nodes undergo **complete resolution**, these patients need only **observation**. Nodes that persist are likely to be malignant and treated accordingly. **Metastatic nodes** as mentioned above are treated by **radical surgery**.

Q. 26. What is the treatment for advanced cancers?

Advanced primary tumours **fixed to the bone** are rare. They are treated by **palliative radiotherapy**. A **small number** may need **urinary diversion**.

Fixed metastatic nodes are more **common**. In addition, involvement of the **internal iliac** and **obturator nodes,** as detected on **imaging studies**, suggests **inoperability. Palliative chemoradiation** is the line of treatment for this group of patients. **EBRT** along with **Cisplatin** is the drug often used for palliation.

Q. 27. What are the causes of death in penile cancer?

Recurrent urinary infection can lead to renal failure. **Secondary nodes** may erode the **femoral vessels** leading to **exsanguinating haemorrhage**.

Box 15.12	Treatment of regional nodes

• No nodes (including US) – Sentinel node biopsy
• Infected nodes – Antimicrobials – Resolution – Observation
• Metastatic nodes – Positive sentinel node on biopsy
  ▪ Nodes persisting after antimicrobials
  ▪ FNAC positive nodes – Hard and mobile
• Ilioinguinal radical lymphadenectomy.
• Superficial, deep inguinal and external iliac nodes along with fat, fascia over the femoral triangle.
• Terminal part of the long saphenous vein.
• Fixed nodes - Palliative EBRT.	

In general carcinoma of the penis being a **squamous cell tumour** behaves like a **locoregional tumour**. The **five year disease-free interval** is more than **90%,** except in the last group mentioned above.

■■■

Skin and Soft Tissues

16

COMMON SUBCUTANEOUS SWELLINGS

EPIDERMOID CYST

Setting

- Surgical ward.

Chief Complaint

- **Swelling** in the **sole of the left foot**.

Occupation

- Manual labourer.

History of Present Illness

- A **52-year-old man** was **admitted** to the surgical wards with the **complaint** of **swelling** in the **sole of the left foot** of **two years duration**. The **swelling** was **noted** by the **patient** around the **middle** of the **sole** of the foot **two years** ago. It was **small** initially and over a **period of time** it had **gradually increased in size**. He did **not** have any **pain.** The patient had **difficulty in walking**

due to the **size** of the **swelling,** but he was **able** to **continue with his occupation**. He was used to **walking without** any **footwear**. There was **no history** of **minor trauma**. There was **no history** of **fever**. He **did not complain** of **similar swellings** in **other parts** of the body.

- **Past, family and personal histories** were insignificant.

Treatment History

- He had **not taken** any **treatment** for this condition.
- **General physical examination** was within normal limits.

Local Examination

Inspection

- **Gait:** The patient was **walking** with the **foot inverted** to avoid the swelling coming in contact with the ground.

- A **swelling** was present in the **sole** of the **left foot**. It was **extending** from the **middle of the sole** to the **base of the toes. Horizontally,** the extension was from the level of the **third metatarsal** to the **medial border** of the foot.

- It was **oval** in **shape**. The **size** was **6 cm by 4 cm**. The **margins were distinct**.

- The **surface** was **lobular.** The **skin** appeared **stretched** over the swelling.

- The **surrounding area** was **normal.**

Palpation

- It was **not warm or tender**.

- The **size and shape** were confirmed. The **borders** were distinct.

- The **consistency** was **soft.** It was **fluctuant** but **not transilluminant.**

- The **skin** over the **swelling** was **adherent** to the **swelling** at the **periphery.**

- **Mobility. Restricted mobility** was present both in the **horizontal** and **vertical directions.**

- The **anatomical plane** was **subcutaneous.**

- **Movements** of the **toes** were **not restricted**.

- Examination of the **subtalar** and **ankle joints** did **not** show any **abnormality.**

- **Examination** of the **circulatory, nervous and lymphatic systems** in the limb did **not** show any **abnormality**.

- The **inguinal lymph nodes** were **not palpable.**

- **Clinically** all the **other systems** were normal.

Box 16.1:	Points regarding history

- Swelling – Site – Sole of the foot.
- Duration – 2 years – Rate of growth – Slow.
- Associated symptoms - None.
- History of trauma - Absent.

Box 16.2:	Points regarding the clinical findings

- Site and extent – Sole of the foot – Distal half – Medial aspect.
- Size and shape – Borders.
- Surface – Skin over the swelling – Surrounding area.
- Consistency – Soft – Fluctuant – Nontransilluminant.
- Mobility – Thick plantar skin – Restricted.
- Plane – Subcutaneous.

Q. 1. What was the clinical diagnosis?

(*a*) Sebaceous cyst.

(*b*) Epidermoid cyst.

(*c*) Ganglion.

The **diagnosis is (*b*).**

Since **sebaceous glands** are **not** present in the **sole of the foot**, the swelling **cannot** be a **sebaceous cyst. Ganglions** occur in relation to the **synovial sheaths** of the **tendons**. They are **more common** around the **wrist.** In the **foot** they are seen on the **dorsal surface**. They are not only **cystic,** but also **transilluminant.** They **lose** their **mobility** when the **tendon** is put on **contraction** against **resistance. Epidermoid cysts** are seen frequently in the **sole of the foot** amongst **our patients** since many **walk bare feet**. The swelling is **cystic.** It is **free** from the skin and is in the **subcutaneous plane**.

Q. 2. Is the presence of an epidermoid cyst an indication for treatment?

The answer is yes. The patient had **mechanical difficulty** in **walking** due to the **location** and **size** of the **cyst. Infection** is a known complication resulting in the formation of an **abscess.** The **abscess** has to be **drained** under **antimicrobial cover** and the **removal** of the cyst needs a **second operation**.

Q. 3. What is the content of an epidermoid cyst?

The cyst contains **pultaceous material.**

Setting: 4 days later.

Q. 4. How was this patient treated?

Excision of the **cyst** was **performed.** A **vertical incision** was made over the **summit** of the swelling (**avoiding** the **weight-bearing area** of the sole of the foot). The **medial** and **lateral skin flaps** were raised. In some areas the **skin** was **firmly adherent** to the swelling. The **cyst** was **dissected off** from the **deeper structures**. The incision was **closed** with **interrupted sutures**.

He was **discharged** from the hospital the **next day.** He reported to the OPD **10 days** later for **removal of sutures**.

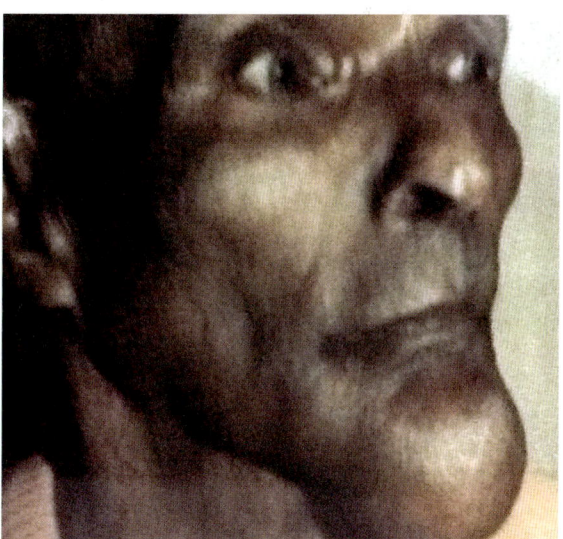

Fig. 16.1: Epidermoid cyst in the submental region.

3 weeks later he was seen at the **OPD** again. The **incision** had **healed well**. He was advised to **use footwear** before going back to work.

Q. 5. What is an epidermoid cyst?

It is a **cyst** formed by the **epidermal cells** when they are **buried** in the **deeper tissues**. It is an **inherent character** of **skin cells** in that when they are **placed** into the **deeper layers**, they **curl amongst themselves** to form a **cyst.**

Q. 6. What are the two types of epidermoid cysts?

1. **Sequestration epidermoid cyst:** The cyst is of **congenital origin**. During **fusion** of **two dermatomes, skin cells** are **sequestered (isolated)** into the **deeper tissues** resulting in **cyst formation.** Hence they are **seen** only at **specific sites** of **embryonic fusion.** The **commonest site** is an **external angular dermoid** seen **above and lateral** to the **outer angle** of the **eye.** During **development** of the **face,** the **fusion** of the **frontonasal process** and **maxillary process** occurs at this **site.** Despite its **congenital origin,** the cyst **often presents in adults** since the **rate of growth** is very **slow.**

It manifests as a **globular swelling** in relation to the outer angle of the eye. It is usually about 2 **cm in diameter,** being **fluctuant and nontransilluminant.** The **skin** can be **lifted off** the swelling. It has **transverse mobility.** If a **cyst** has been present for **several years,** it may **cause erosion** of the **outer table** of the **skull bone.** This clinical sign is **detected** by **displacing the cyst laterally** and **feeling the medial border.** As the **finger traces the border,** it may **dip in** indicating a **depression** in the **bone. Treatment** is by **excision.**

Most of the **remaining sequestration dermoid cysts** tend present as **midline swellings.**

2. **Implantation epidermoid cysts:** This is an **acquired condition.** As a result of **minor trauma,** like a **thorn** or a **needle prick, viable epidermal cells** are **deposited** in the **subcutaneous plane.** In **many patients,** a **history of trauma** may **not** be **available.** These **cells multiply** giving rise to a **cyst.** In our patients the **sole** of the **foot** is the **commonest site.** It is also

described in the **palm and fingers**, especially in **tailors**. **Treatment** is by **excision.**

Box 16.3:	Points regarding epidermoid cysts

- Results from deposition of skin cells into the deeper layers.
- Sequestration type – Congenital – Lines of fusion of dermatomes.
- External Angular – Commonest – Asymptomatic swelling – Bony erosion.
- Others – Midline swellings.
- Implantation type – Acquired – Viable skin cells placed deep to skin.
- Minor trauma – Thorn or needle prick – Often forgotten by the patient.
- Sole of the foot or fingers.
- Treatment – Excision.

Q. 7. What is a sebaceous cyst?

It **is a retention cyst of the sebaceous gland**. The **duct draining** the gland is **blocked** by **inspissated sebum**. The **contents** are **retained** within the **gland** resulting in the **formation** of the **cyst**. Hence the **content** is **sebaceous material**.

Q. 8. What are the clinical features of a sebaceous cyst?

The **scalp** and the scrotum are the **common sites of occurrence**. At these sites they are often **multiple**. But they can occur at **other sites** as well, **except** the **palm** and the **sole** of the **foot**, since **sebaceous glands**

are **absent** at these two sites. They **present** as **asymptomatic swellings** of **several years** duration. They may **assume a large size**. They are **cystic and nontransilluminant**. At the **summit of the swelling**, the **blocked opening** of the **duct** may be **visible** as a **black or brownish black spot** known as the **punctum.** In the **coloured population**, the **punctum** may **not** be **easily recognized**. Since the **sebaceous gland** is present in the **skin**, the **swelling** is **always adherent** to the **skin** especially near the **summit or the punctum.** In the case of **large cysts**, the **skin** may be **free** at the **periphery**.

Q. 9. What are the complications of a sebaceous cyst?

Infection is a **frequent complication.** Once the **punctum** is **breached**, the **bacteria** have a **free access** to the **cyst**. The **cyst becomes painful and tender.** There may be **redness** of the **overlying skin**. **Spontaneous rupture** leads to a **foul smelling discharge**. **Incision** and **drainage** under **antimicrobial cover** is necessary. All the **contents are curetted** out. **No attempt** is made to **excise the cyst** at this stage. **Inflammation increases** the **vascularity** and the **cyst wall** is **very friable**. If a **portion** of the **cyst wall** is **retained, recurrence is likely**. Once the **incision has healed,** it is safer to wait for a **period of three months** before the cyst is **excised.**

When a **sebaceous cyst** in a **hairy scalp** gets **infected,** it can lead to a **rare complication** called **Cock's peculiar tumour**. **Spontaneous rupture** leads to the formation of a **proliferative granuloma**, which **resembles** a **squamous cell carcinoma** with **raised edges**. But there is **no induration**. The **word tumour** is a **misnomer** in this situation, since it is only an **infective granuloma** probably **caused** by **repeated minor trauma** while **combing the hair**. **Treatment** is by **excision**. A **large defect** may need a **rotation flap** for a **primary closure.**

Q. 10. What is the treatment of a sebaceous cyst?

Excision is the treatment. An **ellipse of skin around the punctum** is **excised** to **reduce** the **chances** of a **recurrence**. This is to **ensure** that the **ductal epithelium** is **removed** along with the cyst. In **most instances,** it is a **simple operation** done under **local anaesthesia.**

Box 16.4:	Points regarding sebaceous cysts

- Retention cyst – Blockage of the duct – Sebaceous material.
- Scalp and scrotum common sites – Not seen in palm and sole of foot.
- Asymptomatic swelling – Several years – Cystic – Nontransilluminant.
- Infection – Common – Rupture – Foul smelling discharge.
- Incision and drainage – Excision 3 months later.
- Infection in a cyst – Hairy scalp – Cock's peculiar tumour – Infective granuloma – Simulates squamous cell carcinoma – Excision.
- Treatment – excision with an ellipse of skin around the punctum

Q. 11. What is a lipoma?

It is a **benign tumour** arising from the **adipocytes.** It is the **most common benign tumour** seen in the body.

Q. 12. What are the clinical features of a subcutaneous lipoma?

Lipoma appears as an **asymptomatic swelling**. It can be seen in **any part** of the **body.** The **back** is a **common site**. The **rate of growth** is **very slow**. The **duration** is always mentioned in **years.** Hence it is **not uncommon** to see **huge lipomas** in **our patients.**

The **shape** is **oval**, and the **size** is **variable**. The **margins** are **well defined**. The **surface is**

lobular. On palpation it is **soft** in consistency. It is **fluctuant** since **fat** is said to be in a **liquid state** at **body temperature**. It is **mobile** in both directions. The **classical sign** of a lipoma is that the **edge slips** under the **palpating finger**.

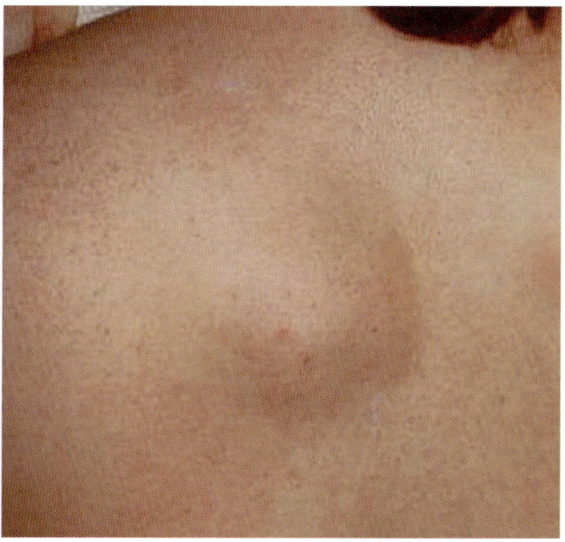

Fig. 16.2: Lipoma over the shoulder region.

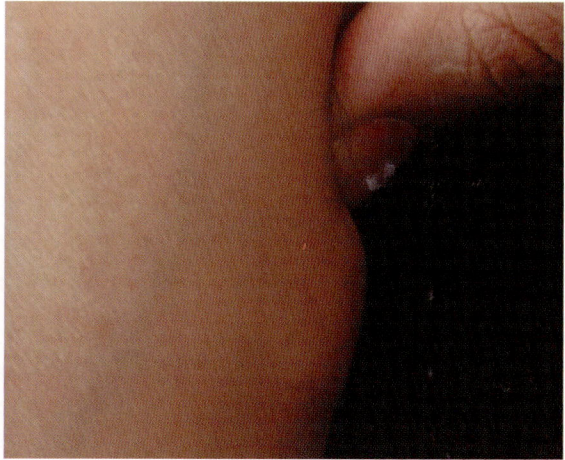

Fig. 16.3: The "slip sign" being demonstrated in a lipoma.

Q. 13. What are the other sites where lipoma can occur?

This tumour has been described at the **following anatomical sites**.

(*a*) Subfascial.

(*b*) Inter or intramuscular.

(*c*) Intra-articular.

(*d*) Intraosseous.

(*e*) Extra or subdural and subarachnoid in relation to the spinal cord.

(*f*) Subserous or submucous in the bowel.

(*g*) Retroperitoneal.

(*h*) Extension of retroperitoneal fat along the spermatic cord is known as lipomatosis of the spermatic cord.

Depending upon the **site,** these produce **different clinical pictures**. A **submucous lipoma** may cause an **intussusception.** Lipomas in relation to the **spinal cord** may cause **pressure symptoms**. **Intermuscular** or **intramuscular** lipomas may be **difficult** to detect **clinically.** A **retroperitoneal** lipoma **may not be detected** until it reaches a **large size.**

Q. 14. What are the investigations needed in these cases?

CECT or **MRI scans** of the **region** are performed to identify these lesions.

FNAC preferably under **image guidance** is done if **malignancy** is suspected.

CT chest to rule out **secondaries.**

Q. 15. What are the complications?

The **rate of complication** is rather **low.**

Infection can occur in a **subcutaneous lipoma**.

A **lipoma** that has been **present for several years** can undergo **calcification**. This is seen in **lipomas** occupying the **anterior abdominal wall.**

A **retroperitoneal lipoma** has the **highest risk** of a **malignant change**. A **recent rapid increase in size** along with symptoms due to **involvement** of the **adjacent structures** like **bowel or ureter** may suggest **malignancy.**

Q. 16. What is the treatment of a subcutaneous lipoma?

Enucleation from **within the capsule** is **easily performed**. **Small tumours** can be removed under **local anaesthesia**. The rate of **recurrence** is practically **zero.**

Box 16.5:	Points regarding lipomas

- Benign – From adipocytes – Most common – Subcutaneous – Oval – Lobular – Fluctuant – Slip sign.
- Deeper – Various sites – Clinical features – Depending on site.
- CECT – MRI-guided biopsy – CT chest.
- Enucleation for subcutaneous lipoma.

A CASE OF MALIGNANT MELANOMA

Setting

- Surgical OPD.

Chief Complaint

- **Blackish lesion** in the **sole of the right foot**. Duration: **6 months**.

- A **44-year-old man** presented to the OPD with the complaint of a **blackish growth** in the **sole of the right foot** of **6 months duration**. He had noticed a **small black mole** at that site **several years** ago.

- For the **last six months** he had noticed that the **mole** was **rapidly increasing** in **size.** It had **ulcerated** after a period of 2 months, and was associated with a **foul smelling discharge**. There were **two episodes** of **bleeding** from the ulcer.

- He had **difficulty** in **walking.** But there was **no pain**.

- He had noticed a **swelling** in the **right groin** about 2 months ago and this was also **rapidly increasing in size**.

- He had **no fever**. He did not complain of **chronic cough** or **chest pain.**

- There was **no loss of weight or appetite**.

- **Past history and family history** were not significant.

Personal History

- He was a smoker and used to consume alcohol regularly.

Treatment History

- He had applied **several ointments** locally **without consulting** any **doctor.**

- **General physical examination** was normal.

Local Examination

Inspection

- **Gait:** The patient was **walking** with the **heel** of the right foot **raised** off the ground.

- A **proliferative blackish ulcer** was present occupying the **calcaneal region of the sole** of the **foot**.

- It was **6 cm by 5 cm in size** and was **irregular** in **shape.**

- The **margins** were irregular.

- The **floor** consisted of **blackish tissue** with areas of **slough** in between. Few areas of **reddish nodular tissue** were also seen.

- The **surrounding** area appeared **swollen.**

Palpation

- It was not **warm or tender**.

- The **site**, **size** and **borders** were **confirmed** as on inspection.
- The **edges** were **raised**. There was **no induration**.
- The **ulcer** was fixed to the **calcaneum,** which formed **the base**.
- No **thickening** of the **bone** could be made out.
- There was **no bleeding** from the ulcer during palpation.
- Both **inversion and eversion** were **restricted** and **movements** at the **ankle joint** were also **restricted.**
- There was **no evidence** of any **satellite or transit nodules**.
- **Examination of the inguinal region** revealed **multiple enlarged lymph nodes** belonging to the **superficial inguinal** group. They were **2 cm to 3 cm** in **size, soft and nontender**. All the nodes were **mobile.**
- **External iliac lymph nodes** were **not palpable.**
- Examination of the **abdomen** did **not** reveal any **hepatomegaly.**
- **Chest** was clinically normal.

Box 16.6:	Points to be noted in history

- Presence of a black mole – Several years – Sole of the foot.
- Recent increase in size – Ulceration.
- Foul smelling discharge.
- Pain – Absent.
- Difficulty in walking.
- Swelling in the groin.

Box 16.7:	Points to be noted in inspection

- Site and extent – Sole of right foot – Margins.
- Size and shape.
- Floor – Blackish with slough and reddish nodules.
- Discharge – Purulent – Foul smelling.
- Surrounding area - Swelling.

Box 16.8:	Points to be noted during palpation

- Site and extent.
- Size and shape.
- Edge – Raised and everted.
- Base – Fixed to bone – Calcaneum.
- Absence of induration.
- Neighbouring joints – Subtalar and ankle – Restricted.
- Satellite and transit nodules.
- Inguinal nodes.

Box 16.9:	Points regarding the rest of clinical examination

- External iliac nodes.
- Abdomen – Hepatomegaly.
- Chest

Q. 1. What was the clinical diagnosis?

The clinical diagnosis was a **malignant melanoma**. The features were typical of a melanoma. The patient had a benign naevus that later turned into a malignant melanoma. The **signs** also supported the same diagnosis.

Q. 2. What were the investigations done in this patient?

Edge biopsy.

X-ray of the foot AP and LAT views showed **erosion** of the plantar surface of the **calcaneum.**

US abdomen. External iliac nodes were not enlarged. **Liver** was normal.

Chest X-ray was normal.

Setting: Four days later.

Biopsy report was a **malignant melanoma**.

Q. 3. **What was the treatment carried out for this patient?**

A **below-knee amputation** was performed.

Two weeks later he underwent an **ilio-inguinal radical lymphadenectomy.**

Q. 4. **What was the postoperative treatment?**

Patient was given a course of **DTIC.**

Q. 5. **What could be the outcome for this patient?**

The **outcome** would be rather **poor.** Once lymph node metastases develop, the **long-term survival** figures are **low.** Despite **chemotherapy** the chances are high that he would develop **fatal secondaries in the lung or liver**.

Q. 6. **What is the incidence of malignant melanoma?**

Malignant melanoma is an **uncommon** but **aggressive tumour**. It is responsible for only about **3% to 4%** of all **malignant skin tumours**. In the **developed countries,** a **significant increase** in the incidence has been reported. **Lifestyle changes** with an **increased exposure** to the **ultraviolet rays** of the sun have been blamed for this increase. It is **less frequently** seen in the **coloured population** as compared to the Caucasians. It arises from the **melanocyte** present in the basal **layer** of the **epidermis**. These **cells** are derived from the **neural crest**. Melanomas are also seen in the **mucous membrane** of the **oral cavity** and **anal canal** as well as the **choroid plexus** in the eye.

Q. 7. **What are melanocytes?**

These are **neuroectodermal** cells present in the **basal layer** of the epidermis. These cells are derived from the **neural crest**. They secrete the pigment **melanin,** which is an **antioxidant** and a **free radical scavenger**. Hence it helps to protect the **skin cells** as well as the **melanocytes** themselves from the **harmful effects of UV** rays

Q. 8. **Name the common types of naevi found in clinical practice.**

A **naevus** means a birthmark in **Latin**. Though **pigmented lesions** arising from **connective and vascular tissue** have been described, the **word** is commonly referred to **lesions arising from melanocytes**. The following are the common varieties.

(*a*) **Blue naevus:** This is **very common** especially in the **Asian population**. Their **size** varies around **6 mm.** They are **blue** or more often **bluish black** in colour. They may be **slightly elevated**. The risk of **malignant change** is **very low**.

(*b*) **Hairy naevus: (CNN)**. It is said to arise from **melanoblast** cells. These are the **precursors of melanocytes** that have **migrated** from the **neural crest**. They are most often seen at **birth**. These are **blackish lesions** covered by **hair**. Some of them are **large** and are described as **giant CNN**. The origin is **embryological**. The lack of **maturation** of these cells during **foetal life** allows them to **persist** and give rise to this **naevus**. Hence the term **congenital naevomelanocytic naevus** (**CNN**) is used to describe this lesion. Lesions present in the **face** may be associated with **melanocytic lesions intracranially**. **Symptomatic children** may need a **MRI** scan. The risk of **malignant transformation** is high. Thus they need to be **treated**

during infancy. The **risk** of malignancy **decrease** as **age advances**.

(*c*) A **dysplastic naevus** is one where **certain changes** suggestive of **malignancy** are present and hence **should always be excised**.

(*d*) **Junctional naevus:** It extends from the **epidermis** to the **dermis**. Their **malignant potential is high** when they are present in the **mucous membrane** or the **external genitalia**.

Q. 9. Name the conditions that favour the development of a melanoma.

The **following conditions** favour the development of melanoma.

1. **Caucasian** (White ancestry).

2. **Fair skin, light hair** and **light coloured eyes**.

3. A history of **intense, intermittent sun exposure** especially in **childhood**.

4. Presence of **more than 100 naevi** in the body. (Average is about **30**)**.**

5. **Large irregular naevi**.

6. History of a **melanoma in** close **relatives**.

7. **Xeroderma pigmentosum** predis-poses not only for **melanoma** but also for other types of skin cancers.

Box 16.10:	Points regarding general characteristics and aetiology

- Tumour arising from melanocytes present in the basal layer of the skin.
- Biologically aggressive tumour.
- Responsible for 3% to 4% of all skin cancers.
- Common in the White races.
- Lifestyle changes – Increased exposure to UV rays of the sun.
- Presence of pre-existing naevi.
- Xeroderma pigmentosum – Known premalignant disease.

Q. 10. What are the common features of a melanoma?

The tumour may occur as a **complication** of a **pre-existing benign naevus** or arise **de novo. Minor trauma** or **repeated mechanical irritations** to a mole may result in a **malignant transformation**. Some of our patients have a habit of trying to **scrape** the **mole** from the skin using a **razor blade**. This is one of the **surest method** of **inducing** a **malignant change**.

The most **common site** in **this part of the world** is the **sole of the foot,** as opposed to **the West** where **exposed areas** such as the head and neck as well as the **trunk** have a **higher incidence**. This is due to the fact that many **Indians** do **not use footwear,** exposing **moles in the sole of the foot** to repeated **minor trauma**.

Age: A disease of the **older age group**, it can also be seen in the **young.**

Gender: It is more common in **men,** but in the **younger age group** there is a **female preponderance**.

Changes in a pre-existing naevus. This part of the history is **most significant,** but it depends on the level of **education** and the powers of **observation** of the patient. Unfortunately, both these factors are **lacking** in many of **our patients,** and hence most of the **information** garnered from the **books** is of very **little relevance in our country**. It includes the **classifications** based on the **depth of the tumour**. The **large scale efforts** in the **West** to identify **early cancers** and thereby improve the **prognosis** are of limited **practical value** in **our patients**. It is hoped that in the future with **improved health care facilities**, our patients will also reach the hospital **early in the course of the disease.**

Q. 11. What are the changes that suggest malignancy in a naevus?

The **changes** described below are **useful** to **detect** a malignant transformation.

(*a*) **Rapid increase** in size of the mole.

(*b*) **Change in colour.** The naevus may become **lighter** or have a **brownish** tinge. Development of a **"halo"** around the naevus.

(*c*) **Fissuring, scaling and ulceration.**

(*d*) Symptoms like **itching and pain.**

(*e*) Changes in the **surface** like **nodularity.**

(*f*) **Redness** or a **new swelling** beyond the border.

(*g*) **Bleeding**

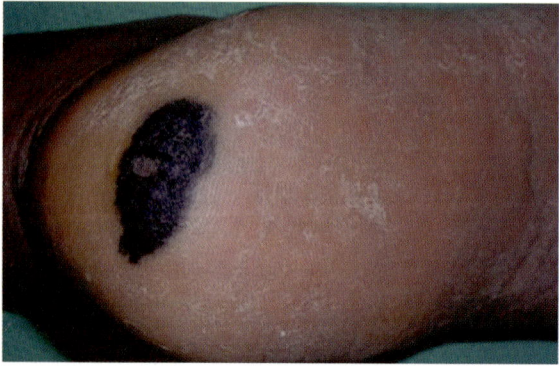

Fig. 16.4: Melanoma of the sole of the foot.

Q. 12. Describe the local signs of a melanoma.

1. The classical **ABCDE** signs are as follows:

   A. **Asymmetry** where a **portion** of the lesion looks **different.**

   B. **Border** may be **irregular, ragged, notched** or **blurred.**

C. **C is for colour: Benign** moles have a **uniform colour.** The colour may **become lighter** or assume shades of **brown, red, white** or even **blue.** The presence of a **"halo"** at the margin is significant.

D. **Diameter:** If the lesion is **more than 6 mm** in diameter, the risk of **malignancy** is very high. Most of **our patients** present with **lesions** that are **several centimetres** in diameter.

E. **Evolving tumours** presenting with any of the changes mentioned above. **Elevation** of the tumour is also a **sinister sign.**

2. **Ugly Duckling sign:** When a **particular mole** looks different or **"funny"** as compared to others, the suspicion of **malignancy is high.**

3. **Ulceration: Majority** of our patients have an **ulcerated lesion** at presentation. The **ulcer** has raised and everted edges. But **induration** unlike in a squamous cell carcinoma is **conspicuous by its absence.** It indicates the

lack of **host versus tumour** reaction. It also explains the biological **aggressive nature** of the tumour.

4. **Vertical growth of the tumour:** Melanoma is unique in that not only the **radial growth** as measured in **millimetres** or **centimetres** is **vital,** but the **prognosis** depends mainly on the **vertical growth (depth).**

Box 16.11:	Points regarding local signs – ABCDE
A – Asymmetry – A part of the tumour looks different.	
B – Border – Irregular or blurred.	
C – Change in colour – Lighter or brown – Halo at the border.	
D – More than 6 mm – Suggestive of malignancy.	
E – Evolving tumour. Elevated tumour.	

Box 16.12:	Points regarding other clinical findings
• Ugly duckling sign – One particular mole looks different.	
• Vertical growth – More important than radial growth.	
• Depth of the tumour determines the outlook.	
• Absence of induration.	
• Presence of satellite nodules.	
• Presence of transit nodules.	
• Amelanotic melanoma.	

Q. 13. What are the two common classifications of a melanoma?

The **two** basic classifications depending on the **depth of the** **tumour** are the ones described by **Clark and Breslow. Clark's staging** refers to the various layers of the **skin. Breslow's** method employs the **depth** in terms of **millimeters.**

Clark Staging of the tumour.

Level 1: Melanoma confined to the **epidermis.**

Level 2: Invasion into the **papillary dermis.**

Level 3: Invasion limited to the junction of the **papillary and reticular dermis.**

Level 4: Invasion into the **reticular dermis.**

Level 5: Invasion into **subcutaneous fat.**

Box 16.13:	Points regarding Clark's classification
Level I: Confined to the epidermis.	
Level II: Invasion of the papillary dermis.	
Level III: Invasion limited to the junction of the papillary and reticular dermis.	
Level IV: Infiltration of the reticular dermis.	
Level V: Extension into the subcutaneous fat.	

Breslow Classification (depth of the tumour).

Stage 1: Less than or **equal to 0.75 mm.**

Stage 2: 0.75 mm to **1.5 mm.**

Stage 3: 1.5 mm to 2.25 mm.

Stage 4: 2.25 mm to 3 mm.

Stage 5: More than 3 mm.

Box 16.14:	Points regarding Breslow's classification
Stage 1: Depth less than 0.75 mm	
Stage 2: Depth between 0.75 mm and 1.5 mm.	
Stage 3: Depth between 1.5 mm and 2.25 mm	
Stage 4: Depth between 2.25 mm and 3 mm	
Stage 5: Depth more than 3 mm.	
Deeper tumour – Incidence of nodal metastases high.	

Breslow classification is also a **good predictor** of **lymphatic spread**, with **deeper** tumours having **more chances** of **metastatic nodes**. If the tumour **depth** is more than **4 mm**, the outlook is **very poor**. The **base of a melanoma** of the heel as seen in our patients is often formed by the **calcaneum**. Thus the **depth** of the tumour is measured in **centimetres.**

Q. 14. What is an amelanotic melanoma?

A **small number** of tumours arising from the **melonacytes** are so **undifferentiated** that they **lose the capacity** to **produce melanin** pigment. They present as **proliferative tumours** without the **characteristic black colour**. They may easily be **mistaken** for a **squamous cell carcinoma**. But the **absence of induration** should help to **distinguish** between the two. The **anal canal** is a **common site** for this kind of cancer. Since they are **more anaplastic** in nature, their **outlook** in general is **worse** than that for the **pigmented tumours**.

Q. 15. What are satellite nodules?

These are **pigmented elevated nodules** with **irregular borders**, seen within **2 cm to 3 cm** of the borders of the **main lesion**. They are the **result** of **retrograde spread** of **malignant cells** along **blocked dermal lymphatics**.

Q. 16. What are transit nodules?

These are present along the **lymphatic pathway** of the primary tumour. If the lesion is in the **medial part** of the foot, **transit nodules** are seen along the **long saphenous vein**. They occur at the sites of **valves** inside the lymphatic vessels. These valves tend to **block the passage** of **malignant cells,** thereby allowing them to **proliferate,** and hence the term **transit nodules**. Both **satellite** and **transit nodules** are indicators of a **poor outcome**.

Q. 17. What are the modes of spread of a melanoma?

1. **Direct spread:** The tumor spreads both laterally and vertically. The vertical spread involves the subcutaneous tissue, muslce tendon and bone.

2. **Lymphatic spread:** Being an aggressive tumour, the cancer **spreads** to the regional lymph **nodes early** in the course of the disease. The lymph **nodes** are **soft** to **firm** in consistency, **nontender and mobile** to begin with, but later are **fixed** to each other or to the **deeper structures** due to **extracapsular** spread. Since the **lower limb** is the **commonest site** of melanoma in our country, the **inguinal nodes** show enlargement. At a **later stage**, the **external iliac group** is also involved. **Ulceration** of these nodes occurs if **treatment is** either **delayed** or inadequate. A small group of patients present with a **swelling** in the **inguinal region** as the **chief complaint**. The **primary** melanoma may not be **manifest** at this stage. A **meticulous search** for a primary site includes the **subungual** region, the **external genitalia** and the **anal canal**. The **primary** tumour may be much **smaller** and **insignificant** when compared with the **massive lymphadenopathy**.

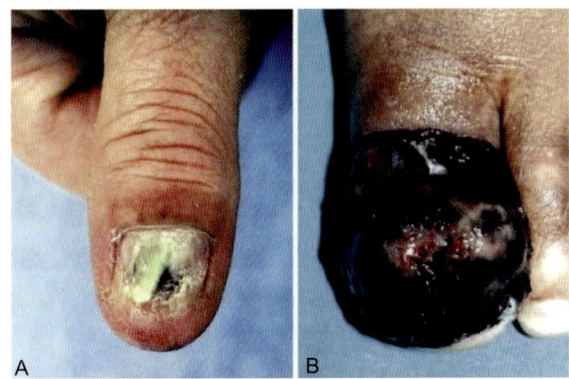

Fig. 16.5: Subungual melanoma.

3. **Blood spread** is also **common**. **Metastases** occur in the **liver, lungs and brain**. They are seen in the **late stage** of the disease. These **secondaries** usually occur **after** the primary has been **recognised and treated**. But an **occasional patient** may have at the **time of presentation**, a **primary tumour** with **secondary lymph nodes** as well as **distant metastases**.

Box 16.15:	Points regarding the spread of melanoma

- Direct spread.
- Lymphatic spread.
- Early – Nodes soft and mobile.
- Extracapsular spread – Fixed nodes.
- Ulceration through the overlying skin.
- Nodal enlargement – Presenting symptom.
- Primary sites – Subungual region, anal canal.
- Blood spread – Liver and brain common sites.

Q. 18. What are the clinical types of melanoma?

(*a*) **Superficial spreading melanoma** is the most **common type (70%).** It spreads **laterally** along the **epidermis** for **several months** before **penetrating** into the **deeper layers** of the skin. The melanoma appears as a **slightly raised lesion** with **irregular borders. Variations** in **colour** are usually seen. **Darkening** of an existing mole or **appearance** of a **new one** in close proximity are signs of a **malignant transformation.**

(*b*) **Nodular melanoma** is responsible for about **15% to 20%** of these cancers. It grows **deeper** more **quickly** than other types. The **trunk** and **head and neck** are the **common s**ites. It appears as a **blue-black** dome-shaped **nodule.** But the colour may be **reddish or pink**. This type is more often seen in **men.**

(*c*) **Lentigo maligna melanoma** arises from a pre-existing **lentigo (a small sharply circumscribed pigmented macule)** rather than a **mole.** The incidence is about **5%.** A disease of the **elderly**, it takes **many years** to develop. It is usually seen in the **areas** exposed to the **sun.** The size may be **large** and the tumour may have **varied colours.**

(*d*) **Acral lentiginous melanoma** comprises of less than **5% of** all tumours. This is the **most common** type seen in the **coloured population. Extremities** are the common site and are seen in the **palms, soles** and the **subungual** region. A history of injury leads to a **delay in diagnosis** with a mistaken impression of a **subungual haematoma.** They are in general aggressive tumours with vertical growth being a common feature.

Box 16.16:	Points regarding the clinical types of melanoma

- Superficial spreading. 70%. Lateral spread more than vertical. Flat slightly raised lesions with change in colour.
- Nodular type. 15% to 20%. Common in men.
  - Vertical growth is more. Bluish dome appearance.
  - Trunk, head and neck common sites.
- Lentigo maligna type. 5%. Elderly men.
  - Arises from a lentigo.
  - Exposed areas.
- Acral lentiginous. Less than 5%.
  - Coloured population - More common.
  - Extremities – Palm, sole and subungual regions.

Q. 19. What are the methods employed to diagnose melanoma clinically?

Since **majority** of **our patients** present **late** in the course of the **disease**, the diagnosis is **easy.** But to **differentiate** an **early malignancy** from a **benign mole** can be a **daunting task.** Clinicians use a Dermascope (also known as a **dermatoscope)** to look at these lesions. This instrument affords **adequate magnificat**ion so that **subtle changes** suggestive of **malignancy** can be identified. Even **interpretation** of biopsy results needs a dedicated and experienced **pathologist.**

Q. 20. How are these patients investigated?

1. **Biopsy:** If the **intent is to cure** as in early cases, **incisional biopsy** is **absolutely contraindicated.** The **procedure** will allow **local dissemination** of malignant cells. **Excision biopsy** is ideal and the extent of the **tissue** to be **removed** is discussed in detail later. **Brush biopsy** is an alternative if **facilities** for **adequate studies** are available. Hence edge or **incisional biopsy** is performed only when **palliative treatment** is being planned.

2. **FNAC** of enlarged nodes is **not** very **informative**. A **positive** result will **help** in the **management**. But a **negative** result **does not rule** out **secondaries** in other nodes. Most often **palpable nodes** are presumed to be **malignant.**

3. **Chest X-ray** is taken to detect **secondary deposits**. A **CT chest** is more accurate since blood spread is common.

4. **Ultrasound study** of the abdomen may pick up **liver metastases**.

5. **MRI** scans are needed only if **secondaries** are suspected in the **spinal cord** or **brain.**

6. **Immunohistochemistry** may be needed if the **pathological type** cannot be defined accurately by **histopathology.** Further, in advanced centres, tests for **mutations in the BARF gene** are performed. This kind of mutation is seen in about **50%** of patients. These are useful in the **development** of specific **monoclonal antibodies.**

7. **Sentinel node biopsy** is needed in patients **without palpable nodes**. This group represents a very small percentage in **our**

country. The **advantage** of this investigation is to **avoid** the **morbidity** associated with a **radical dissection** of the **nodes.** For example, an **inguinal block dissection** carries significant morbidity associated with **lymphoedema.**

Box 16.17: Points about the investigations

- Use of a dermascope – Improved clinical results.
- Biopsy. Early cases – Excision (therapeutic) biopsy.
- Incision biopsy – Contraindicated – Local spread - Brush biopsy.
- Advanced cases – Palliation – Incision biopsy.
  - Edge biopsy – Ulcerated lesions.
- US abdomen – Lymphadenopathy and liver metastases.
- Chest X-ray – Secondaries lung. CT chest if needed.
- Sentinel node biopsy – Avoids morbidity.
- FNAC of enlarged nodes – Limited value.
- MRI scan – Secondaries brain.
- Immunohistochemistry – Accurate typing.
- Genetic studies – Mutation of BARF gene.
- Development of monoclonal antibodies.

Q. 21. How are melanomas staged clinically?

Stage 1A) Primary tumour less than **1 mm thickness with or without ulceration**

1B) Primary tumour between **1 mm and 2 mm** in thickness **without ulceration.**

Stage 2A) Primary tumour between **1 mm and 2 mm** with **ulceration.**

2B) Primary tumour between **2 mm and 4 mm without ulceration**.

Stage 3A) Primary tumour of **any thickness** with palpable **1 to 3** regional lymph **nodes.**

3B) Primary tumour of any thickness with **satellite or transit nodules**.

Stage 4 Presence of more than **3 enlarged lymph nodes** and or **blood** borne **metastases.**

Box 16.18: Points regarding the staging of melanoma

I A) Pr. tumour less than 1 mm thickness with or without ulceration.

I B) Pr. tumour between 1 mm and 2 mm without ulceration.

II A) Pr. tumour less than 2 mm with ulceration.

II B) Pr. tumour between 2 mm and 4 mm without ulceration.

III A) Pr. tumour – Any size with 1 to 3 nodes.

III B) Pr. Tumour – Any size with satellite and transit nodules.

IV) More than 3 nodes or blood spread metastases.

Q. 22. What are the principles of treatment?

A **wide excision** of the tumour is both **diagnostic and therapeutic** in nature. The incision is made **2 cm** beyond the **margin on all sides**. In certain **anatomical**

locations, such as the face, the safety margin is reduced to **1 cm** without **compromising** the **oncological clearance**. In a **small number** of patients, a **primary closure** is feasible after a wide excision. In the remaining group a **split-skin graft** or more sophisticated **plastic surgical reconstruction** is needed. Since the **common site** in our patients is the sole of the **foot** which is a **weight bearing area**, a **cross leg flap** or a rotation flap based on the **dorsalis pedis artery** is performed.

Patients presenting with **advanced local disease**, where the primary is fixed to the **bone** need a **proximal amputation**.

Patients in whom **no nodes** are detected **on clinical examination or US,** need a **sentinel node biopsy**. If the **frozen section report** of the node or nodes is **negative, no further surgery** is indicated. But a positive report demands a **radical lymphadenectomy**. This approach **avoids** the **morbidity** associated with **removal of lymph nodes**.

Enlarged palpable mobile nodes are removed by a **radical lymphadenectomy**. For a **lesion** in the **foot**, the patient needs an **ilioinguinal radical lymphadenectomy**. The **structures** removed **include fat** and **fascia** over the **femoral triangle** and the **femoral sheath**. The following **groups of lymph nodes** are removed. They include the **superficial horizontal** and **vertical group**, and the **deep inguinal as well as the external iliac lymph nodes**. Since the **terminal part** of the **long saphenous vein** is **intimately related** to the **nodes,** it is also **excised**. All the **structures** mentioned above are excised **en bloc.**

If the **primary tumour** is in **close proximity** to the nodes, an **in continuity block dissection** is performed, wherein the **primary tumour** is **excised** along with a **radical lymphadenectomy** A typical example would be a primary in the lower part of the face with metastatic nodes in the neck.

Chemotherapy is routinely given to all patients with **metastatic nodes. Dacarbazine (DTIC)** is the standard drug. **Interferon Alfa** and **Interleukin 2** have shown good response, but have **serious side effects**. A monoclonal antibody**, Ipilimumab** is also being used in the treatment with **encouraging results.**

Box 16.19: Points regarding treatment

- Direct spread.
- Wide surgical excision – Incision 2 cm beyond the margin of the tumour.
- Primary closure – Possible only in a small number. of cases.
- Split-skin graft or flaps – Depending on the location.
- No nodes clinical or US – Sentinel node biopsy.
- Negative – No surgery. Positive – Radical lymphadenectomy.
- Palpable nodes – Radical surgery.
- Nodes close to primary Tumour – In continuity dissection.
- Post op. chemotherapy – DTIC.
- Advanced cases – Palliative – Surgery or DTIC.
- Recent advances – Interferons, Interleukins and Ipilimumab.

Q. 23. What are the survival rates in a melanoma?

In **stage 1 and 2** adequate treatment results in a **ten-year survival** of more than **90%.** It drops down to about **1% to** 2% in **stage 4** of the disease. **Females** in general and patients below 70 years of age have a better prognosis. Unfortunately, **melanomas** occurring in the **coloured population** and located in the **palms or soles** have a **very poor outcome.** These are usually **very aggressive tumours.**

Thickness of more than 6 mm, **size of more than 1 cm**, **ulceration,** and the presence **of satellite or transit nodules** and **palpable nodes** are all indicators of a **poor prognosis**. In addition a **high grade tumour** as shown by **mitotic studies** confirms **the same**.

SOFT TISSUE SARCOMA

A CASE OF RHABDOMYOSARCOMA

Setting

- Surgical OPD

Chief Complaint

- **Swelling** in the **lower part** of the **right arm** of **3 months** duration.
- She was a **student** at a local government secondary school.
- A **16-year-old girl** presented to the OPD with complaint of a **swelling** in the **lower part** of the **right arm** of **3 months** duration. She had noticed a **slight fullness** on the **back** of the **right arm 3 months** ago. She was **not sure** about the **size at onset**. But she **felt** that the **part** of the **arm** was **bulkier compared** to the **left side**. Over a period of **three months** she noticed that the **swelling** had **rapidly become bigger**.
- The **arm** felt much **heavier,** but there was **no pain** over the site of the swelling. But she could **continue to do** her **work** as a **student** during this time.
- There was **no history** of **trauma.**
- She did **not** give any **history** of **similar swelling** in **other parts** of the body.
- Patient did **not** give any history of **fever.**

- There was **no history** of **respiratory symptoms.**
- She had **not lost weight** during this period. There was **no history** of **loss of appetite**.
- **Past and personal histories** were insignificant.
- **No other member** of the **family** had **similar problems**.
- Her **menstrual history** was normal.
- **General physical examination** showed a **healthy young girl.** There was **no pallor, jaundice or clubbing of fingers**.

Local Examination

Inspection

- A **diffuse swelling** was seen in the **posterolateral aspect** of the **lower one-third** of the **right arm**. Its **margins** were **ill defined**.
- The **size** was **15 cm by 12 cm**. The **shape** was **irregular.**
- The **skin** over the **swelling** was **normal. No dilated veins** were visible over the swelling.
- The **limb below** the elbow appeared **normal** on inspection.

Palpation

- The **swelling** was **warm** but **not tender.**
- It was **larger on palpation** measuring **18 cm by 14 cm.**

- The **shape** was **irregular.**
- The **skin** was **free** from the swelling.
- It appeared to be **deeply placed** and was probably **arising** from the **lower half** of the **triceps muscle** with **ill-defined borders**.
- The **consistency** was **firm.** It had **restricted transverse mobility**. This **disappeared** when the triceps **muscle** was put on **contraction** against **resistance.**
- **Movements** of the right **elbow joint. Terminal flexion** was **restricted.**
- **Pronation** and **supination** were **normal.**
- The **motor power** in the **extensors** of the **wrist** and **fingers** was **normal.** There were **no areas** of **sensory loss** on the **dorsum** of the **forearm or** the **hand.**
- **No dilated veins** were seen in the distal limb.
- **No lymphoedema** was seen.
- **Radial pulsations** were normal.
- **No lymph nodes** were palpable in the **right axilla.**
- The **respiratory system** was clinically normal.
- **Other systems** were clinically normal.

Q. 1. What was the clinical diagnosis?

The **clinical diagnosis** was a **soft tissue sarcoma.** A **rapidly growing soft tissue tumour** with **fixity** to the **surrounding** **structures** made the diagnosis easy. **No other condition** can be considered in the **differential diagnosis**. Since it appeared to be **arising** from the **triceps** muscle the possibility of the **type** being a **rhabdomyosarcoma** was **high.**

Q. 2. What were the investigations done in this patient?

A **core needle biopsy** (CNB) was performed.

Chest X-ray was normal.

MRI scan was done. It **confirmed** the **origin** of the **tumour** from the **triceps muscle**. It showed **infiltration** of the **surrounding soft tissues**. The **radial nerve** was seen in **close proximity** to the tumour. There was **no infiltration** of any **vital structures**. The **axilla** showed evidence of **multiple discrete lymph nodes**.

CT chest was normal.

Setting: A week later.

CNB report was a **rhabdomyosarcoma** of the **alveolar type.**

Q. 3. What was the treatment strategies planned for this patient?

The **size** of the tumor and the presence of **metastatic nodes** along with the **type** of **rhabdomyosarcoma** all indicated a **poor prognosis**. The **nature** of the **disease** and the **possible outcome** was **explained** to the **relatives** in detail. A **palliative resection** followed by **chemoradiation** and **sorafenib** was the **treatment** suggested for this **patient.**

Q. 4. What was the operation performed on this patient?

She underwent a **palliative wide excision. Most of the tumour** with **involved muscle and adjacent soft tissues** was **excised.** The **radial nerve** was **conserved**. But **some parts of the tumour** in close proximity of the **nerve** were **left behind**. Thus it was a **R2 resection**, with **macroscopic tumour** tissue left **behind** at the **end of the operation**. A **wrist drop** was observed **after surgery,** probably resulting from **neuropraxia** due to **traction** on the **radial nerve** during **surgery.** This was expected to **recover** over a **period of time**. A **splint** was to be used till the **function** of the **extensors** returned.

Q. 5. What was the histopathology report?

It showed a **high grade alveolar type of rhabdomyosarcoma.**

Q. 6. What was the clinicopathological staging?

It was **T2B, N1, M0 and G3. Final staging III**

Q. 7. How was this patient managed postoperatively?

The patient was **discharged** after the **sutures** were **removed**. She was asked to **return** after **three weeks**. She was asked to attend the **physiotherapy department** for **exercises** involving the **extensors** of the **wrist and hand.**

She underwent **concurrent chemoradiation**. **Ifosfamide and Doxorubicin** were used as **combination chemotherapy**. **EBRT** was used in the dose of **50 Gy** given over a period of **5 weeks**. At the end of **6 cycles** of chemotherapy she was discharged from the hospital with an advice to take **oral sorafenib.**

Q. 8. What could be the possible outcome for this patient?

The **outcome** is likely to be very **unfavourable.** The **size** of the tumour and the presence of **metastatic nodes** are indications of a **poor prognosis**. In addition the **alveolar type** of **rhabdomyosarcomas** are **aggressive tumours**. The tumour was also of a **high grade** pathologically. **Metastases** in **lung** or at other sites are likely to develop within a **short time**. **Death** is the result of **metastatic disease**.

Q. 9. What does the term soft tissue sarcoma mean?

Soft tissue sarcomas (STS) form a **heterogeneous group** of tumours arising from the **mesenchymal cells**. They are **rare tumours** being responsible for about **1% of** all **cancers**. **Histopathology** was used in the **past** to **classify** these **cancers**. But it was **inadequate** because, as these **tumours** became more and more **undifferentiated** their **cellular characters** were **lost,** making **identification** of their **origin** more **difficult**. The **modern classification** is based on **immunohistochemistry** and **molecular genetics**. This has helped in better **understanding** of the **disease** and an **improved outcome**. But there still **remains a group** where the **cell of origin cannot** be **identified**.

Q. 10. What are the important aetiological factors?

Most of these cancers arise **spontaneously**. In a **small number** of patients the following **aetiological factors** may be **important**.

1. Patients with **Li–Fraumeni syndrome** have **mutations** of the **TP53 gene**. They are **susceptible** for developing **STS, breast, bone** and **other cancers**.

2. **Children** surviving a **retinoblastoma** are **prone** to have **STS later in life**.

3. **Chronic lymphoedema** predis-poses to **Kaposi sarcoma**.

4. **Gardner's syndrome** with **mutation** of the **APC gene** is associated with **malignant fibrohistiocytoma**.

5. Patients with **multiple neuro-fibromatosis** are likely to **develop malignant peripheral nerve sheath tumours (MPNST)**.

6. A **higher incidence** has been reported in **patients** following **radiotherapy** for **cancers** like that of **breast** or other **sites**.

The **risk** of developing **STS increases** as **age advances**, and it is **slightly** more **common** in **men**.

Box 16.20:	Points regarding aetiology

- Aetiology – Most cases not known.
- Risk is higher in the following conditions.
- Li-Fraumeni syndrome.
- Children surviving retinoblastoma.
- Gardner's syndrome.
- Familial adenomatous polyposis.
- Long standing chronic lymphoedema.
- Previous radiotherapy.
- HIV patients.

Q. 11. What are the common clinical features of STS?

The **symptoms and signs** depend upon the **site** of the **tumour.** When they occur in the **extremities** the **picture** is **different** from that of lesions in the **abdomen** or **head and neck**.

Tumours located in the **limbs** present as a **swelling** of a **few months duration**. The **common sites** are the **arm and leg.** They are **painless** during the **early stage**. **Extension** to the **adjacent structures** may result in **pain.** The **rate** of **growth** is **rapid. Huge tumours** are **frequently seen** among **our patients** because of **minimal symptoms**. The **consistency** is often **variable,** with **firm** and **hard** areas. But **liposarcoma** and **synovial sarcomas** are **soft**. The **borders** are **ill defined.** They have **restricted mobility** or they may be **fixed** to the **deeper structures.** **Occasionally** a patient **presents** with an **ulcerated tumour.** The **haematogenous route** is the **common mode** of **spread.** Hence a patient may **present** with **symptomatic secondaries**. But **some** of these **cancers** often spread to the **regional lymph nodes. Synovial, clear cell** and **angiosarcoma** belong to this **variety.** The **nodes** are **soft** to **firm** in consistency. **Additional symptoms** and **signs** appear when the **adjacent structures** like the **nerves and vessels** are involved by the **tumour**.

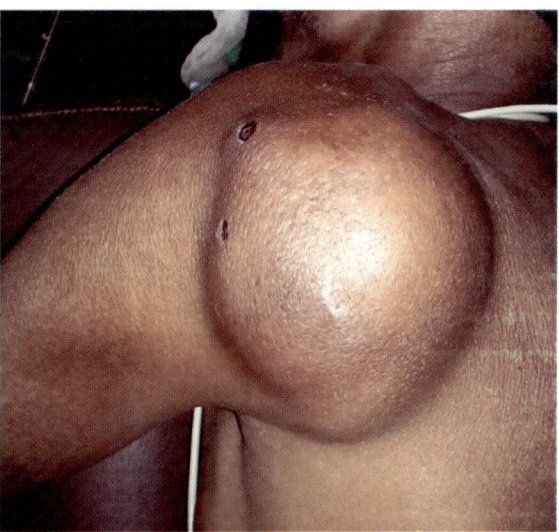

Fig. 16.6: Soft tissue sarcoma over the scapula

Box 16.21:	Points regarding the clinical features of extremity STS

- Rapidly growing swellings – Painless initially.
- Huge swellings are common.
- May be ulcerated at presentation.
- Pain is due to infiltration of adjacent nerves.
- Blood spread is common - Secondaries in lung, brain.
- Lymphatic spread – Uncommon – Seen in synovial, clear cell and angiosarcomas.
- Presentation with metastatic disease – Uncommon.

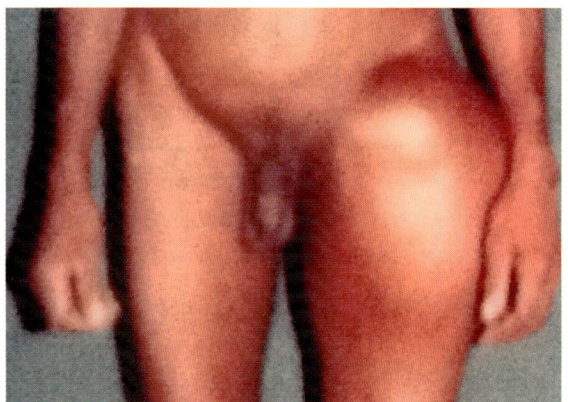

Fig. 16.7: Soft tissue sarcoma thigh.

Abdomen: **Retroperitoneal liposar-comas** are the most **frequent type** (GIST is not included in this group). Since they are **asymptomatic** till a very **late stage,** they are **detected** only when they are **large in size**. **Deeply located** tumours are **difficult** to **palpate**. They are usually **fixed** and **nontender**. **Extension** into **adjacent viscera** may lead to **obstructive** and **other symptoms**.

Chest wall: These **tumours** present as **painless swellings** and hence the **patients** present rather **late** to the **hospital. Rate** of **growth** is **rapid. Infiltration** of the **nerves** causes **pain. Tumours** located close to the **scapula** or the **shoulder** may cause **limitation of movement** of the **neighbouring joints**. **Invasion** through the **chest wall** occurs at a **late stage**. **Blood spread** is the **common** route of **dissemination.**

Box 16.22:	Points regarding clinical features of abdominal STS

- Retroperitoneum – Common site – Liposarcoma.
- Large size – Before recognition.
- Symptoms – Involvement of gastrointestinal or urinary tract.
- Deeply located – Difficult to palpate.
- Fixed, soft-to-firm in consistency.

Box 16.23:	Points regarding chest wall STS

- Huge size before presentation.
- Pain – Late symptom.
- Spread into the thoracic cavity at a late stage.
- Firm to hard tumours.
- Restricted mobility or later fixed.
- Ulceration at a late stage.

Q. 12. What are the investigations in STS?

1. **Core needle biopsy (CNB)** is **preferred** to a **FNAC,** since **immunohistochemistry and genetic studies** are **not possible** with the **quantum of tissue** obtained with **FNA.** For **deeply located lesions,** **CNB** is performed with the help of **CT.**

If **CNB** is **inconclusive** (an **uncommon** situation), an **incision biopsy** is advised. **Skin flaps** are **not raised** during this procedure and **absolute haemostasis** is **secured** before **closing** the **incision**. The **incision** is placed in **such a manner** that the **area** will be **included** when **excisional surgery** is performed at a **later date.** These **measures reduce** the **risk** of **seeding** and **local recurrence**.

2. **Chest X-ray** is **not adequate** to **identify** the **metastases** since the **lungs** are the **most common site** for **secondary deposits**. Hence a **CT chest** is **mandatory. Multiple secondaries** appear like **cannon balls** and a **solitary** deposit is known as a **coin shadow.**

3. **CECT abdome**n defines the **extent** of **retroperitoneal tumours** and the possibility of **curative resections**. It also identifies **secondaries** in the **liver**.

4. **Most tumours** also need a **MRI scan**. In **tumours affecting the extremities**, **involvement** of the **adjacent nerves** and **vessels** is **made out** by this **scan**. The possibility of a **radical curative resection** is often **decided** by the **MRI findings**.

5. PETCTscanis**replacing**many of the **other investigations**. It has the **advantage** of **identifying** the **morphologic** and the **functional status** of the **tumour** and the **metastases**. It is **very useful** in **assessing** the **effectiveness**

of the **treatment** as well as in **detecting metastases** before symptoms appear.

Box 16.24:	Points regarding investigations in STS
1. Biopsy. FNA NOT DONE – Tissue obtained not adequate for immunocytochemistry and genetic studies. • CNB – Standard mode of biopsy. • Deep seated tumours – CT-guided CNB. • Incision biopsy – Only if repeat CNB inconclusive. 2. CT chest – Always needed. • CECT abdomen – For retroperitoneal tumours. • MRI scan for extremities tumours. • PET CT becoming more popular.	

Q. 13. What is the pathological classification of soft tissue tumours?

Soft tissue tumours, both **benign** and **malignant,** are usually **classified depending** on the **cell of origin**. But in **certain cancers** this is **not possible. Clear cell sarcoma** cannot be **traced** to any **particular cell**. It must also be **stressed** that the **histologic appearance** and the **clinical behaviour** may **not** always **correspond** with **each other**. All soft tissue tumours are **divided** as follows depending on their **clinicopathological behaviour**.

1. **Benign tumours:** They are **encapsulated** and do **not metastasise. Lipoma** is a classic example.

2. (*a*) **Intermediate (locally invasive)**. These have an **infiltrative** and **locally destructive** pattern. Hence **despite a wide excision**, **local recurrences** are known to **occur**. The **typical lesion** in this category is a **desmoid tumour** or aggressive fibromatosis.

(*b*) **Intermediate (rarely producing metastases)**. Tumours belonging to this group are **locally aggressive** like 2(a), but have a very **low risk** of producing **distant metastases (2%)**. **Plexiform fibrocystic tumour** is an example for this variety.

3. **Malignant:** Most **sarcomas** belong to this **type**. In addition to **being locally invasive,** they **spread** by the **blood stream** producing **distant metastases**. The **lung** is frequently the site of **secondaries**. When a **soft tissue tumour** spreads to the **lymph nodes**, the **outlook** is much **worse** as **compared** with a **carcinoma** with nodal metastases.

Box 16.25:	Points regarding the basic classification of soft tissue tumours

1. Benign – Encapsulated – Removal – Cure eg.lipoma.

2. Intermediate:
   A) Uncapsulated locally invasive – Hence high chances of recurrence – Desmoid tumour.

   B) Rarely metastasising – Plexiform fibrocystic tumour.

3. Malignant. Blood spread common mode.

   Certain tumours – Lymph node spread – Poor prognosis.

Q. 14. Describe the TNM classification of STS.

T Primary tumour.

TX Primary tumour **not accessible**.

T 0 No evidence of primary tumour.

T 1A Primary tumour **less than 5 cm** in size and **superficial** to the **deep fascia**.

T 1B Tumour **less than 5 cm, deep** to the **fascia.**

T 2A Tumour **more than 5 cm, superficial**.

T 2B Tumour **more than 5 cm, deep** to the **fascia.**

N Lymph nodal status.

N X Nodal status **cannot** be **assessed**

N0 No regional palpable lymph **nodes.**

N1 Palpable lymph **nodes.**

M Distant metastases.

MX Metastatic status cannot be assessed.

MO No distant **metastases.**

M1 Distant metastases present.

Box 16.26:	Points regarding the TNM classification
TX – Primary tumour not accessible.	
TO – No evidence of primary tumour.	
TIA – Tumour less than 5 cm in size, superficial to fascia.	
TI B – Tumour less than 5 cm, deep to fascia.	
TII A – Tumour more than 5 cm, superficial.	
TII B – Tumour more than 5 cm deep.	
NO – No palpable nodes.	
N1 – Enlarged regional nodes.	
M0 – No distant metastases.	
M1 – Distant metastases present.	

Q 15. Which are the other factors that are considered in the final staging of STS?

In addition to the **clinical staging**, the **histopathological grading** is **vital** in the **treatment** and **outcome** of the **disease**. The following factors decide the **pathological grade** of the tumour.

(*a*) **Histological type. Desmoid tumour** exemplifies a **low grade** tumour and **angiosarcoma** a **highly aggressive** tumour.

(*b*) **Cellularity and pleomorphism:** The **presence** of **atypical** or **bizarre cells** with a **high degree** of **pleomorphism** indicates a **high grade** tumour.

(*c*) **Degree of mitosis:** A pattern of **more than 50% mitosis** in a given **section** indicates a **poor prognosis**.

(*d*) **Extent of tumour necrosis:** If a tumour shows **extensive necrosis** it indicates a **favourable response** to treatment.

The tumours are **graded** as low **G1,** intermediate **G2** and high grade **G3,** depending on **these factors**

Box 16.27:	Points regarding pathological grading of STS
• Type of tumour.	
• Desmoid – Locally invasive. Angiosarcoma – Highly malignant.	
• Cellularity with degree of pleomorphism.	
• Degree of mitosis – More than 50% – Aggressive tumour.	
• Degree of tumour necrosis – Better prognosis.	
• Tumour grade – GI, GII and GIII.	

Q. 16. Describe the final clinicopathological staging of STS.

Stage I A	T1A N0 M0 G1
	T1B N0 M0 G1
Stage I B	T2A N0 M0 G1
	T2B N0 M0 G1
Stage II A	T1A N0 M0 G2
	T1B N0 M0 G2
Stage II B	T2B N0 MO G2
Stage III	Any T N1 M0 G3
Stage IV	Any T Any N M1 any G

Q 17. What are the general principles of treatment of STS?

The **treatment** of **STS** involves **many modalities**. These include **surgery, radiotherapy** and **chemotherapy**. **Immunotherapy** is also used in the **treatment**.

Surgical treatment. Three dimensional wide surgical excision offers the **best outcome**. But the **operation** may have to be **modified** under the following **circumstances.**

(*a*) **Size and extent** of the **tumour.**

(*b*) **Proximity** or **involvement** of the **neurovascular structures** and **viscera.**

(*c*) The **presence** of **metastases**.

(*d*) The **age** and the **general health** status of the **patient.**

If the **margins** of the **specimen** do **not show** any **evidence** of the **tumour (R0)** on **frozen section** or **histopathology,** the **outlook** is generally **good**. If **tumour tissue** is seen at the **edges** on **microscopy (R1)**, or a **complete excision** was **not possible (R2)**, **additional treatment** is **needed**.

In the **extremities, limb salvage surgery** is being performed **more frequently.** This has been made possible due to **advances** in **reconstructive surgery. Blood vessels, nerves and bones** can be **resected** if **facilities** are available for **reconstruction.** It is now **possible** to **resect** even the **sciatic nerve** with the **cancer** and provide a **functionally active limb** with **tendon transfers** along with **major orthopaedic procedures. Amputation** is the **last option** when all other **measures** have **failed**. It is more **often** performed for **recurrent tumours. Active rehabilitation** forms an **integral part** of **treatment** for all these patients.

Box 16.28:	Points regarding the role of surgery

- Three dimensional wide excision – Best treatment.
- Needs modification – Proximity to neurovascular structures.
- Extensive resections including the sciatic nerve performed.
- Tendon transfer with major orthopaedic procedures.
- Functioning lower limb.
- Proximity to important viscera.
- RO resection – Margins are free – Good prognosis.
- R0 resection – High grade tumour – Adjuvant therapy.
- R1 margins on microscopy – Positive – Adjuvant treatment.
- R2 – Palliative resection – Adjuvant treatment.

Q. 18. What are the indications for radiotherapy in STS?

Basically most **STS** are **radioresistant** in their behaviour. But **advances** in this **mode of treatment** have **increased** its **role. Radiation** is used under the **following circumstances**.

(*a*) **Preoperative radiotherapy** is needed when the **primary** tumour is **unresectable** due to **local infiltration** or **proximity** to **important structures**. If the **size** of the tumour is **reduced,** and it is found to be **resectable** on **imaging studies**, **radical surgery** is performed.

These **patients** are given the benefit of **postoperative radiotherapy**.

(*b*) **Postoperative radiotherapy:** All patients with **R1 and R2** resections are advised **postoperative radiation**. For patients with **high grade tumours** (**G3**), even a **R0 resection** is followed up with **radiation** to **reduce** the incidence of **local recurrence**. The dose is **40 to 45 Gy** for **microscopic** disease and **50 to 55 Gy** for **gross residual disease.**

Q. 19. What is the role of chemotherapy?

The availability of **chemotherapy** has **improved** the **prognosis** in many **STS**. The **best example** would be an **embryonic type** of **rhabdomyosarcoma** seen in **children**. This was invariably a **fatal disease** in the **past**. A combination of **Vincristine, Actinomycin D and Cyclophosphamide** has made this a **curable cancer**. Other drugs like **Ifosfamide and Doxorubicin** are used more **frequently** in the **treatment** of **STS** at the present time. **Chemotherapy** may be used as per the **following regime**.

Neoadjuvant chemotherapy: The indication is the presence of a **high grade localised** tumour which is either **unresectable** or which if operated on would be **associated** with **significant morbidity**. It is usually **combined** with **radiation**. If **down staging** of the **tumour** does take place, as **confirmed** by **imaging studies**, a **surgical resection** is performed. **Postoperative chemoradiation** is **continued** for this group of **patients.**

Adjuvant chemotherapy: It is useful in **patients** who have **undergone** an **R1** or **R2 resection**. It is also **combined** with **radiotherapy.**

Palliative chemotherapy is used for **patients** with **advanced disease**. In these cases the **outlook** is **uniformly poor**.

Box 16.29:	Points regarding indications for radiotherapy and chemotherapy

- Preoperative – Radiotherapy combined with neoadjuvant chemotherapy.
- Unresectable tumours or tumours in close proximity of important structures.
- Down staging – Confirmed by imaging studies – Radical surgery.
- R0 resection – High grade – Post op – Chemoradiation.
- Postoperative – RI and RII resections – Radiotherapy with chemotherapy.
- Palliative chemotherapy – Advanced or metastatic disease.

Sorafenib, an **oral multi– tyrosine kinase inhibitor,** has shown some **promise** in the management of **STS.** It has shown **survival benefits** in patients with **advanced disease.**

Q. 20. **What is the prognosis in STS?**

Prognosis in general is **poor.** The **primary reason** is that **most** of **our patients** present at a late stage. Again many **subtypes** of **STS** are both **chemo- and radio-resistant**. In general the **5 year disease**-free **interval** ranges between **50% and 60%.** These are **Western figures**. But **children** with an **embryonic type** of **rhabdomyosarcoma** have a **success rate** of more than **90%** at the end of **5 years**. At stage **IV level**, the **5 year cure rate** dips down to below **20%**. Our **survival figures** are probably **related** to these **figures.**

Q. 21. **Describe the various soft tissue tumours in relation to their cell of origin.**

Fibrous tissue may give rise to a **locally invasive tumour** like a **desmoid tumour** or a **more aggressive malignant fibrosarcoma.** **Pure fibrosarcomas** are **uncommon** tumours. What was previously diagnosed as a **fibrosarcoma** in **many instances** has been **proved** to be **MFH** on **immunochemistry**.

Desmoid tumour or **aggressive fibromatosis** is the most **frequent**

type seen in clinical practice. Their **association** with familial adenomatous polyposis (**FAP**) is well **documented.** It is **common after** the **age of 40.** The tumour is more **common** in **females** especially **after pregnancy**. The **anterior abdominal wall** is the **most frequent** site, though the **tumour** has been described in the **limbs** also. It is an **uncapsulated** tumour being **locally invasive**. The **origin** is from the **fibroblasts** present in the **fascia** or **aponeurosis,** and may cause **severe morbidity** by **infiltration** of **adjacent structures**. **Histologically** it shows **spindled fibroblasts** arranged in **broad sweeping fascicles separated** by plenty of **collagen.**

These **tumours** present as **slow-growing asymptomatic abdominal masses**. These are **firm** in **consistency** with **ill-defined margins**. .**Symptoms appear** only when the **adjacent viscera** are involved. **Intestinal obstruction** results if the **tumour** involves the **adjacent bowel. Wide surgical excision** with **mesh reconstruction** is the choice of treatment. But the **recurrence rates** are **quite high. Nonresectable** tumours are treated by **EBRT or chemotherapy. Tamoxifen**

in high doses (**120 mg**) has been found to be **successful** in **some** of these **cases.** In general **outlook** is poor in these cases. **Recurrent tumours** may need **extensive resections** including the **bowel** etc. But these carry a **poor prognosis**.

Box 16.30:	Points regarding desmoid tumour

- Uncapsulated – Locally invasive – Females - Multiparous.
- Anterior abdominal wall common site.
- Slow growing asymptomatic tumour.
- Bowel obstruction due to local invasion.
- Firm in consistency, fixed to the abdominal wall.
- Cell of origin – Fibroblasts. Microscopy – Spindle-shaped fibroblasts arranged in fascicles – Plenty of collagen in between.
- Wide surgical excision with mesh placement.
- Recurrences common. Repeat resections with involved structures.
- Nonresectable tumours – EBRT, chemotherapy, tamoxifen (120 mg)
- Outlook – Poor.

Fat Liposarcomas are divided into **well-differentiated** and **myxoid** types. The **latter type** is of the **high grade** variety. **Most** of these tumours **arise spontaneously.** But a **small number** may occur as a **complication** of a **deep seated lipoma.** They are **slow growing** tumours and the **retroperitoneum** is a **common site.** They may **assume** a **large**

size before they are **detected.** Under the **microscope, atypical adipocytes** are seen with **several areas** of **fat** within the tumour.

Box 16.31:	Points regarding liposarcomas

- From adipocytes.
- Divided into well-differentiated and myxomatous types (high grade).
- Retroperitoneum common site.
- Asymptomatic rapidly growing tumour.
- Huge size not uncommon.
- Spread to adjacent structures very early.
- CECT and biopsy. CT chest
- Atypical adipocytes with fat cells on microscopy.
- Most tumours nonresectable.
- Wide surgical excision along with involved structures if feasible.

Malignant peripheral nerve sheath tumours (MPNST). Nearly **50%** of these cancers occur as a **complication** of a **pre-existing benign tumour** in patients with **multiple neurofibromatosis**. They are quite often **missed** in the **early stages** since these **swellings** have been **present** for **many years**. A **rapid increase** in size over a **short period** of **time** and the onset of **pain** may bring the **patient** to the **hospital**. Hence the **outlook** is rather **poor.** The **larger nerves** like the **sciatic** are involved more **frequently**. A **malignant transformation** of the **cells** of **Schwann,** which line the nerve sheath, is the

common histological type. The **fibroblasts** present in the **nerve sheath** can also become **malignant**. The **previously used terms** like **neurofibrosarcoma** and **malignant neurolemmoma (malignant Schwannoma)** have been replaced by the present term MPNST.

Box 16.32:	Points regarding MPNST

- 50% arise from pre-existing neurofibroma (neurofibromatosis).
- Hence delay in presentation.
- Onset of pain and rapid increase in size – Suggests malignancy.
- Pain radiating along the involved nerve.
- Cell of origin – Schwann cell or fibroblast lining the nerve sheath.
- Investigations – CNB, CT chest, MRI.
- Curative surgery – Local wide excision if feasible.
- Needs plastic surgical reconstruction if major nerve sacrificed.

Malignant fibrohistiocytoma (MFH). This forms the **commonest type** of **sarcoma.** The availability of **modern investigations** has helped to **distinguish** this group from **fibrosarcoma**. These tumours typically occur in **late adult life**. The **proximal part** of the **extremities**, the **pelvis** and **trunk** are the **common sites involved.** **Macroscopically,** they have an **irregular contour** with **poorly defined margins**. On **histology,** the tumour is **undifferentiated**

with **marked pleomorphism** and **nuclear anomalies**.

Box 16.33:	Points regarding MFH

- Commonest soft tissue sarcoma.
- Histopathology – Reported as fibrosarcoma in the past.
- Extreme degree of anaplastic changes in the connective tissue cells.
- Macroscopy – Tumour with irregular margins and poorly defined edges.
- Cells are undifferentiated with marked pleomorphism and nuclear anomalies.
- Common in adults.
- Proximal part of the extremities, pelvis and trunk common sites.

Rhabdomyosarcoma is a tumour of the **striated muscle fibre**. A more **accurate definition** would be a **sarcoma** arising from the **primitive mesenchyme,** exhibiting a profound **tendency** towards **myogenesis. Histologically,** they are **classified** as **embryonic** and **alveolar types**. The **embryonic type** is commonly seen in **children, accounting** for **4% to 8%** of all **solid tumours.** It is **uncommon** in **adults.** They are commonly **associated** with syndromes like **Li–Fraumeni etc. Anatomically** they may be located in the **trunk (axial type)** or the **extremities.** The **orbit, parameningeal, paranasal and paratesticular** sites represent the **axial type.** In the **extremities** they manifest as **swellings**

infiltrating the **adjacent structures. Cytologically** these tumours have **embryonal cells** that are **oblong in shape** with deeply staining **eosinophilic cytoplasm** and **bland chromaffin**. As mentioned earlier, these **tumours respond** well to **chemotherapy.**

Box 16.34:	Points regarding embryonic rhabdomyosarcomas

- Cell of origin – Striated muscle fibre.
- More accurate definition – Primitive mesenchyme showing myogenesis.
- Common in children – Association with Li–Fraumeni syndrome.
- Extremities – Rapidly growing soft tissue tumour.
- Axial location – Orbit, parameningeal, paranasal and paratesticular.
- Early infiltration of adjoining structures.
- Microscopy – Embryonal cells, oblong in shape, deeply staining eosinophilic cytoplasm with bland chromaffin.
- Excellent response to chemotherapy – Actinomycin D, Vincristine and Cyclophosphamide.

Alveolar RMS is seen more frequently in **adults.** Histologically, they are characterised by the presence of **round blue cells** lining the **fibrovascular septae** with **loose spaces**, resembling the **alveolar structure of the lung.** They are more **aggressive** in their behaviour, and their **response** to **chemotherapy** is also **worse** compared to the embryonal type. **Additional subtypes** have also been described, but they are **not significant clinically**.

Box 16.35:	Points regarding alveolar rhabdomyosarcomas

- Seen in adults.
- More aggressive tumour.
- Microscopy – Round blue cells lining the fibrovascular septae along with loose spaces resembling the alveoli of the lung.
- Response to chemotherapy poor.

Synovial sarcoma. A **common** type of **STS,** it is **frequently seen** around the **joints, tendons and ligamentous** structures, often in the **distal part** of the **extremities**. Under the **microscope** they show **atypical synovial cells. Flecks** of **calcification** are made out on **histology. Sometimes** these are **large enough** to be seen **radiologically.** Many of **these lesions** are **myxoid** in character.

Box 16.36:	Points regarding synovial sarcomas

- Site – Distal part of the extremities.
- In relation to joints, tendon sheaths and ligaments.
- Microscopy – Atypical synovial cells.
- Flecks of calcification – Diagnostic.
- Myxomatous type also seen.
- Occasionally calcification made out on X-ray.

Smooth muscle: Leiomyosarcoma. The **common sites** involved are the **uterus** and the **abdominal** and **urologic viscera**. But these are **not included** under the term **STS.** These are also **seen** to occur in the **extremities**. The **smooth muscle fibres** present in the **vessel wall** is said to be the **cells of origin**. Their **proximity** to the **blood vessel** make them **spread early** and produce **metastases**. Hence the **outlook** is **very poor. Histologically,** the sections show many **bizarre cells** in a **myxoid stroma**.

Box 16.37:	Points regarding leiomyosarcoma

- Common in organs containing smooth muscle – Uterus, abdominal viscera, urinary bladder – Not included under STS.
- Extremities – Arising from smooth muscle present in the vessel wall.
- Blood spread very early – Proximity to blood vessels.
- Microscopy – Bizarre cells in a myxoid stroma.

Blood vessels. A **group of cancers** have been described **arising** from the **endothelium** of the **blood vessels**. **Haemangioendothelioma** is a

low grade tumour that is **locally invasive,** but **rarely spreads** to **other parts** of the body.

An **angiosarcoma,** commonly seen in the **subcutaneous tissue,** is an **aggressive tumour**. Areas of **haemorrhage** are seen on **macroscopy. Histological** examination shows **tumour cells** with **collections of red cells within the tumour**.

Box 16.38:	Points regarding sarcomas arising from the endothelium of blood vessels

- Haemangioendothelioma.
- Slow growing tumours. Extremities common site.
- Locally invasive.
- Rarely metastases occur.
- Angiosarcoma – Aggressive tumour.
- Subcutaneous tissue is a common site.
- Macroscopy shows areas of haemorrhage.
- Microscopy – Atypical endothelial cells with RBC within the tumour.

Clear cell sarcoma does **not** have a **specific cell of origin**. The **diagnosis** depends on **immuno-histochemistry. Histological** examination shows **multiple cells** with **clear cytoplasm** with considerable **pleomorphism** and **bizarre forms**. These tumours often **contain melanin** but this

may **not** be **detected** on **routine** haemotoxylin and eosin **staining**. **Immunohistochemistry** shows **melanocytic differentiation**. The **common sites** are around the **foot and the ankle**. But **many** of these cancers are **deeply placed** in the **tissues**. They are **highly malignant** and **metastasise** very **early** in the **course of the disease**. Lymph **node spread** is a **feature** of this **sarcoma**.

Epithelioid sarcomas are **uncommon cancers** affecting the **upper extremity**. Clinically they appear as **ulcerated tumours** in the **subcutaneous tissue** of the **fingers, hand and forearm,** and are often **mistaken** for a **benign lesion. Some** of these tumours resemble a **squamous cell carcinoma**. But they are **highly malignant tumours. Histologically,** they show **spindle cells** with **densely eosinophilic cytoplasm** and **atypical giant cells**.

■ ■ ■